Pandora's picnic basket

Pandora's picnic basket

The potential and hazards of genetically modified foods

ALAN McHUGHEN

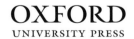

OXFORD

UNIVERSITY PRESS

OXFORD
UNIVERSITY PRESS

Great Clarendon Street, Oxford ox2 6DP
Oxford University Press is a department of the University of Oxford.
It furthers the University's objective of excellence in research, scholarship,
and education by publishing worldwide in

Oxford New York

Athens Auckland Bangkok Bogotá Buenos Aires Calcutta
Cape Town Chennai Dar es Salaam Delhi Florence Hong Kong Istanbul
Karachi Kuala Lumpur Madrid Melbourne Mexico City Mumbai
Nairobi Paris São Paulo Singapore Taipei Tokyo Toronto Warsaw
with associated companies in Berlin Ibadan

Oxford is a registered trade mark of Oxford University Press
in the UK and in certain other countries

Published in the United States
by Oxford University Press Inc., New York

A catalogue record for this book is available from the British Library

Library of Congress Cataloging in Publication Data
(Data available)

ISBN 0 19 850674 0 (Hbk) (Pandora's picnic basket)
      0 19 850714 3 (Pbk) (A consumer's guide to GM food)

Typeset by J&L Composition, Filey, N. Yorks
Printed in Great Britain
on acid-free paper by
T.J. International, Padstow, Cornwall

This book is dedicated to my mentors,
who taught me the love of nature:

Gary Hicks, Dalhousie University, Canada
Lionel Clowes, Oxford University, UK
Ian Sussex, Yale University, USA

and my family, who taught me the nature of love:

Nicola McHughen
Stephanie McHughen
Donna Greschner

Acknowledgements

No man is an island, no one can conduct modern scientific research in isolation. All of my work is built upon the achievements of others, and I hope my results will contribute in helping others in attaining greater heights.

I must especially recognize and explicitly thank some contributors from my students, staff, and colleagues. This book would not have been possible without the excellent service of my lab staff over the years: Marvin Swartz, Robin Browne, Diney Kneeshaw, Ira Borgmann, Gail Thompson, and especially Patti Hayes-Schryer.

A modern university research laboratory is a microcosmic United Nations where people from around the world congregate to learn from one another. Visiting scientists and students gather to learn and exchange ideas. In addition to science, we learn and respect differences in culture, religious and spiritual beliefs, philosophy, and lifestyle. I suspect I've learned at least as much from my students as they have from me. Brian Orshinsky, Dave Williams, Linda McGregor, Mark Jordan, Lesley Boyd (UK), Raman Kapur (India), Tom Warkentin, John Kosir (USA), Sandra McSheffrey, Brigette Weston, Mohamed Koronfel (Egypt), and Teguh Wijayanto (Indonesia) all contributed greatly to my education during their own.

Postdoctoral and visiting scientists also make substantial contributions to our knowledge of nature. Brian Forster (UK), Jin-Zhou Dong (China), Alexy Polykov (Russia), Igor Bartish (Ukraine), Anju Gulati (India), Carsten Köhn (Germany), and Perumal Vijayan (India) were among the talented scientists coming from overseas to share their expertise in my lab.

My local colleagues deserve recognition here. Gord Rowland, my co-developer on the three biotechnology linseed flax varieties (Andro, CDC Normandy, and CDC Triffid) deserves special mention. Also instrumental in developing Triffid were Rick Holm, Ron Bhatty, and Ed Kenaschuk. Others helping in my continuing education include Bryan Harvey, Graham Scoles, and Brian Rossnagel.

International colleagues helped me understand the crucial issues in the commercialization of genetically modified organisms and provided me with much material for this book. Especially important are my associates on the International Biosafety Advisory Committee: Professor Sir John Beringer, former Chair of the UK Advisory Committee on Releases to the Environment (ACRE)— thanks for your dedication and integrity in the many years of underappreciated service to your country, John—Klaus Ammann (Switzerland), Alvarez Morales (Mexico), Supat Attathom (Thailand), Ervin Balazs (Hungary), Simon Barber (Canada), Willy DeGreef (Switzerland), T. Hatanaka and Ken-ichi Hayashi (Japan), Magdy Madkour (Egypt), Terry Medley (DuPont), Michael Schectmann, (USA), Joachim Schiemann (Germany), Blair Siegfried, (USA), Kornelia Smalla, (Germany) Mark Tepfer (France), and Zhangliang Chen (China). Other important contributors include Julian Kinderlerer (UK), C. S. Prakash (USA), Doug Powell (Canada), and Peggy Lemaux (USA). Thank you all for sharing your thoughts and stimulating discussions. I know you don't necessarily agree with all the points I make in this book, but I do know you appreciate the need to conduct vigorous debate based on scientific principles.

Bill Anderson, who 'held my hand' in Japan and displays tireless energy in organizing meetings, deserves special recognition, as does Steve Adkins, who provided me with an office and my family with a homey atmosphere during my sabbatical leave in Australia when the bulk of this manuscript was being compiled. Thanks also to the wonderful people of Brisbane for making us all feel welcome and comfortable.

I wish also to thank the various people and institutions who provided public access, via the Internet, to their information and data. They include the US Patent and Trademark Office (US patent searches), Genbank (DNA sequences), Government of British Columbia (chemical composition of cigarettes). House of Lords (Select Committee report), Rowett Institute (Dr Pusztai's alternate report and data), Royal Society (Report on toxicity of GM potatoes), and the Nuffield Council on Bioethics (Report on the ethical and social issues in GM crops). Most government agencies, companies, and non-governmental organizations (NGOs), and activist groups maintain websites carrying information relevant to the GM debate. Some web addresses are listed in Chapter 16.

Donna Greschner provided excellent editorial, copyediting and proofreading advice in addition to considerable emotional support through the entire process. Special mention goes to Susan Harrison at Oxford University Press, whose encouragement and enthusiasm provided the impetus to transform the initial manuscript, an amorphous mass of words, into the book you now hold.

Finally, this book would not exist if not for the people to whom I dedicate this book and who deserve their own page.

A.M.

Contents

Table d'hôte or á la carte?

Don't take another bite until you read this book. Unless you can properly compare genetically modified (GM) foods with those from conventional or organic production, you are not making informed decisions. Everyone, it seems, is concerned about GM food, but most admit they don't really know much about it. Reading this book will enable you to make an informed choice to support, or reject, GM, conventional, and organic foods.

Where's the public debate on GM foods?

In America, where GM crops cover millions of acres and people consume large quantities of GM foods, until recently there has been scant media attention and the populace seems largely unconcerned. There is no public debate in America because there is no public discussion of the relevant issues. Why should this be?

In the UK, by contrast, no commercial GM crops are grown and people consume relatively small amounts of GM foods. Yet the populace is highly aware and highly suspicious of GM foods. No wonder; the British media subjects us to a daily barrage of intense heat and GM fireworks. Unfortunately, these pyrotechnics may be spectacular but provide little comforting warmth or illumination. This is illustrated by the emigration of a prominent British medical researcher, Dr Roger Gosden, to Canada, citing the UK furore over GM foods. 'Wait a minute' you say 'If he was so concerned about GM food, why would he move to a country where GM foods are far more plentiful and less likely to be labelled?' He didn't emigrate to get away from GM food—he moved to escape the *hysteria* over GM food. As in America, there is no true debate in the UK because there is virtually no rational discussion of the relevant issues.

Genetically modified organisms on the menu

This book is not an accounting or listing of current genetically modified organisms (GMOs) and GM food products, as my intention is not to preach, but to teach. Although such information might be relevant and interesting, it has limited educational value and, in any case, would quickly become outdated. Oh, why not, it'll take only a minute. Here's a recent listing of approved GM foods in the major regulating nations. These do not include the microbial GM food additives, of which there are several. Nor are animals on the list, as no GM meat, poultry, or fish has yet been approved for human consumption. The first will likely be a fish (but not with a tomato gene).

- The US has most approvals, with 44 foodstuffs, including 12 corn (maize), 7 canola (rapeseed), 6 tomato, 5 cotton, 4 potato, 3 soya bean, 2 sugar beet, 2 squash, and 1 each of radish, papaya, and linseed flax.
- Canada has approved 42 GM foods, including 15 corn, 11 canola, 5 cotton, 4 potato, 3 tomato, 2 squash, 1 linseed, and 1 soya bean.
- The UK has approved 19, including 5 rapeseed (canola), 3 tomato, 1 corn, and 1 soya bean. Only five GM products are being marketed.

The GMO I am researching is linseed, approved in the USA and Canada and pending in the UK.

New GM products coming down the pipe are quite different; they carry novel features unrelated to the current types which are mostly pesticide-resistant. But you need to know more than the features of GM products already available or nearing release. This book will allow you to make a thorough evaluation of GM products, now and into the future. Only with this foundation can you make truly informed decisions on whether or not such products deserve your support and custom.

Developments in genetic technology will bring us a constant array of new things—not just products, but conceptually new ideas to discuss and evaluate. This book provides a sufficient background in molecular genetics to enable a fuller, more satisfactory understanding of the issues, to place the new ideas and products in perspective in the context of comparable but conventional products. The public interest is best served in any controversial issue by an informed debate with all salient facts and considerations being presented truthfully and eloquently by skilled and knowledgeable intellectual protagonists. No one is likely to enjoy a mismatch between a professional heavyweight and an untrained lightweight. Instead, I enjoy the excitement of an intellectual debate between well-trained and capable participants, conducted in full public view. The current state of debate over GMOs, especially in the UK, has been of such an appalling standard that, if we had a council to referee, all sides would be declared disqualified.

Why is the public debate in such a dysfunctional state?

That's a simple question with an equally simple answer we have already alluded to—lack of factual information. Being for or against GM and taking a stand requires a solid platform. To build a solid platform we need a stable foundation. A stable foundation is built on accurate information and fact. For genetic technology, much of the factual support is scientific and technical. What appears to be lacking in the public GM debate is the scientifically sound foundation supporting the respective arguments of proponents and opponents.

How do we elevate the GM debate? Only by acquiring the factual foundations, then building on top a platform incorporating sound social, ethical, and other components. Science provides the bedrock granite. Without this firm footing, you might find yourself trying to build on an unstable base. If you're going to take a stand, make sure your footing is adequately supported. Otherwise, you might find yourself with one foot in quicksand, the other in your mouth.

The scientific base of many arguments, both pro and con, is faulty. With just a little effort, however, society could enjoy a healthy and vigorous discussion of the issues. The basic scientific concepts are not all that difficult to comprehend for interested people of normal intelligence.

The public debate on GM technology also suffers from an apparently deliberate campaign of emotional pleadings based on scientific misinformation, misinterpretation, and simple misunderstanding, peppered with occasional invective and sometimes personal attacks by both proponents and opponents. This may make exciting tabloid copy but does nothing to advance the cause of informed public deliberation. The underlying foundation of this debate, GM technology, is scientific. We must, unfortunately, rely on scientists to provide the fundamentals. I say unfortunately because, in general, the public doesn't like to rely on scientists.

Society conducts informed debate on a wide range of contentious and controversial issues—abortion, gun control, euthanasia, universal medical care, and so on. In each case, the protagonists not only put forward and present their positions but stay around to to defend them. The argument may not convince you, but you can still respect the legitimate foundation supporting it. If we can enjoy informed debate on these issues, legitimate informed debate on GM is equally possible. This book is intended to kickstart a real informed and vigorous public debate.

Why does it need a stimulus? Why does the UK lack a legitimate GM foods debate? Many observers in the UK refuse to legitimize the current GM frenzy by calling it a debate. It is more like a childish bun fight. Opponents to GM put forward untenable pseudo-scientific assertions, then run away, unwilling or unable to defend their positions. Proponents trip over their swords, disembowelling themselves in the process—witness Monsanto's advertising campaign of 1998. Independent experts in government, having lost public credibility in the wake of BSE and other regulatory disasters, are ignored or dismissed as incompetent. Experts in academia, those capable of setting the public debate on an even keel, are largely afraid to speak out, or are ignored when they do, or fall into infighting over technical minutia irrelevant to the public. Those that do try to referee, and there are many, spend their time reacting to questionable assertions. They have no remaining time to set a scientifically sound foundation for an informed public debate.

A sensible, rational GM foods debate is not only possible but imperative for true informed choice. We will all be better off if opponents abandon the scare stories and instead fight with real ammunition (it is available), and if proponents are more open and honest with the public in forwarding their case, acknowledging real risks as well as real benefits. Experts working in the public interest must abandon the often paternalistic attitude of 'don't worry—we have everything under control' and instead provide the public with the basic information necessary to allow people to decide for themselves whether to support or reject GM technology. Only then can society enjoy a true informed debate. Only then can consumers exercise true informed choices.

Food safety, labelling, environmental hazards, political and economic control, intellectual property, 'science-based' regulation—all present legitimate and fascinating points for public discourse. What has most motivated me to write this book is the anger elicited by the continued exhortation by the various participants that their own arguments are supported by science, whereas those of their opponents are not. From my perspective as a scientist, the implicit argument that 'science is on my side' is disingenuous. Neither side has a monopoly on science.

This does not mean that science ought to be the exclusive or primary arbiter of GM issues. These are complex questions, requiring input on the ethics, economics, politics, and social impact of GM technology as well as the science. Although I occasionally express my opinion on these other components, my expertise is limited to the scientific issues.

This book is based on my experience as a research scientist and educator, instructing people with differing backgrounds, from farmers and housewives to professional scientists and nine-year-old schoolchildren. The anecdotes and incidents occurred while I was negotiating the scientific and regulatory evaluations required for the commercial release of the University of Saskatchewan's GM linseed in Canada, the USA, Europe, and Japan—several of the petitions are still pending.

The people of Saskatchewan pay me to conduct research into and provide advice on the benefits and risks of these 'new genetic technologies'. The university breeds and develops its own new crop varieties, but on occasion we collaborate with a private company wishing to develop a product we deem of public benefit. The companies don't need my help selling and competing with each other in the marketplace, and I do not endorse any specific product. I am reluctant to comply when people ask me which specific product they should buy, preferring instead to provide information to allow an independent assessment and decision. I take the same approach here.

I share with you my view that genetic engineering is in many respects like any other new technology. It ought to be approached with neither fear nor complacency, but with caution, to enable an informed objective assessment of risk management and utility. You will learn about genetics, especially molecular genetics, in such a way as to understand and critically evaluate the increasing media coverage of the subject. We will explore some of the current GMOs, discussing not only the reported but overstated hazards, but also the real but largely ignored risks associated with the products. We'll learn how GM products get into our food and on to the market. We'll see how public and regulatory attitudes vary in different places. We'll expose mistakes made by activists opposed to GM technology; for example, their scaremongering about some GM products that don't exist. We'll see some mistakes made by proponent companies, especially in their approach to marketing GM technology. Mistakes also abound in regulatory theory and practice.

You will learn how to make up your own mind whether you wish to buy or deny GM technology.

I disclose no confidential business information. Over the years I have had various dealings with most of the big companies involved in the GM game, and the technical details and business aspects of these routinely required my oath of confidentiality. There is no need to break these confidences. There is plenty of relevant and interesting information in the public domain without resorting to unethical disclosures. In any case, the confidential information revealed to me by the companies usually pertains to their relationships and competition strategies *vis-à-vis* their competitors. Although business executives find such information highly sensitive and interesting, it invariably and immediately puts the rest of us to sleep.

This book explores the science behind GM based on my personal experience, with scientific discovery and the commercialization of resulting new crop varieties. In addition to presenting the largely undisputed basics of the relevant science, I also share my opinion or interpretation on many issues and aspects of genetic modification. These opinions and interpretations are of course open to dispute and debate. There are three reasons for my sharing my opinion:

1 To appeal for a sensible discussion and debate. The present state of public debate is disgraceful. Even some activist groups are now calling for a return to rational debate.
2 Like any human, I am not infallible, nor do I know all there is to know on these important issues. New information and perspectives emanating from the ensuing debate might convince me to re-evaluate my position on a given topic.
3 I include a story of how a particular GM crop variety was developed and made its way into the international marketplace. The history is largely dependent on my interpretation of both the scientific and political processes.

The interpretations are therefore germane to understanding the overall processes. I share many of the questions I asked myself *en route*, and some of the solutions. In pondering these questions, you will no doubt come up with different, even opposing, but perhaps equally legitimate answers.

I am not trying to sell you my opinions; such an objective would be contrary to the fundamentals of education. My purpose is to inform and advise, then encourage a vigorous and vital informed debate. I have more respect for an informed dissenter than I do for an uninformed blind follower.

Make no mistake: I am in favour of an orderly and appropriately regulated introduction of some GMOs into the environment and marketplace, and I adamantly oppose others. There are good reasons to ban certain products of genetic technology, and good reasons to allow, with management, certain others; some may require no extraordinary regulation at all. If your opinion differs from mine after reading this book, I hope you will be able to justify, if only to yourself, why we disagree. My philosophy is to be sceptical, be critical, even cynical of claims by business interests, government agencies, and activist groups. But also keep an open mind and then decide for yourself.

CHAPTER 1

Hors-d'œuvres and entrées

- Are you concerned about fish genes in tomatoes?
- Will brazil nut genes in soya beans result in potentially lethal allergic reactions?
- Will rapeseed plants resistant to herbicides become uncontrollable superweeds?
- Will genetic engineering really eradicate starvation and malnutrition?

As a molecular geneticist, I create genetically modified organisms (GMOs). As a consumer, I'm concerned about threats to health and the environment. On first hearing of the examples listed above, I sought factual information to assess them for myself. Unfortunately, I didn't find it with the proponent biotechnology companies; their advertising didn't reveal many facts and just told me the positive aspects. I didn't find it with the opposition activists, either—their negative interpretations of equally sparse facts were hardly informative, they were scary. And the public media seemed more interested in covering the battle between the proponents and the opponents. So I went to the sources, the peer-reviewed scientific literature, the patent documents, the government offices charged with approving such products. Most importantly, I contacted directly the men and women involved, the scientists using GM techniques to create the controversial genetically modified organisms (GMOs) and those who evaluate them.

The factual information does exist but, unfortunately, not in a form readily accessible to the general public. My position as an academic scientist representing the public interest, and as a developer of an approved GMO (in the USA and Canada, so far) allows me a unique opportunity. In this book I share an inside look at the technology behind GM and explore the risks and benefits in non-technical terms. Along the way, I consider the facts behind the examples given above and discuss many more issues and examples relevant to a rational public discourse of the merits and demerits of not only GM, but also conventional and organic foods production systems.

In the course of forty thousand years, humanity has introduced any number of new technologies, some beneficial and still with us in various forms, some ephemeral or less beneficial and now dropped by the wayside. For the first time, however, we humans now have the ability to modify life in its most fundamental form. According to the opposition activists, with genetic engineering technology we can now unleash potentially self-perpetuating and uncontrollable monsters of unimaginable terror. Meanwhile, the proponents of genetic engineering argue we have unlocked secrets revealing the means to eradicate malnutrition and produce food on a scale to make the Green Revolution of the last generation look like a mere skirmish. We may now, or in the near future, overcome hundreds or even thousands of disabling and terminal diseases; the recent announcements of 'ageing' genes suggest that we may be able to cheat death itself.

Society has a cultural history of assessing new technological developments. We debate the hazards and benefits, weigh pros and cons, and, via governments, regulate the orderly introduction of the technology, while generally the marketplace determines the degree of adoption or cession. Rarely is a technology successfully banned outright. Once Pandora's box is open, the technology escapes. Sooner or later, someone somewhere inevitably, perhaps covertly, practises the craft. Not too many years ago we feared the possible adverse effect of excessive speed in trains. According to the argument, the human body was not designed to travel faster than, say, twenty-five miles per hour and society had to consider the long-term effects of such travel before allowing the 'bullet trains' of the day. Over time, either the technology is seen as less threatening or we become inured. If there is commercial value, it makes its way into the mainstream to be tolerated, if not embraced. Traditionally, probably out of inertia, people have been satisfied to defer to government to arrange bureaucracies and regulators to maintain society's personal and environmental safety interests.

This deference is no longer good enough. Public credibility in bureaucrats and government scientists continues to deteriorate as a result of science policy disasters such as those surrounding the 'mad cow' BSE fiasco. Such debacles result from political interference, overwork, and, on (thankfully rare) occasions, plain old incompetence and corruption. Public confidence in political leadership is rarely enhanced by cabinet ministers owning major stakes in biotechnology companies, like Lord Sainsbury in the UK, or government agencies employing experts with intimate ties to the industry, like the Food and Drug Administration (FDA) in the USA. Is it any wonder the populace is confused and suspicious?

If the government experts lack credibility, who can we entrust to evaluate new genetic technology, regulate it appropriately, or ban it altogether? If we believe the 'suits' from the multinational corporations, molecular genetic technology is simply an extension of past, acceptable technologies and we have no reason to fear it. If we instead believe the anti-technology activists we can expect widespread environmental destruction and pandemics of cancer and novel untreatable diseases, along with the concomitant substantial increases in profits for and power of multinational companies. We seem faced with a choice between confused, inappropriate regulation, little or no regulation, or disabling regulation.

Even the most resolute anti-technology activist admits that recombinant DNA (rDNA)—GM technology—is among us and will almost certainly continue to grow and spread. Our best chance to ensure we maintain political and regulatory control is to acquire the knowledge to enter informed dialogue and press legitimate concerns. One major problem with the current state of public debate on this vital topic is the widespread misunderstanding and misinformation, particularly in the UK but evident everywhere. Recent surveys show many people simply don't have the basic understanding of genetics required to engage in informed debate. For example, only 40% of respondents in the UK correctly recognize that ordinary, non-GM tomatoes contain genes. In fact, all microbes, plants, and animals contain genes and other DNA. To the more than half the population who are either uncertain or believe that food is normally devoid of genes, biotechnology appears to be adding an alien contaminant—DNA—to our foods. Putting the debate on a rational footing requires us to start at the beginning.

What *is* genetic modification? What *are* GMOs?

Defining our terms is often the most logical way to initiate a rational debate. Unfortunately, there is no common definition of the terms GM and GMO. Few scientists use these expressions when they communicate with one another. The term 'biotechnology' itself suffers a similar lack of formal definition. It is bandied about, but generally refers to any application of technology to living systems. In this broad respect, humans have been eating products of biotechnology for forty thousand years. In popular usage, the term is restricted to products of 'modern' technologies, comprising genetic engineering and a whole range of other 'recent' but undefined technologies.

Genetic modification (GM), also known as **genetic engineering** or **rDNA technology**, is actually a collection of many technologies. These begin, perhaps, with the molecular identification and analysis of genes and DNA. They include extraction and isolation, then 'cloning' or multiplying fragments of DNA or genes. They include gene-splicing, cutting pieces of DNA, and connecting together fragments from different sources. They also include shifting the DNA from test tube to Petri dish,* or from bacteria to other bacteria. They may involve subtle or substantial directed alteration of the DNA along the way. They could also include transferring or inserting the DNA into the cell of a higher plant or animal, then recovering a complete new organism. Only this last stage is what most of us consider when defining 'genetic engineering'. Yet each of these stages requires different technical expertise, and no scientist is adept at all of them. Few scientists describe themselves to other scientists as being a 'genetic engineer'.

The application of GM techniques results in a **genetically modified organism**

---

* A Petri dish, named after the German bacteriologist Richard Julius Petri (1852–1921), is a flat round glass dish with a loose-fitting glass lid—one of the most common pieces of laboratory glassware.

(GMO), also known as a **transgenic** or **genetically transformed** organism. The GMO might be a soya bean (soybean in the North America) with a new piece of DNA originally isolated from a bacterium. Some refer to GMOs as gene-altered, mutant, or even 'Frankenstein foods'. For simplicity, I use GM and GMO to refer to the general set of technologies and the resulting organisms, respectively.

Not surprisingly, we lack a common political definition of GMO on which to base regulatory policy. Lacking a standard scientific benchmark, each jurisdiction defines GM and GMO according to local political expediency. In the EC Novel Foods Regulation GM food is defined as '. . . a food which is, or which is made from, a genetically modified organism' and which contains genetic material or protein resulting from the modification. In contrast, the USA uses a product-based, not process-based, definition. Canada carries the product further, basing their regulatory oversight on the novel features of a product, regardless of method of origin. That is, a product is regulated as a GMO if it carries some trait not previously found in the species, even if it was generated using traditional breeding methods.

The Convention on Biological Diversity (CBD) is an international political body attempting (among other things) to reach consensus on a common definition. One proposal is to use the term **living modified organism** (LMO) to encompass all products of rDNA, including the actual transformed organism plus anything produced from it, even non-living derivatives with no DNA or protein. These differing definitions across major trading partners causes considerable political and economic turmoil. Unfortunately, we cannot carry a unified set of definitions to the next step—defining the issues.

Popular concerns over GM technology and GMOs fall into one of two broad categories: ethical (including theological, social, economic, and political) issues, and scientific issues. The ethical components are raised in this book only on occasion and then briefly. A superb analysis and report by the Nuffield Council on Bioethics on the ethical and social issues in GM crop technology is available on the web (*http://www.nuffield.org/bioethics/publication/modifiedcrops/index. html*). The report is essential reading and highly recommended. Although it is written from the British standpoint, the ethical considerations are common to everyone.

The rational GM debate often turns on 'scientific' arguments and premises. The final decision on accepting or rejecting GM technology demands consideration of social, ethical, political, and other aspects. But because so much of the debate is founded on science and scientific interpretation, this book concentrates on the scientific issues. With the scientific and factual basis, you may then incorporate the other aspects to build your position, confident in a stable and solid foundation.

Entrées

According to recent surveys, most ordinary consumers, even those holding a strong opinion on GMOs, admit they don't know much about GM. An encouraging number add that they'd 'like to learn more' about the technology. But where does an interested layperson gain the objective information needed to meaningfully debate genetic engineering issues and evaluate GM products? Certainly, genetic engineering is taking a gene from one organism and inserting it into another. And we can see that, apart from ethical and social concerns, the scientific issues fall into two general areas:

1   First, is this GM product safe for the environment? That is, will it disturb local environment, disrupt natural ecological processes, displace or infiltrate wild species or natural populations? How will we control an 'escape' of the genetic material into the environment?
2   Second (but no less important), is this GM product safe for human food and animal feed? How can we be sure the GM product won't poison us? Is meat from animals raised on GM feed safe for human consumption?

We can't pursue these questions to acquire the information necessary to conduct a proper assessment until we gain further knowledge. What's the next step? Let's see.

Comparing recipes

When we debate these and other questions about the environmental and food safety of a GM product, we need to consider the differences between the closest conventional version and the GM product. Are there environmental or health safety differences between, for example, a tomato supplied with new genes from a distant relative inserted using traditional breeding methods and a tomato with the same genes inserted using molecular genetic technology? The only apparent difference is the method used to transfer the genetic information. The final product in each case, the one grown by farmers and eaten by consumers, is identical. The environmental and food safety issues ought to be identical. Then what about a tomato genetically modified with genes from bacteria as opposed to a tomato modified with other tomato genes? Now we have to consider potential risks of the GM to both health and environment. Will the bacterial genes escape from the GM tomato to wreak havoc in the environment? Is the new DNA toxic; is it safe to eat?

We also need to consider the three basic types of GM product: intact GM tomato, GM tomato paste, and oil extracted from GM seeds. Each presents a different set of potential hazards requiring a different regulatory approach.

- An intact GM tomato requires scrutiny for both environmental and food safety issues.
- Now consider a GM tomato destined exclusively for processing into paste. As long as we only import the final paste product, we shouldn't be too concerned over gene escape into the wild. Or ought we? Are the genes still capable of escape after being squished and cooked? We also need apply different food safety questions. What is the difference between eating a fresh GM tomato and a cooked or processed GM tomato? What does cooking and processing do to the novel DNA?
- Finally, what about ingredients derived from a GM crop? A GM tomato might be processed to extract the small amount of oil. Similarly and more commonly, GM soya produces commercial vegetable oil. Is it different from regular soya oil? The extraction process removes all but trace amounts of DNA and protein from the oil; further refining can remove even those. GM sugar beet is processed to provide pure sugar, devoid of DNA and protein— novel or otherwise. What environmental or health safety questions, if any, are raised concerning refined oil from GM soya, or sugar from GM sugar beet?

All of these examples involve GMOs, each with its own potential concerns, but the public debate almost invariably lumps them together as if they were equally hazardous. They are not. We'll explore the differences and the real hazards in more detail later.

The prix fixe menu: course outline

Each chapter of this book is a course in itself. The book starts with a primer of the technology before delving into the issues and, possibly, the solutions. At the head of each chapter is a set of questions answered, or at least addressed, in the chapter. The questions are those most often asked of me and set the tone for the book.

As a starter, you will learn that the science behind rDNA, the technology of genetic engineering, is not beyond all understanding, and that the GM debate is open to all. After this starter, Chapters 2 and 3 explain, in plain English, the basic concepts of molecular genetics and why genetic engineering is technically feasible. We continue with how to acquire individual genes (you'll be amazed at how simple and inexpensive it can be!) and then how to transfer these genes into another organism. Lest you think this is too far above your head, let me say that these technical chapters are based on lectures initially developed for interested and intelligent non-scientists, including schoolchildren. Their ability to grasp the concepts, if not the details, reinforced my belief that anyone with a reasonable interest can understand the basics of genetic modification. However, if you find you can't wait for dessert, at least eat the meat. Don't try to devour the technical details, satiate yourself instead with the concepts. Given a taste of molecular genetics, anyone can enter and contribute to an informed debate on the future of these awesome technologies.

After these basics, we place the controversial issues in context by considering classical or current technologies in Chapter 4. What is ordinary classical breeding and how do new food crops get to the table?

In Chapter 5 we take a close look at food, critical to all of us. Is our food contaminated? If so, are GMOs responsible? Discover how much GM DNA and novel protein products we are actually eating. Learn some of the other things in our foods we might prefer not to know about. Organic products are a safe and viable alternative to GM foods. Or are they? Let's find out.

We deliver the meat of the matter, discussing the underlying issues in the GM debate in Chapter 6, and, among other things, try to determine why public attitudes are so different on either side of the Atlantic.

Numbers are constantly bandied about, from industry, from activists and from governments, each vying for our support in the 'battle of the statistics'. What do the numbers mean? Chapter 7 provides a simple primer. Then we clarify the relationship between science and regulatory policy in Chapter 8. We explore some of the biosafety issues, evaluations regarding the real risks posed by GMOs to human and other animal health as well as to the environment. All regulatory agencies are concerned with the two major concerns of GMOs, environmental protection and health safety. All claim to take a 'science-based' approach to evaluating GMOs. If this is true, why is regulatory approval for a given GMO straightforward in one jurisdiction and near impossible in another? Large amounts of public money are spent on largely irrelevant government-sponsored GM environmental calculations. What are these wasteful programmes and what can we do about them?

What are the real risks of GMOs? Chapter 9 exposes some that might have been overlooked or ignored. A void in public credibility and trust stifles meaningful debate, pro and con. How can ordinary people obtain factual and objective information on the issues? Is there anyone we can trust? Yes, there is. We dish up the sources in Chapter 10. GM technology supporters often complain of scaremongering. Chapter 11 exposes some of the myths or misunderstandings.

Many consumers are demanding mandatory labelling on GM foods to enable an informed choice. As a consumer advocate, I believe everyone has the right to know what is in the package and how the product was made. But in Chapter 12 you'll learn why mandatory labelling for GM food will not enable informed choice; it will not satisfy our demands to know what is in each package of food and how it was produced.

You have no doubt heard that over 60% of processed foods carry GM ingredients. Is there any way we can avoid GM foods? Your best bet for a GM-free meal is covered in Chapter 13. This leads on to Chapter 14 on an associated and similarly contentious issue, intellectual property protection. In Chapter 15 I make my predictions for the direction of the GM industry in the coming years, along with my recommendations on the evaluation of GM products.

Having finishing your meal, decide for yourself if and how you wish to engage in the debate, or at least be satisfied that you are now better able to evaluate the (often confusing and contradictory) media accounts.

An example of healthy scepticism

At the start of this chapter I asked if you were concerned about a fish gene in tomatoes, a Brazil nut gene in soya beans, or herbicide-resistant superweeds. All are commonly cited examples of genetic technology gone berserk. I, too, was very concerned about each one of these when I first became aware of them. I strove to find the full story behind them. The beans and weeds can wait until later chapters. This is what I found on the fishy tomatoes.

The tomato in question is often cited as the now defunct Flavr-Savr™ tomato, the first entire GM food product on the US market. Since the mid-1980s it has been a frequent target for the popular press and opposition activists. When I first heard of the fish gene in a tomato, a question popped into my suspicious mind: What is a fish gene doing in a tomato? What genetic information might a fish contribute to a tomato to make it 'improved' enough to be a commercial success? It must have some marvellous feature to overcome people's natural apprehension of such a product. My curiosity was piqued, but the activist newsletters and press clippings did not provide enough dispassionate information to provide an answer. Some mentioned that the modified genes were supposed to provide long shelf life. The tomatoes could be picked ripe (instead of green, as commercial outfits do now), sent to market, and purchased by you to sit on the kitchen work-top for weeks before being discarded.

Understanding why tomatoes with freshness staying power might be attractive to some consumers, I formulated a new question: What is a fish doing with a gene for long shelf life? I've never considered fish to be a food with a long shelf life. Maybe the fish gene just gave the tomatoes a distinctive smell, to let us know as fish do that they are past their prime. Surely they could have found a source for such a gene in, say, tofu. Tofu seems to last months in the fridge before being thrown out, still looking as it did on day of purchase.

Surely the scientific literature would answer the questions.

It didn't. Peer-reviewed science journals contained no reference to the denizen-of-the-deep-cum-red-coated fruit. Perhaps the company was developing this super tomato in secret, not wanting to release any scientific information on it. These trade secrets work well for some products. No one outside company head office knows for sure what's in Coca-Cola or Kentucky Fried Chicken, because the recipes have been maintained as trade secrets for years. However, trade secrets do not work so well for self-reproducing products like tomatoes. To start a competing production line, an unscrupulous competitor need acquire only one specimen of the 'real thing', scoop out and plant the seeds. The only way to protect the intellectual and genetic property in this wonder fruit effectively is through a patent.

In searching through the US patent office database, I was able to find no patent reference to tomatoes with fish genes. (If you have an Internet connection, you can search for yourself; *http://patent.womplex.ibm.com/*). Nothing came up in searches of other world patent offices, either. No proponent can place a new product on the market in total secrecy. This tomato–fish story was beginning to smell, well, fishy. The search was now limited to the notoriously unreliable articles in the popular press.

Eventually, I managed to trace the fish gene story back to California in the mid-1980s, when Calgene was developing the delayed-ripening Flavr-Savr™ tomato. Calgene was a small start-up company with a handful of superb scientists developing creative ideas, like the slow-ripening tomato, on a shoestring budget. Being cash poor and idea rich, Calgene looked like a tasty morsel ripe for consumption. Biotech behemoth Monsanto didn't like the upstart competition and took the first bite out of Calgene, acquiring a minority ownership in the smaller company. (A few years later, Monsanto completed its takeover of Calgene. It was the first of several exercises of Monsanto's competitive philosophy that continued for years: if you can't beat 'em, eat 'em.)

About the same time as Calgene was developing the Flavr-Savr™, other possible genes were being mentioned as candidates for transfer to crop species by Calgene and other small companies looking for venture capital investors. One of these genes was the Arctic flounder anti-freeze gene, which allows the fish to live and thrive in the icy waters of the Arctic. The conceptual idea was that transferring this gene to a crop would allow the crop to survive unseasonable frosts (a good idea in theory, but it hasn't worked in practice). I suspect that the journalist who originally wrote the story combined the two distinct but related stories to warn the world about a tomato with a fish gene, but could as easily have confused us by having a tomato gene in a fish. Although the scientific community has discredited the fish-in-the-Flavr-Savr™, the story is so captivating it seems to have taken on a life of its own. Even now, when I read some of the horror stories of GMOs, I see references to the fishy tomato, sometimes complete with the same spelling errors as in earlier reports. It would be amusing if it weren't so harmful to non-critical readers.

The Flavr-Savr™ tomato did not have an inserted fish gene. It acquired its longer shelf life from an inserted, inverted tomato gene. This particular GM product is well documented in the scientific literature and the information is available to anyone. The tomato is no longer on the market, but not because the genetic modification didn't work. Other GM tomatoes with extended shelf life that have also been to the market include Zeneca's GM tomato paste, at one time available at Safeway and Sainsbury's in the UK. Flavr-Savr™ did not fail because of public outrage and boycott of the GM product. Rather, it failed because Calgene was strong on science, but weak in the basic crop production, marketing, and distribution systems. It was a mistake other biotech companies would come to know well.

This fishy story illustrates one of the difficulties ordinary consumers have in evaluating GM food and GM technology. In cases like this they're basing their opinion on a widely publicized urban myth. Inserting a fish gene into a tomato is not a technical problem. It can be done, and probably has, in some lab somewhere, but I'm not aware of any fish–tomato product being developed for the market. 'Fish gene in tomato' has all the standard characteristics of an urban myth—it's scary and it sounds 'too good to be real'; it's based on the weird, yet is entirely plausible. I can always tell when a reporter writing up a story on GM foods didn't dig very far, by the references to the fish gene in the Flavr-Savr™ tomato, the brazil nut gene in soya bean hospitalizing people from unexpected allergic reactions (see Chapter 5), or the superweeds completely immune to herbicides (see Chapter 6). I chose the tomato story here because it is commonly cited but easily corrected. Not all activist news releases, newsletters, and websites are as blatantly erroneous, nor are the industry 'fact sheets' devoid of misinformation. We'll encounter some examples of those later.

The critical underlying issue with this incident is that the media helped incite public fear by creating an unnecessary scare out of shadows and inadvertently diverting attention from legitimate safety concerns with GM products. In retrospect, the substantive story of the fish-gene-in-the-tomato, was that it turned out as a metaphoric tomato gene in a fish: the first GM red herring.

CHAPTER 2

Cooking school primer: molecular genetics for everyone

- Why can't scientists speak (or write) English?
- How 'safe' is 'safe'?
- What is DNA? A gene? A protein?
- What are the four foundational pillars of molecular genetics?
- Do humans naturally share any genes with other creatures?
- Do genes have parts?
- What happened to Mendelism ('traditional' genetics)?
- How are genes acquired for genetic engineering?
- What is a 'gene bank' and how does it work?

The 'incomprehensible' vernacular of genetics

Geneticists (like other scientists) use arcane terminology—words and expressions, often sprinkled with Latin or Greek, that can be totally alien to ordinary, otherwise intelligent and educated people. Of course scientists do need specialized words to provide accuracy as well as precision in communicating required detail to other scientists. For example, there is no common English name for the microbe *Agrobacterium tumefaciens*, but the Latin name is understood by scientists of all nationalities. Scientists sometimes need the precision and accuracy of these technical names to evaluate data properly. An easily genetically modified crop known as oilseed rape, or rapeseed, or (outside the UK) canola, is often in the news because of its predilection for mating with similarly promiscuous but non-GM crops or weeds growing across the road. To assess the data on inappropriate mating, scientists need to know which particular species is cited—*Brassica napus*, *Brassica rapa* or, less likely, *Brassica juncea*. All of them can produce the vegetable oil so popular in our kitchens, but, like humans, have very different degrees of promiscuity and mating preferences.

This kind of arcane scientific nomenclature or terminology is only a small component of the confusion, because at least it is unambiguous. You might not know exactly what the word 'blastocele' means, but at least you don't confuse it with a word in common usage. It doesn't often come up in casual conversation.

The ambiguous terminology of science

A greater problem in communication between scientists and laypeople arises over the different meanings given by scientists to common, ordinary words. The words thus become ambiguous and lead to gross miscommunication and misunderstanding. An example is a phrase familiar to all developers of GM crops, and never fails to strike fear into every scientist: 'Prove that the GM plant (or microbe, or animal) is safe'.

As a sceptical consumer, this is the first phrase that comes to my mind when I am told of an impending new GM foodstuff. While keeping an open mind, I want reassurance that this product isn't going to cause harm to me, my family, community, or environment before I'm prepared to accept it. Every consumer ought to have the same thoughts about a new product. Why then, do the developers and scientists have so much difficulty with such a simple, reasonable demand?

The question is threatening to the scientists not because they are concerned that their new plant isn't safe (although that might be part of it, too), but because of the differing definitions of safety.

What does this mean? Let's look at the construction of 'Prove that the GM product is safe'.

Proof

The word **proof** has at least four distinct meanings, even if you exclude its association with alcoholic content (the measure of which is itself ambiguous as it varies across the Atlantic). The legal community, no stranger to arcane and often misleading use of language, splits the definition of 'proof' according to criminal law ('beyond a reasonable doubt') and civil matters ('on a balance of probabilities'). To scientists, on the other hand, a proof leaves no doubt whatsoever—it is an absolute. Because of the stringency of an absolute, there are relatively few 'proofs' in science. To the common user, proof is usually defined somewhere between the extremes provided by the scientists and the more relaxed approach of civil law. Scientists, then, interpret the demand for 'proof' to be so onerous as almost certainly beyond compliance, when, in terms of ordinary language, they are being asked to provide assurances that the new product is at least as safe as current, similar, foodstuffs.

GM

Next in the phrase comes **GM**. Again, the definition differs according to where you are. As we saw in Chapter 1, there is no internationally accepted definition of a GMO. A new GM crop in the USA might not be classed GM in Canada, and vice versa. This might not make too much difference, except that foodstuffs are highly travelled commodities. They may be produced and evaluated in one jurisdiction under one definition of GMO, but transported for consumption to another jurisdiction with perhaps a different view of their provenance. Nations might distinguish between a **whole GM organism** (like a soya bean with a bacterial gene), a **processed GMO** (like tofu made from the GM soya bean) and a **by-product of a GMO** (oil or lecithin from a GM soya bean). Also, few countries have a regulatory policy and competent regulatory infrastructure to evaluate the GM products properly.

Plant

Then we grapple with **plant** (but the request could equally be made for a microbe or animal.). You might think the definition of a plant is obvious, but it is not. For example, does a shipment of the oil processed from a GMO oilseed crop, devoid of DNA, constitute a GM plant for regulatory or labelling purposes? Some jurisdictions have resolved the question, but others have not. The definition is under intense international debate, thus presenting a moving target. Developers might properly conduct the required experiments and tests of the GM product under one definition of GM plant, only to discover the definition changed part way through the process. They then have to conduct evaluations under a different set of criteria, ones that don't necessarily contribute to a greater knowledge of the products' safety or hazard characteristics.

Safe

Finally, what is 'safe'? That is a very subjective issue. The major stated concerns with GMO safety relate to environmental safety and food safety. Often, though, the 'safety' criticisms are not specified. Safe for whom or what? Children? Pregnant or nursing women? Smokers? Safe for the environment? Relative to what other environmental components? Or is safety an absolute? If it isn't absolute, it has to be relative to something. Safe as a foodstuff? Relative to what other foods currently on the market? Or, again, is it absolute? We also must recognize that some products might be perfectly fine for environmental release, yet toxic to humans as foodstuffs. Many natural as well as non-GM products come into such a category. Similarly, some products might be suitable for consumption, yet present an ecological risk in at least some environments. For most people, in common usage, safe relates to what is currently considered safe. To a scientist, however, it appears to be a near-unattainable absolute.

'Safe' is further complicated by the subjective nature of the word. Whenever there is a question of safety, an emotive cloud darkens rational illumination. It evokes an emotional response, whereas scientists try to avoid emotive components. All scientists and all regulators are reluctant to say 'I believe this product is "safe"', because it appears to give an emotional and absolute proclamation of safety. They are apprehensive of someone coming back, saying 'But you said this product was safe' after suffering some misfortune, whether caused by the GMO or not.

Proving a negative

Finally and perhaps most important: Underlying the original phrase 'prove the GM plant is safe' is implied 'prove this won't ever cause harm'. **Science cannot**

prove a negative. It is not scientifically valid to say 'I have proved there is no risk associated with this product'. It could well be, and often is, a politically valid or legally valid statement, but it is not valid in the realm of science.

Other terms are also ambiguous, even if we associate them with modern science. 'Biotechnology' is a term often used by laypeople, rarely by scientists. Scientists avoid it because it has lost any semblance of specific meaning. Genetic engineering is not ambiguous when it refers to the application of recombinant DNA (rDNA) technology, but has gained a somewhat emotive negative public image, so scientists tend not to use it. As we saw in the previous chapter, governments cannot agree on what is meant by GM, GMO, or even a living modified organism (LMO). Because of the international negotiations and mass confusion about 'official' definitions, we face the possibility of having to regard a bottle of vegetable oil as a living, if modified, organism. Scientists generally refer to genetically engineered organisms as 'transgenic' or 'genetically transformed', or simply 'transformed'.

The universal language of DNA

Fortunately, unlike English (or any other human language), DNA is a universal language. There is no ambiguity, although there are certain usage preferences within some species; these might be thought of as accents, not even dialects, of the same language. We've all heard about DNA and the genetic code, the 'blueprint' or 'language of life' which most people interpret as a metaphor. It's actually a real language in that it is truly a medium of communication.

The molecular genetics primer

Several years ago, my daughter came home from school and excitedly asked me (or rather, in the inimitable style of a nine-year-old, instructed me) to partake in a 'parents' work' lecture to her class. My immediate reaction was that nine-year-olds have interests well beyond molecular genetics, but deferring to her perseverance and confidence I reluctantly contacted the teacher. The teacher, I was sure, would pursue someone else, a police officer, perhaps, or an engineer, and so let me off the hook with my daughter. Thwarting my expectations, the teacher instead enthusiastically welcomed the plan, assuring me that the important feature was the personal appearance, not the content. Furthermore, fifteen minutes was my maximum commitment, as that was the limit of their attention span.

My next task was how to fit even a simple lesson in molecular genetics into a fifteen-minute time slot. Eventually I decided to go with an easy and relatively common human genetic trait: hair on the mid-digit of each finger, and the story behind how it was discovered. It combines a readily detectable genetic trait with a fun 'man-on-the-bus' story of scientific discovery, and the children could each test their own fingers for mid-digit hair. I thought this could fit, with a few minutes left over for questions.

The day arrived. I described how a student first noticed the trait while on a bus, sitting behind a very hirsute man, who was covered in dark hair except for the middle portion of each finger. Within a few minutes, twenty-eight sets of juvenile mid-digits were dutifully inspected. Fortunately, some of the pupils had the trait, other didn't. A couple of quick questions, and the fifteen-minute job was over. However, the questions continued—most were surprisingly insightful and probing. Only a few children were quiet or raised simplistic queries. Soon the chalkboard held a diagram of the molecular structure of DNA, as I tried to explain how DNA carried genetic information and how the information was translated into mid-digit hair. The class permitted my retreat after an amazingly short two hours, on the negotiated condition that I return the following week for another hour.

I was pleasantly astonished to learn that nine-year olds could grasp simplified but nevertheless accurate concepts of molecular genetics. My guess is that they were not yet socially conditioned to regard 'molecular' anything to be beyond their grasp. Although they were clearly a bright group, this was not a special school with exceptional pupils. It made me realize that the basics of molecular genetics, the fundamental concepts of life, could be grasped by anyone of reasonable intelligence and an interest in making the effort to learn them. Much of the content of the first part of this book, the basic concepts of molecular genetics, grew out of those initial lessons with nine-year-olds.

What is DNA?

Everyone knows what DNA is. Or do they? The well-known abbreviation for deoxyribonucleic acid is even accepted by my computer spellchecker these days. People have learned that DNA is the 'blueprint', the 'language of life' in a thread-like, double-helix molecule first described by James Watson and Francis Crick in Cambridge less than fifty years ago. The problem with this is that most of us associate the idea of a blueprint with a sketch or diagram. I recall thinking in undergraduate lectures that molecules, any molecules, were so small they didn't really exist in physical form, or if they did, they were exempted from normal laws of observational physics, such as gravity or tensile strength. A cotton thread has a certain degree of tensile strength; if you pull the ends hard enough, the thread will snap. But will a thread of DNA snap? Is DNA really a physical entity subject to the ordinary laws of physics? How might one grasp a DNA thread to test its strength? Eventually, I learned that DNA is not a blueprint; it is a physical entity. It can and does break when, for example, it is pushed too forcefully through the narrow bore of a syringe held by a trembling novice technician.

DNA consists of four small chemical bases: thymine, guanine, adenine, and cytosine, abbreviated T, G, A, C (or t, g, c, a), respectively. They are linked together in long chains supported by a chemical 'backbone'. The strands form the famous 'double helix' of Watson and Crick. See Figure 1.

DNA looks rather like a twisted plastic ladder, where each pair of bases (A–T or C–G) is a rung and the strand backbone is one of the two side rails. One base on one strand, say a T, always pairs with A on the other strand. Similarly, G always pairs with C. The two strands are said to **complement** each other, in that they don't have identical base sequences, but they are complementary. If you know the base sequence of one strand, you can easily deduce the sequence of the other.

DNA is ubiquitous in life, contained in every living cell.* DNA is teeming inside every lettuce leaf, every bacterium, and every cell of every water buffalo. That fresh salad you ate for lunch is full of DNA, whether it came from the organic market or a big multinational corporation's cellars.

RNA (ribonucleic acid), a close relative of DNA, is also present in every cell and is far more active than DNA. Physically, RNA differs from DNA primarily in having one different base: uracil (U), instead of thymine (T), so U complements A in RNA, as T does in DNA. RNA also differs in usually being single-stranded, as opposed to the normally double-stranded structure of DNA. DNA has one job— to carry genetic information. The more versatile RNA also carries genetic information but has other duties as well. RNA, not DNA, is the 'genetic material' in most viruses, but DNA is the genetic information carrier in all higher organisms, like humans and liverworts. RNA, in addition, conveys information from the DNA to the cell machinery to make proteins, helps organize the protein synthetic machinery, collects and conveys the appropriate amino acids during protein synthesis, and can even act as an enzyme, facilitating chemical reactions. DNA may be head of the house, but RNA does most of the work. DNA, however, like the head of the house in human society, gets almost all the attention.

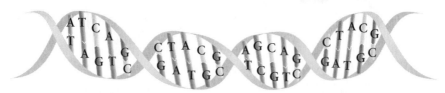

Figure 1   A simple diagram of the molecular structure of DNA consisting of pairs of the bases A, T, C, and G between two 'backbones'.

---

* There are a few cell types lacking DNA, your red blood cells being the most conspicuous.

The relationship between DNA and genes

Think of DNA not as a blueprint but as a set of instructions; a cookery book where the recipes are laid end-to-end as in a long scroll. A gene is not a physical entity the way DNA is; rather, it is a unit of biological information. Ink and paper may provide a physical vehicle for a recipe, but the fundamental nature of a recipe is non-physical information. Think of a gene as one of the recipes contained in the DNA. The entire complement of genetic information of an organism is called the **genome**. Think of it as an encyclopaedia of genetic recipes. Each gene is a recipe for how to make a particular protein, just as in human language a recipe informs a cook how to make a particular dish. Sometimes in the popular press I see reference to a gene being a type of protein. It is not. A chocolate cake is not a recipe, it results from the ingredients and actions described by the recipe. In the same way, a gene describes how to make a particular protein. The physical gene itself is a stretch of DNA.

Identical twins have identical genomes, identical recipe books. Different individuals can have different genomes or recipes, yet have many in common. For example, a Thai recipe book will contain many recipes that are similar, perhaps even identical, to those in a Burmese recipe book, but some recipes in each will be unique.

The cell housing the DNA performs the duties of the cook in preparing each recipe. The ingredients are amino acids, twenty different small peptide molecules floating around in every healthy cell. The specific amino acids become connected together in the orderly sequence directed by the recipe, forming a chain of amino acids (called a **polypeptide chain**) not unlike a string of pearls, where each pearl is one of the twenty different amino acids. The final product of each recipe is a protein, often an enzyme, which facilitates chemical reactions. Its characteristics are determined by the specific sequence of amino acids and any subsequent physical or chemical modifications. The presence or absence of a particular protein gives each individual genetic characteristic to the human, the plant, or the bacterium.

The genetic code: the relationship between genes and proteins

How does the cell know how to make proteins from the DNA recipe?

The sequence of the chemical bases in the DNA carries the genetic information, just as a sequence of English letters can convey an idea, a recipe, or alternatively be total nonsense, depending on the arrangement of the letters into words. The

DNA language has two important features:

1 Although there are twenty-six letters in the English alphabet, DNA uses only the four base chemical 'letters' (CATG) to make words.
2 Whereas English words can be any number of letters long, DNA 'words' are always three bases (letters) long.

For example, the DNA base sequence ATGGCCCTG, when read and 'expressed' by a cell, results in the amino acids methionine (from the first three bases, ATG), then alanine (from the next three bases, GCC) and then leucine (from the next three bases, CTG) being brought together in a short chain. The continuation of this process results in a long polypeptide chain of successive amino acids following the gene's recipe from the DNA sequence. This polypeptide chain, or **gene product**, forms the basis of the resulting protein. Simple proteins may be functional without subsequent modification, but most polypeptide chains are processed further by other enzymes before they become fully functional. Human insulin, the protein that regulates our blood sugar levels, is a good example. The amino acid chain resulting from the insulin gene DNA recipe needs to be modified by splicing out segments, then rejoining the resulting smaller sections together. Many important proteins are composed of several polypeptide chains configured together in a particular manner.

What are proteins?

In any cell, there may be 20 thousand different proteins, each with a different job, each one the product of a gene recipe. Some are simply structural, providing physical characteristics such as keratin or collagen contributing solid structure in the skin, hair, and nails. Most, however, are **enzymes**, which regulate chemical reactions among the various chemical building blocks or nutrients in the cell.

Enzymes are important because they control almost all the work in the cell. They are biological catalysts, in that they facilitate a chemical reaction, either by bringing chemicals together to make a new chemical (an **anabolic** reaction), or by breaking a complex chemical down to its basic parts (a **catabolic** reaction). Both types of reaction are necessary to normal functioning. Growth is only possible when enzymes build structures anabolically from constituent parts. Digestion, on the other hand, is the breakdown of complex nutrients. Our bodies do not benefit directly from starch, for example. A group of enzymes, amylases, break down complex carbohydrates (e.g. starch) to simpler carbohydrates (sugars). Our bodies can then use the sugars for energy.

Enzymes can be highly specific. They work with target chemicals, called **substrates**. The common analogy, very appropriate here, is the 'lock and key', where the enzyme is a key, and the 'substrate' is the lock. Just as a key will work only in certain locks, an enzyme may work only on certain substrates. These can be highly specific, such that any change to the amino acid sequence of the enzyme might alter its activity or even entirely disable it, just as modifying the shape of a key will probably change its ability to open the lock. Other times, changing some of the amino acids will have no effect on the enzyme activity—this is analogous to, say, filing a notch in the handle of the key, as opposed to filing a notch in the teeth. Some enzymes are less specific, much like master keys that can open a series of different but related locks. Some can work with a wide range of substrates, and we could compare them to skeleton keys.

The human genome, the total complement of genetic information in a human, consists of about 60 thousand to 90 thousand different genes or recipes, so human cells have the capacity to make that many different proteins. Identical twins have identical DNA base sequences; the rest of us differ slightly by relatively minor differences in the DNA base sequence.

How does it all fit together?

How do DNA, RNA, chromosomes, genes, and proteins all work together in operating an organism? Let's look at a typical organism we all recognize: a plant. Follow the diagram (Figure 2). If we take a close look at a leaf with a magnifying glass or microscope we easily see cells, usually rectangular or spherical structures, all packed together. The entire leaf is composed of them; in fact, the entire plant is composed of them, as are all organisms. All living things are composed of cells and cell products. The cells may look somewhat different, from tissue to tissue or organism to organism, and they may perform different physiological or anatomical functions, but they're all basically the same. Remember, some organisms (like bacteria) consist of only one cell, others, like humans and our plant, consist of many cells.

Let's look at the next step of magnification of our leaf. Inside each cell is a spherical structure, the **nucleus**. The nucleus is home to the **chromosomes**; these are the X-shaped structures. They are composed of DNA wrapped up in protein. A linseed plant has thirty of these chromosomes; humans have forty-six. There's no firm relationship between complexity and number of chromosomes. Wheat plants have forty-eight chromosomes. Simple organisms like bacteria do not have nuclei or chromosomes like these: although it's still called a chromosome, the DNA in these simple organisms floats around the cell naked, without the protein covering.

With another step of magnification, inside the chromosome we see the coiled DNA. If we could remove the DNA from one cell and unwind the coils, we would have a long thread of DNA. That thread would be about 20 centimetres long if we took the DNA from a cell of linseed plant, about 2 metres if from a human cell.

Magnifying another step shows the arrangement of the genes. We notice that not the entire DNA is part of a gene recipe. In a higher organism (and invariably and perhaps chauvinistically we include ourselves in this category) less than half

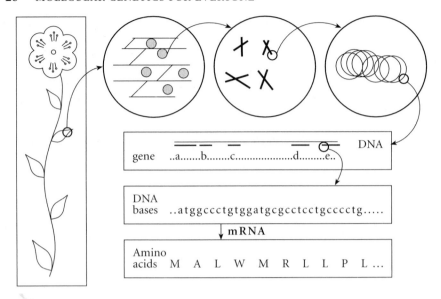

Figure 2   The secret of life condensed onto one page.
Starting with the stylized plant on the left, we encounter a series of magnifications to see, in progression, the arrangement of cells, each with a round nucleus. The second step magnifies the nucleus of one cell to view the chromosomes, the X-shaped structures, composed of DNA wrapped in protein.

The next step shows the coils of DNA within a portion of one of the chromosomes. Magnifying a tiny portion of the DNA we can see, in the first horizontal panel, how the genes are arranged on the DNA molecule. Only five genes (a, b, c, d, and e) are shown here, out of perhaps 25 thousand in a typical plant cell. Notice that adjacent genes are not always abutting; there is often considerable DNA space between genes, as indicated between genes c and d here. Any cell taken from an organism will have the same genes, in the same arrangement, as any other cell from the same organism.

The middle panel shows the DNA base sequence, a magnification of the start of gene e. All DNA, whether part of a gene or not, is made from the same four bases (A, T, C, and G). Only a few bases are shown from this gene. In real life, the average gene is about a thousand bases long. Like all genes, gene e provides a recipe for a protein. The machinery of the cell follows the recipe in order, generating a string of amino acids which, when complete, constitute a particular protein. It is the presence or absence of a specific protein that gives a trait or characteristic to an organism.

The last panel how the cell machinery uses messenger-RNA (mRNA) as a template to begin assembling the specified amino acids, normally found floating around the cell as common nutrients. The DNA bases, read three at a time, call for particular amino acids.

In our gene e, for example, the first three DNA bases, atg, specify the amino acid methionine (Met, or M). The next three bases, gcc specify alanine (Ala, or A). The cell 'cook' brings a molecule of Ala and chemically attaches it to the Met. The next three bases in the recipe, ctg, call for leucine (Leu, or L). Again, the cell finds a molecule of Leu and attaches it to the Ala. The process continues, with an ever-increasing chain of amino acids, until the recipe is completed. The resulting amino acid chain, now called a polypeptide chain, may be further modified to enable a functional protein. With this new protein, the organism 'expresses' a specific trait associated with the gene. Other amino acids shown are tryptophan (Try, or W), arginine (Arg, or R), and proline (Pro, or P).

The four foundational pillars of genetics

Anyone who has completed a biology course in school will be able to comprehend the basics of molecular genetics. With the following four simple points, all of the salient concepts in genetic engineering are made understandable. For those of you who have not taken such a course, or who need a refresher, here they are:

1 All organisms are made of cells and cell products. Some organisms—bacteria and the amoebae, for example—consist of one cell. Most plants and animals consist of many cells. Most cells are not quite large enough to be visible to the naked eye.

2 Each cell in an organism contains the same set of genes (referred to as the 'genome'). Each of your liver cells contains the same DNA sequence, the same genetic information as each of your skin cells. The difference is that many of the recipes are not read or 'expressed' in any given type of cell. That is, your liver cells will not make proteins used only by skin cells, and vice versa, even though the recipes are present in every cell.

3 The genome contains all the genetic information needed to make the entire organism. Theoretically, we might take a mature cell from, say, the liver of a mouse, and have it grow an entire new mouse, a genetically identical clone of the parent mouse donating the liver cell. This cloning is done almost routinely in some plants, but the technology is still crude in animals. Dolly the sheep made headlines because she grew from a single mature cell. The first plant clones from single mature cells were generated over fifty years ago. The resulting carrots weren't given names, nor did they attract much media attention.

4 All organisms share the same genetic language. The basis of all genetic engineering is the common language of DNA. A gene from a mouse can be read and properly understood in a human cell or, for that matter, a plant cell. Take an example of a short DNA base sequence, ATGGCCCTG. All organisms from bacteria to humans will read this information and construct the same amino acid sequence, resulting in the same polypeptide chain (protein). This real-life DNA sequence is the start of the gene recipe for the protein insulin. The human gene recipe for insulin was inserted into bacteria by scientists at Genentech Inc. Since 1978, the bacteria have been making genetically engineered human insulin, injected by everyone diagnosed with diabetes in recent years. Not only does this technology save cattle, pigs, and sheep from sacrifice to provide insulin, the amino acid sequence of the genetically engineered insulin is better suited to human usage because it is so, well, human. It is so good, in fact, that the first users switching from animal insulin had to carefully monitor and adjust their dosages to account for the 'perfect fit'.

of the DNA is part of a gene recipe. Most the DNA bases serve regulatory functions, to turn genes on or off as appropriate, or simply as spacers between genes and even within parts of genes. Physically, each gene is a portion of DNA. A typical plant carries about 20 thousand to 25 thousand genes; we do not yet know the number for certain.

By increasing our magnification one more step, we see how the DNA chemical bases (A, T, C, and G), are arranged in long sequences. An average gene is composed of about a thousand of these bases. A simple plant or animal can have DNA composed of 100 million bases in each cell.

To return to the cookery book analogy, we can think of each of our chromosomes as an individual volume in an encyclopaedia of recipes. Just as a major encyclopaedia is too long to fit into one volume, so is our DNA too long to fit into one chromosome. Human cells (with a couple of exceptions) carry twenty-three pairs of chromosomes, forty-six in total. These are explored wonderfully in Matt Ridley's book, *Genome* (see Chapter 16, for more information).

Bacteria are not as complex as humans are; they don't need as many proteins, they don't have livers, muscle, or other specialist tissue, so they don't need different cell types. Their genes fit into one long DNA molecule, freely floating around inside the single bacterial cell. They also lack an important genetic safety back-up system. As noted above, each human cell has twenty-three pairs of chromosomes. Each of the corresponding partners in a pair is called a **homologue**. The pairing of chromosomes is important and fortuitous because, for example, if a gene on one chromosome mutates or is otherwise incapacitated, the homologous gene on the homologous chromosome usually provides the necessary protein to fulfil the duties of the trait and the organism carries on normally. However, when a bacterium suffers a mutation in a critical gene, it's out of luck. It dies.

However, the corresponding genes in homologous chromosomes of higher organisms are not always identical, just as the recipes for chocolate cake may differ somewhat between two different cookery books. They may perform the same function, but be distinct from each other.

An important distinction in our chromosome–cookery book volume analogy is that cookery books are usually arranged in a logical order. All recipes for entrées are grouped together, as are those for soups, desserts, and so on. Not so in nature's chromosomes. A recipe for a liver enzyme might be adjacent to a recipe for a blood protein.

In the 1990s, British scientists made a stunning observation, one to my mind equivalent to the discovery of the biological ubiquity of DNA. Mike Gale and his colleagues at Cambridge were investigating the arrangements of gene locations in cereal crop species. The linear order of genes along the chromosome was not well known then, but maps were being constructed showing the general location of a particular gene on a particular chromosome. It was not surprising that genes regulating completely different functions were located adjacent to each other, as there was already some evidence of this. What was fascinating was the particular gene arrangement on a chromosome was virtually identical in chromosomes of other cereal species. Conceptually, you could take chromosomes of wheat, rice, or maize, for instance, and line them up. The corresponding homologous genes would be aligned as well. This commonality of gene arrangement is called **synteny**.

There is no need for such alignment in organisms, any more than there is need for a common DNA language. The most likely explanation for the shared alignment is that there was an ancestor common to all cereals, and this was the gene order in the ancestral chromosome. However, the observation came as a complete surprise, making it that much more delightful. Similar gene alignment in chromosomes of different species is being observed elsewhere. The alignment of genes in major sections of human chromosome 21 appears to be almost identical to that in mouse chromosome 16. Not only is DNA and its language universal, but even the ordered arrangement of genes in chromosomes can be shared across different species. Organisms are more closely related than we previously thought.

This synteny does not imply that the chromosomes are interchangeable. I would not recommend a chromosome transplant between a mouse and a human (or vice versa) because the individual genes will have continued to evolve over the aeons. Although the genes from the different species might be homologous and the proteins retain similar functions, they are likely to be sufficiently different that there may be some difficulties, especially with enzymes and immunological reactivities. That is, the genes on the transplanted chromosome would likely make a protein sufficiently different from the local type to activate an unpleasant immune reaction.

Also, minor differences between homologous genes of different species might have greater consequences in practice. There were some initial problems in diabetic treatment when genetically engineered insulin was first approved to replace animal insulin. Patients previously using the animal insulin suddenly had to contend with human insulin, albeit produced by bacteria reading the human gene recipe. Adjustments in dosage and treatment regime were required because the GM human insulin worked better in humans than did animal insulin. Any change in therapeutic treatment, GM or non-GM, demands careful monitoring and possible adjustment.

The DNA base sequence of several genes from different species has been elucidated, but the 'holy grail' of DNA sequencing is to determine the complete DNA base sequence from humans. A massive international effort is grinding out the human ATCG sequence; it will be completed over the next few years. The complete sequence has already been elucidated for some single cell organisms, mainly bacteria and yeast. Work is also being conducted to sequence the entire genome of a higher plant, *Arabidopsis* (thale cress), which will serve as a 'recipe reference library' for crop plants. The complete DNA genome sequence has also been elucidated for one multicellular animal. It is a tiny nematode worm—the adult has less a thousand cells—technically known as *Caenorhabditis elegans* but usually abbreviated to *C. elegans*. It is such an insignificant worm that it doesn't have a common name. Its only claim to fame, other than being the first animal to be completely DNA sequenced, is that its parasitic relatives are responsible for some $80 billion in crop losses each year. The completed DNA sequence analysis from a second animal, the common fruit fly (*Drosophila melanogaster*), has just been announced. Details should be available soon.

The DNA of *C. elegans* consists of 97 million ATCG base pairs carrying the genetic recipes for fewer than 20 thousand genes. Many of these genes seem to be unique to this species of worm (and probably serve to give the organism its characteristic 'worminess'), but a great many, almost 7000 of the 20 thousand in total, are homologous to known counterpart genes in humans. On this basis, one could justifiably conclude that these insignificant creatures are one-third human.

Similar information continues to pour in concerning our genetic relationship with other organisms. Apparently, we share about 99% of 'our' genes with chimpanzees. This comes as an astounding revelation to those chauvinists among us who think humans are unique. Even if the number is exaggerated, and the real value is more like 97% or even 93%, we must abandon any claim to both uniqueness and, especially, haughty superiority.

Clearly, since we share so many genes with other species, we do not possess 'our' genes. Rather, they 'own' us, as we are simply their ephemeral corporeal manifestations. 'Our' genes were in existence long before any one of us came along and will probably continue to thrive long after we are gone. We are simply their carriers through a small portion of their evolution.

I noted above that the little worm has about seven thousand genes in common with humans. But if the human genome is not yet sequenced, how do we know we have seven thousand genes in common with the worm? **Gene banks** are international databases keeping track of DNA base sequences along with associated protein amino acid sequences. The largest and most comprehensive database is the American gene bank, called, appropriately enough and complete with typical American spelling, Genbank. Although there are several, we usually say we're going to 'the bank' as if there's only one. Gene banks are wonderful resources for molecular biologists.

Although the complete human genome has not been fully sequenced, a substantial portion of it has, and the information from these portions is deposited in the gene banks, along with information acquired by similar sequencing projects for other species in labs around the world. The gene banks are searchable by computer and able to identify similarities in DNA sequences between different organisms, which is fortunate, because few humans would be capable of searching thousands of records per second. For example, to make the amino acids lysine, valine, and isoleucine, plants need acetolactate synthase (ALS). The gene providing the recipe for this enzyme (*als*)* is common in plants but the *als* gene

---

* By convention, we abbreviate gene names in lower case italics (e.g. *als*); the resulting protein is in upper case (e.g. ALS). DNA base sequence can be either upper case (ATCG) or lower case (atcg).

never has exactly the same DNA base sequence. (The *als* gene is not present in animals although we do need the amino acids to make our proteins. We acquire these particular amino acids by consuming organisms that do make them.)

Parts of a gene

Every cell contains every gene for the entire organism, so each cell needs to know which of the genes it should read and express (i.e. activate the recipe to make a protein). There can be no cell specialization or different tissue types if every cell expresses every gene. Although all cells express genes controlling common basic and necessary living functions, a given tissue will also express a set of genes related to the special functions of that tissue type. A liver cell will express the basic survival genes (called 'housekeeping' genes) in addition to liver function genes. All the other genes are present in the liver cell, but they are not expressed. How does a cell know which genes to express?

Each gene has at least three basic parts:

1 a **promoter**, a sequence of DNA serving as a switch
2 the part of the DNA sequence that is to be translated into an amino acid sequence
3 a simple tail, or ending sequence, the **terminator,** to signal termination of a gene.

Higher organisms (**eukaryotes**) have more complicated cellular structures than lower organisms such as bacteria (**prokaryotes**). Eukaryotes are higher organisms, easily distinguished from the low-life prokaryotes by having a nucleus to store their chromosomes. Not so easily noticed is an additional feature of the genes. Eukaryotes such as humans, trees, and flatworms have **introns**, DNA sequences within a gene but not translated into amino acids. When a eukaryotic gene is expressed, these intron sequences are removed or spliced out during the translation to make a functional protein. Bacteria, as prokaryotes, have no introns in their genes. A bacterium cannot read and express a gene containing introns. Although the DNA code remains the same, and a bacterial gene can be read and expressed by a eukaryote, a gene containing one or more introns cannot be properly expressed to make a functional protein in a bacterium. In order to get a bacterium to make a eukaryotic protein, such as insulin, any introns must be stripped from the eukaryotic gene.

These 'non-coding' regions of a gene are part of the genetic regulatory system. They do not directly contribute to the final amino acid sequence of the functional protein, but assist in determining when and where a particular gene is expressed. Sometimes these regulatory regions occupy a large proportion of DNA bases. Even a small simple protein like insulin requires far more DNA bases than those needed solely to code for the amino acids in the amino acid sequence of the insulin protein itself. The insulin gene in humans is several thousand DNA bases long, enough to code for over a thousand amino acids, yet the coding portion accounts for just over a hundred amino acids, which are processed to a final protein of only fifty amino acids. We'll take a closer look at insulin later.

Many regulatory sequences, such as the terminator regions, are almost interchangeable between genes and between species. The introns are a bit trickier, in that the processing enzymes in the host cell must be able to identify exactly which parts of the sequences are intron sequences to be spliced out. Prokaryotes have no such intron splicing capability, which is why genes with introns are not functional in bacteria or other prokaryotic organisms. This point is worth noting when discussing the possibility of inadvertent transfer of genes from GM crops or animals to bacteria. Bacteria are unable to make use of genes carrying introns.

The most important and specific regulatory DNA sequence, the promoter, is the switch that activates protein synthesis, causing the gene to be 'expressed'. Few cells in the human body actually produce insulin, but all cells carry the gene. The promoter is what makes the few cells in the pancreas synthesize insulin. Every gene DNA sequence begins with a promoter. Promoters have some similar features, but also some unique features, allowing them to be activated by different stimuli. Some promoters are **constitutive**, meaning they are always actively producing more of the protein. These are found on common genes necessary to maintain basic life processes in every type of cell. If the function required a large quantity of the protein, the promoter is said to be a **strong constitutive promoter**. Other genes might require a constant but lower production of protein; these have **weak constitutive promoters**. Other promoters may be activated by light, heat, moisture, or the presence (or absence) of particular chemicals, or only at specific developmental stages or only in particular mature tissues (such as insulin in the pancreas).

The end of the gene is a more simple DNA sequence called the terminator. It simply tells the cell 'cook' that the recipe is finished.

The parts of a gene, then, are (reading from left to right, as is standard scientific parlance referring to the chemical structure of DNA):

- a **promoter**, to activate protein synthesis when required
- the **coding region**, the DNA sequence to be translated into the amino acid sequence in the ultimately functional resulting protein
- optional **introns** in eukaryotic genes, located within the DNA coding region but spliced out during processing to make the functional protein
- a **terminator** region, indicating the end of the gene.

How does this relate to the genetics learnt in school?

Most people learn something of genetics in school, focused on Gregor Mendel, the father of genetics, and his various laws of genetic inheritance. So far, we've been dealing with molecular genetics. There doesn't seem to be an obvious connection. How does the 'traditional' genetics of Mendel fit with modern molecular genetics?

A few years ago I was honoured with an invitation to speak at a conference in Brno (in what was the Austrian Empire in Mendel's day, then Czechoslovakia, now the Czech Republic). In this city Mendel conducted his experiments on, among other things, simple traits like height and seed colour in garden peas. While in Brno I made the required pilgrimage to the enjoyable museum bearing Mendel's name, and observed a pleasant display of the early history of genetics. Planted in a couple of small flower beds outside the main doors, a series of rows of begonias illustrated the principles of crossing and progeny segregation first

---

The law of independent assortment

Remember, human cells have forty-six chromosomes: two pairs of twenty-two chromosomes plus the two 'sex' chromosomes: X and X for females, X and Y for males. The paired chromosomes don't have names, just numbers: the largest pair was numbered 1, the smallest was numbered 22.* It's not a creative or imaginative system, but it's easy to remember.

Not every cell in your body always has forty-six chromosomes. Just before an ordinary cell divides, it makes a copy of its chromosomes, so there are actually ninety-two chromosomes for a short time, until the cell divides and each of the two resulting 'daughter cells' (sexist term, perhaps, but traditional usage; there are no 'son' cells) receives a normal assortment of forty-six in the process called mitosis.

Gametes, the 'sex' cells of sperm or eggs, undergo a reduction in chromosomes to have twenty-three chromosomes in the cell. This process is called meiosis. A normal egg cell contains twenty-three chromosomes, and a normal sperm cell contains twenty-three chromosomes. When they hybridize together at fertilization, the resulting embryo cell then contains the normal forty-six chromosomes, twenty-three from each parent.

The important feature of these chromosome processes is that when the cell divides, each daughter cell gets one of the two of any given pair of chromosomes. For example, no normal daughter cell ends up with both the paternal chromosomes 6, leaving the other daughter cell with no paternal chromosome 6.

---

*   They got it wrong. Recent measurements show the smallest is actually chromosome 21.

described by Mendel. Coming across the display, I thought, 'What a great educational and illustrative idea!' but on closer inspection I became perplexed; I couldn't figure out what traits were being depicted. Perhaps this was intentional, to show the confusing results Mendel sometimes had to contend with, but I doubt it. Most presentations of Mendel's teachings were, and are, unnecessarily confusing.

During secondary school biology lessons on Mendel and his laws, I recall being confused by the 'law of independent assortment'? 'Independent assortment' sounds like an obstreperous collection of liquorice allsorts. What is it?

The law of independent assortment says that each of the chromosomes separate independently of other pairs during mitosis and meiosis. For example, the paternal chromosome 6 (i.e. the one that comes from the father's gamete), will migrate during mitosis to one of the daughter cells independently of paternal chromosome 7, 8, or any other. Consequently, the maternal chromosome 6 will find itself in the other daughter cell, along with a mixture of the other chromosomes, some of which will have originated from the father, some from the mother. Each of the daughter cells will end up with twenty-three chromosomes; some will have originated from the father, the others from the mother. (See Box.)

This is a good law, because it allows us to have some genetic properties from each of our grandparents, and keeps siblings born years apart from potentially being identical twins.

What about dominant and recessive genes?

Dominant means powerful, and the recessive cowers in the presence of a dominant, right? Perhaps in ordinary English, but not in the scientific lexicon. Novice genetics students often ask, 'Why aren't dominant genes more, well, dominant? Why don't they eventually take over and push the recessive genes into the oblivion of extinction?'

They don't do this because they aren't dominant in that sense. There's no such thing as a recessive gene. A recessive gene is simply one that is non-functional or doesn't work properly, but is occupying the place in the recipe book (in genetic parlance, the locus) dedicated to a particular gene. Cystic fibrosis is a disorder caused by a defect in a gene (*cftr*) located on human chromosome 7. The protein from the normal *cftr* gene regulates sodium and calcium flow between cells. Suppose a spontaneous mutation (i.e. a change in the DNA) changes a single base in the DNA of the *cftr* gene. That mutation can result in a partially impaired or even completely non-functional protein. The gene itself is still located on chromosome 7, but has become 'recessive' because it no longer produces a functional CFTR protein.

The term 'recessive' is used by traditional geneticists, sometimes called Mendelian geneticists, but molecular geneticists find it superfluous or confusing.

In molecular genetics, all functional genes (like the normal *cftr* gene) are dominant. All non-functional genes (like a mutated *cftr* gene) are recessive. There's no point inserting a recessive gene into an organism because it would have no effect; it's non-functional. It is a piece of DNA that simply doesn't code for a functional protein.

How, then, do we give an organism a 'recessive' appearance?

We can't 'turn off' a dominant gene by inserting a recessive gene and hoping for 'recessive' segregation in the progeny. And we can't remove a functional gene using molecular techniques, at least not simply. That objective is much more easily accomplished using classical mutation breeding. However, it is possible to use molecular techniques to inactivate a dominant gene, giving the resulting organism a 'recessive' appearance.

We do this by making a copy of the gene in question and reinserting it into the organism. In some cases, there is conflict or interference between the two copies of the gene, resulting in a dramatic reduction in function of that gene. Also, re-inserting the gene backwards, or inverted, can have the same effect. The Flavr-Savr™ tomato is a famous example of taking a normal gene and inserting it back into the organism, but in reverse orientation, to achieve the equivalent of a recessive appearance. In normal tomatoes, this gene codes for an enzyme called polygalacturonase, which is responsible for ripening the tomato. When there is interference between the functional gene and the inserted version, polygalacturonase is not synthesized, ripening slows to a crawl, and the fruit appears to remain 'fresh' longer.

How do we obtain genes for transfer in genetic engineering?

Currently, there are several ways of obtaining genes; the easiest is to get them from a gene bank. Before there were banks, though, it was much more difficult. The process took years of hard, tedious work employing several techniques, most of which were still in rudimentary form.

Bacteria

Most of the first real genes were acquired from the simplest organisms such as bacteria. Microbiologists have had long experience dealing with bacterial genetics, because the simpler organisms have simpler genetic characteristics and can also be mutated more easily.

Bacteria are clever creatures. They have evolved genes to allow them to live in the most inhospitable environments: the ancient frozen ice banks of Antarctica, the depths of the oceans, boiling geysers. They have even evolved genes to enable them to thrive in the human bowels. Despite being the 'bottom feeders' on the food chain, these organisms have some truly remarkable skills. If you need a gene to do a dirty job, chances are some bacterium somewhere will have beat you to it, living and flourishing in the filth. Let's take a closer look at these fascinating creatures.

Bacteria come in a multitude of different species and may be round, rectangular, or spiral, but all are single-celled. Their genome is naked DNA. In addition to one long naked piece of DNA serving as the main chromosome, bacteria may have **plasmids**—small circular pieces of DNA. Plasmids often carry special purpose genes, such as an antibiotic resistance gene, which generates a protein enabling the bacterium to withstand an ordinarily lethal antibiotic. The plasmid is composed of several functional DNA components. The gene is a segment of the plasmid DNA. In addition to the gene, the plasmid also needs an **origin of replication**, a starting point for its own duplication. Every time the bacterium divides, each daughter cell needs at least one copy of the plasmid. Otherwise, the antibiotic resistance (or whatever the special gene does) is lost from that daughter cell. Some plasmids are present in many copies; other types may have only one copy per bacterial cell. Plasmids are extremely useful because they allow the bacterium to live in the presence of a specific antibiotic or other unpleasant circumstances. However, in the absence of the antibiotic or other stress agent, plasmids are undesirable excess genetic baggage and may be eliminated within a few generations. The presence of a plasmid slows down the growth of a bacterium when the genes on the plasmid are not being used. That is, in the absence of the relevant antibiotic, other bacteria quickly outgrow the plasmid-carrying ones and so come to dominate the bacterial population.

All of these different bacteria have something genetic to offer us. We don't need to artificially synthesize any genes, as is implied by the term 'genetic engineering'. In most cases, bacteria will have done the engineering for us. All we have to do is find the right bacterium and extract the desired gene. If we're lucky, the desired gene is on a plasmid, as plasmids are especially easy to isolate and characterize. If the desired or otherwise interesting gene cannot be found on a plasmid, we can always mutate the main DNA in the bacteria. How?

Scientists start with a uniform population of bacteria and then mutate them by exposure to a nasty toxic chemical or radiation or some other mutagenic agent, anything to cause a change in the DNA. They then look for differences in surviving bacterial populations. Suppose you found a population of bacteria capable of growing in a high concentration of salt water. You mutate part of a population of the saline-loving bacteria, keeping another part as a control group. Then you check the mutant colonies to see if any have lost the ability to grow in the highly saline conditions (see Box for details). Although the incidence of getting the right mutation (i.e. destruction of the gene enabling the saline survival) is small, the advantage of working with bacteria is that you can grow zillions* of them easily. It doesn't matter if the right mutation only occurs in one in a million bacteria if you have a trillion bacteria to work with—you'd have thousands of colonies to choose from.

This all takes a long time and effort, and doesn't usually work as easily as indicated in the Box. Remember, you only ever read or hear about the success stories or dramatic failures. The usual and mundane failures don't often get reported. Everything that can go wrong will go wrong. Perseverance is the key.

Getting genes from the gene bank is much easier, but not many genes were available from the bank in the early 1980s. The first plant genes were just being isolated then. Most of the available genes were from bacteria, and those didn't offer too much in the way of improved traits for crop species.

Finding suitable mutants

After identifying the population with the inability to grow on saline media, you extract the DNA from the original population (always keeping some bacteria alive and happy on the saline culture medium) and use enzymes to cut the extracted DNA into pieces. You can then separate the DNA pieces according to size, using a technique called electrophoresis, and feed each piece (fragment) to the mutant bacteria. Certain bacteria can be treated to take up DNA from their surroundings. Then you replace the mutant bacteria on a saline medium. With luck, a colony of mutant bacteria will grow on saline medium, while the other groups of mutants remain unable to grow. You then determine which DNA fragment was fed to the 'transformed' bacteria with the reacquired ability to grow on saline. Say it was fragment 81. This tells you the gene responsible is likely on fragment 81. The you repeat the experiment of feeding the DNA to the mutant bacteria to confirm that it wasn't a fluke result, or a labelling mistake, or another mutation, or any of the other myriad reasons these things happen. Once you're convinced that fragment 81 is the right one, you repeat the feeding experiments using only DNA fragment 81, but this time you use different enzymes to cut fragment 81 into smaller pieces. Eventually, you end up with the smallest fragment that will successfully transform the mutant bacteria to once again be able to grow on saline.

An agronomically useful gene from bacteria

In the early 1980s, Monsanto was making a huge amount of money from their popular herbicide, Roundup™. Their scientists knew all about the chemistry of the active ingredient in Roundup™, glyphosate. This herbicide attacks EPSP synthase,

---

* No, this is not a technical term but it is a convenient way of describing an unimaginably large number.

a crucial enzyme in plants and microbes. Animals, including humans, lack this enzyme, hence the relative safety of the chemical. EPSP synthase helps make the amino acids tyrosine, phenylalanine, and tryptophan within the plant and microbial cell. If EPSP synthase is inhibited by glyphosate, the cell can no longer make the amino acids. Lacking the essential amino acids, the organism starves to death, unable to make proteins requiring these amino acids. This is why Roundup™ is most effective as a herbicide when applied during active plant growth.

Glyphosate is a very powerful but non-selective herbicide, meaning it inhibits ESPS synthase in all plants. Most herbicides affect only certain plant species and are used on non-sensitive crop species (i.e. ones that don't respond to the chemical) to control sensitive weeds (i.e. ones that do respond, usually by dying) in the crop. Because most fields have a number of different plant species as weeds, weed control often requires applications of several different herbicides to kill or suppress all the different non-crop plants. If a crop species could be made resistant to glyphosate, then farmers could spray that crop with one herbicide, glyphosate, and have complete weed control without damage to the crop plants.

Many scientists around the world, recognizing that Monsanto's patent on glyphosate was nearing the end of its legal lifetime, were trying to find plants with natural Roundup resistance or to develop mutant plants, with little success. Monsanto scientists were engaged in the same race, looking to extend their monopoly by finding and patenting genes conferring resistance to glyphosate. The task was difficult because EPSP synthase is a crucial but delicate enzyme, and any modifications to it to reduce the inhibition by glyphosate would simultaneously reduce the effectiveness as an enzyme in making the amino acids.

Calgene, the small California biotech firm, was a mouse taunting the Monsanto lion. Calgene found and patented a gene conferring resistance to Roundup™. Until this time, no one had ever found a plant or microbe able to withstand lethal doses of glyphosate. The bright brains at Calgene, instead of joining the masses in futile exercises by investigating plants, looked to other organisms. Bacteria usually develop resistance to chemicals far sooner than plants or animals, so they went looking to see if any bacteria were growing in chemical dumps containing glyphosate. They found such bacteria and analysed them to see why they were able to withstand the effects of glyphosate. The Calgene scientists found, isolated, and cloned (copied) the gene responsible. Monsanto, of course, was not happy with this development, as they had a clear patent on glyphosate itself and, if anyone were to find a biological resistance, they felt it should be them, not some upstart company in California. Unfortunately for Monsanto, Calgene took out a patent on their bacterial glyphosate resistance gene. This caused particular annoyance to the giant company because it forced them to try to find a similar resistance gene from higher organisms, which are far more difficult to work with. Depending on your lawyer's interpretation of the patent awarded to Calgene, even that might have constituted an infringement, as it is not clear whether a resistance gene isolated from higher organisms would be protected.

Eukaryotes

Sometimes it is preferable or even necessary to obtain a gene from a higher organism, despite the greater complexity of eukaryotic genes.

The basic method used to isolate a gene from bacteria also works with higher organisms, but is much more difficult because of the far greater amount of DNA and number of genes in higher organisms. Monsanto scientists were satisfied that no one had been able to find or create a plant resistant to glyphosate through mutation work. However, they and others were able to generate plant cell lines capable of surviving a greater dosage than would ordinarily kill the cells. In investigating why these cell lines had greater tolerance to glyphosate, they found the cells did not alter the structure of the EPSP synthase, but rather produced more of the sensitive enzyme than normal cells. By increasing the amount of target enzyme, the effect of a given dose of the herbicide was effectively diluted.

How did the cells acquire these additional quantities of enzyme? Gene promoters evolved different mechanisms to activate protein synthesis for their respective gene. For important cell nutrient components, such as essential amino acids, the genes responsible are active when protein synthesis is taking place. When the cell starts running low on these building supplies, the gene promoter gets a message—'we need more of your amino acid'—and synthesis of the enzyme responsible for making more of the amino acid is induced. Protein synthesis makes the enzyme from the gene recipe, the enzyme synthesizes more of the amino acids, the supply becomes satisfactory, and the promoter shuts off the gene. No need to continue using energy making a product for which there is no current demand.

In the presence of small, sub-lethal amounts of glyphosate, the EPSP synthase is constantly under attack, but not sufficiently to shut down amino acid biosynthesis completely. In this situation the plant is in a growth phase, needing ongoing protein synthesis. The cell is constantly calling for more amino acid. The gene is in constant production, continually producing more EPSP synthase, much of which, but not all, is then attacked and inactivated by the glyphosate. The gene is running flat out, producing as much EPSP synthase as quickly as possible, but still has insufficient amino acid resources to sustain growth. What's a poor cell to do?

Herbicide dose and amount of enzyme

Let's assume that one molecule of herbicide will combine with (inhibit) one molecule of enzyme. A killing dose would have an at least as many herbicide molecules as there are enzyme molecules. If more than the usual number of enzyme molecules were present, the standard dose of herbicide would be insufficient to inhibit all the extra enzyme molecules. A higher dosage of herbicide would be required to inactivate the extra EPSP synthase enzyme in the cell.

As always, nature eventually finds a way around every obstacle. Using a semi-tolerant petunia cell culture, Monsanto scientists took a closer look and discovered the cells were producing more EPSP synthase enzyme by duplicating and reduplicating the gene over and over, until there were thousands of copies, each producing more and more enzyme. Although genetic duplication requires the expenditure of a lot of energy, the cells survived because the effect of the glyphosate was constantly being diluted by the excess EPSP synthase enzyme.

Fortunately for the plant, and unfortunately for Monsanto, this genetic multiplication is reversible. When the herbicide was withdrawn, the genes returned to their normal number. This is good for the plant because it cannot afford to continue wasting energy maintaining thousands of unnecessary genes. It is not so good for Monsanto because the method is not a suitable mechanism to use in crops. The degree of tolerance it afforded was insufficient for commercially use, and the gene multiplication took too long, as it developed over a period of time of sub-lethal exposure to the glyphosate. A single application of glyphosate in the field, instead of a gradual exposure, would kill the plants before they could respond with the gene multiplication.

The clever scientists at Monsanto—Robb Fraley, Rob Horsch, and others, many of whom are still there—did not give up. They took advantage of the fact that the petunia cells had so many copies of the EPSP synthase gene that it became easier to find and extract. Ordinarily, finding one single gene among up to 25 thousand other genes in a plant genome is like looking for a specific needle in a needle stack. They're all made of sequences of DNA, they all look much the same. However, having a cell line with thousands of copies of the desired gene makes identifying and isolating the gene much easier. The Monsanto scientists were able to isolate and clone the petunia EPSP synthase gene. Having it isolated meant they could make some alterations more easily, put the altered gene back into a plant and observe how the modified plant would react to glyphosate. Soon enough, but still taking considerable time and effort, they came up with a modified EPSP synthase enzyme less recognized by glyphosate, but still functional in its usual duty of helping make the aromatic amino acids. Monsanto had their first 'herbicide-tolerant gene'.

Gene banks

In recent years, banks internationally have been decreasing service while increasing service charges, and yet recording record profits. You must make deposits before you make withdrawals, and withdrawing more than was previously deposited is frowned on; the bank manifests its disapproval either by massive service charges or by outright refusal. You might be able to borrow from a bank, but usually only if you can prove you don't have to. Even borrowing comes with a hefty price (the interest on the loan), and an obligation to repay the principal.

(a)

Amino acid sequence for rat (top line) and human (lower line) insulin. Differences are shown in bold.

Rat: *start* MALWMR**F**LPLLALL**VLWE**P**K**PA**Q**AFVKQHLCG**P**HLVEALYLVCGERGFFYTPK**SR**

Human: *start* MALWMR**LL**PLLALL**A**LW**GPD**PA**A**AFVNQHLCG**S**HLVEALYLVCGERGFFYTPK**TR**

Rat: RE**V**ED**P**QV**P**QLELGGGP**E**AGDL**Q**TLALE**VAR**QKRGI**V**D**Q**CCTSICSLYQLENYCN*end*.

Human: RE**A**ED**L**QV**GQ**VELGGGP**G**AGSL**Q**PLALE**GSL**QKRGI**V**E**Q**CCTSICSLYQLENYCN*end*.

(b)
```
2401 tcccagatca ctgtccttct gccatggccc tgtggatgcg cctcctgccc ctgctggcgc
2461 tgctggccct ctggggacct gacccagccg cagcctttgt gaaccaacac ctgtgcggct
2521 cacacctggt ggaagctctc tacctagtgt gcggggaacg aggcttcttc tacacaccca
2581 agacccgccg ggaggcagag gacctgcagg gtgagccaac cgcccattgc tgccctggc
2641 cgcccccagc caccccctgc tcctggcgct cccacccagc atgggcagaa gggggcagga
2701 ggctgccacc cagcaggggg tcaggtgcac tttttttaaa agaagttctc ttggtcacgt
2761 cctaaaagtg accagctccc tgtggcccag tcagaatctc agcctgagga cggtgttggc
2821 ttcggcagcc ccgagataca tcagagggtg ggcacgctcc tccctccact cgccctcaa
2881 acaaatgccc cgcagcccat ttctccaccc tcatttgatg accgcagatt caagtgtttt
2941 gttaagtaaa gtcctgggtg acctggggtc acagggtgcc ccacgctgcc tgcctctggg
3001 cgaacacccc atcacgcccg gaggagggcg tggctgcctg cctgagtggg ccagacccct
3061 gtcgccagcc tcacggcagc tccatagtca ggagatgggg aagatgctgg ggacaggccc
3121 tggggagaag tactgggatc acctgttcag gctcccactg tgacgctgcc ccggggcgggg
3181 ggaaggaggt gggacatgtg ggcgttgggg cctgtaggtc cacacccagt gtgggtgacc
3241 ctccctctaa cctgggtcca gcccggctgg agatgggtgg gagtgcgacc tagggctgag
3301 gggcaggcgg gcactgtgtc tccctgactg tgtcctcctg tgtccctctg cctcgccgct
3361 gttccggaac ctgctctgcg cggcacgtcc tggcagtggg gcaggtggag ctgggcgggg
3421 gccctggtgc aggcagcctg cagcccttgg ccctggaggg gtccctgcag aagcgtggca
3481 ttgtggaaca atgctgtacc agcatctgct ccctctacca gctggagaac tactgcaact
3541 agacgcagcc tgcaggcagc cccacacccg ccgcctcctg caccgagaga gatggaataa
3601 agcccttgaa ccagc
```

Figure 3   A sample of an entry from Genbank: (a) The human amino acid sequence and the comparable amino acid sequence of the rat insulin gene. Note only one of the first 10 amino acids differs between rat and human insulin. Of the total of 102 amino acids, only 19 are different between rats and humans. This sequence uses the single-letter codes for amino acids: A, alanine; R, arginine; N, asparagine; D, aspartic acid; C, cysteine; Q, glutathione; E, glutamic acid; G, glycine; H, histidine; I, isoleucine; L, leucine; K, lysine; M, methionine; F, phenylalanine; P, proline; S. serine; T, threonine; W, tryptophan; Y, tyrosine; V, valine.

(b) The DNA base sequence of the insulin gene, located on human chromosome 11, was provided to Genbank by Dr G. I. Bell of the University of California, San Francisco. The complete entry consists of over four thousand bases and can be found at the public access Genbank website (*http://www.ncbi.nlm.nih.gov/ Web/Genbank*). The sequence coding for amino acids starts with atg (shown in bold) at position 2424, and runs to position 3615.

Now imagine a bank that allows deposits and withdrawals, as with conventional banks. In this bank, however, you can make withdrawals before making any deposits, and you can withdraw more than you ever deposit. In fact, you need never make any deposits at all. You don't even need an account! Borrowing is obsolete (that concept generates true interest!). Why borrow when you can simply withdraw without any obligation to repay?

Flight of fancy? No, this bank is real. It's a gene bank. It works because of the generosity of thousands of scientists around the world who voluntarily deposit the fruits of their labour with little or no direct reward, other than the recognition and appreciation of those of us who make withdrawals. The other remarkable feature is that a withdrawal does not diminish capital. The 'original' deposited material remains in the bank; what you get on withdrawal is like a photocopy of the original capital. Downloading a gene, or a portion of a gene, provides a copy of the DNA base sequence.

Figure 3 shows a record for a withdrawal from the US Genbank, a portion of the human insulin gene. You may notice that the base sequence is only given for one strand. This is the 'sense' strand, the one the cell uses as the recipe. The other strand isn't included, but is complementary, so you could figure it out if you wanted, but no one bothers.

Also provided is the deduced amino acid sequence. The names of the different amino acids are now abbreviated to single letters (A for Alanine, M for Methionine, etc.) to save space—this is the convention molecular biologists generally use. Observe how similar the amino acid sequence is between humans and rats. This similarity, called **homology**, allows us to calculate how closely related we are to rats. It also allows diabetic humans to use cow, pig, or sheep insulin, because it is so similar to our own. Nowadays, of course, diabetics use genetically engineered human insulin, because it is exactly like our own.

The careful observer will have also noticed another oddity. Earlier I said each 3 bases on the DNA is a code word for one amino acid. The DNA sequence for insulin is over 4000 bases long, which means there should be over 1300 amino acids in the protein, but in fact there are just over 100: What is happening here? The answer is that not all of the DNA bases code for amino acids. These additional bases form the other parts of the gene—the promoter, introns, and so on—as discussed earlier. Some of them provide instructions, just as in our cookery book. Recipes give preparation instructions as well as calling for ingredients. The basic list of ingredients isn't sufficient to make a protein. We also need to know the instructions, just as in preparing a recipe.

Genbank listings

The information in the gene bank listing allows me to do a number of things.

- I can use it to reconstruct the physical DNA using a 'gene machine', which artificially synthesizes the DNA from bottles of purified ATCG bases (one base per bottle). Each base is chemically added one at a time and stuck together in the appropriate order according to the recipe acquired from the bank.
- Alternatively, I could use the information to synthesize **primers**, short stretches of DNA from the recipe that are used to 'fish out' the homologous gene from my species of interest.

Primers are effective because of two important features of genes:

1 First, many genes are common to many or most species; they are said to be 'conserved' because they provide a recipe for a protein critical to a common life process. For example, organisms must maintain genes coding for proteins that help synthesize DNA, others that repair DNA, and so on. Because the duties are so similar, the genes for those proteins are also homologous across different species. Look again at the diagram of the human insulin gene in comparison with the rat version (Figure 3). Both mammals require sugar control, and insulin provides it. (Strictly speaking, this protein is not the final, functional product. It is not unusual for cells to take the polypeptide chain and modify it before it becomes functional. Such is the case with our example, properly called 'preproinsulin', as the cell modifies the amino acid chains to make mature, functional human insulin.)

2 The second feature exploits the fact that DNA is composed of two strands (the double helix). Ordinarily, one strand is composed of the bases providing the instructions for the recipe; the other fills in with complementary bases to maintain the double-strandedness and also protects the information sequence bases. For example, if the coding sequence reads ATTCG, the complementary (second) strand would read TAAGC, because A always pairs with T, and G with C; these are the complementary pairs. We usually ignore the non-coding or second strand; if we need to we can figure it out just by filling in the complementary bases from the sequence of the coding bases, A with T, C with G. The two strands fit together rather like a zipper. If we apply energy, usually in the form of heat, the two strands separate from each other, but the bases don't separate from their adjacent neighbours; each individual strand remains intact. If we apply too much heat, the strands explode into bits and pieces, just like a real zipper. However, unlike a real zipper, the bits and pieces of DNA may be recycled into another strand. When we reduce the heat, the two strands recombine, with complementary bases seeking each other out. A sequence of TGCC will only reunite with a sequence of ACGG, so the DNA once again become double stranded, and all down the line, a T on one strand is across from A on the other, complementary, strand, while G is across from C.

Copying genes: the polymerase chain reaction (PCR)

The **polymerase chain reaction** (PCR), because of its power and simplicity, has revolutionized work in molecular genetics. Before it was developed just a few years ago, isolating a gene took years of painstaking work. One of my students took three years to isolate a relatively simple gene from a very simple bacterium. Now, with the gene bank and PCR, we can do it in a few days. Conceptually, PCR is like taking a computer with search capability and hooking it up to a photocopier. If we return to our analogy of the genome being an encyclopaedia of

The polymerase chain reaction

How can we copy genes? We can exploit the complementary magnetism of DNA. We add a pair of short stretches of DNA synthesized according to the gene bank recipe to a test tube containing DNA extracted from our species of interest. Then we apply a bit of heat to separate the double strands into single strands. We reduce the heat but, in the process of the complementary sequences finding each other, our synthesized DNA gets in the way, binding to any complementary DNA sequences on the extracted DNA. It competes with the second strand of the original double-stranded DNA. Then we add enzymes to the test tube to fill in the gaps between our two artificial stretches. Suppose the first of our synthesized short sequences of DNA is complementary to a sequence near the beginning of a gene on the extracted DNA, and the second is complementary to a sequence near the end, several hundred DNA bases away. When we reduce the heat, complementary sequences find and bind to each other. There will be a gap between the two synthesized primers, representing the intervening sequence of bases. The enzymes fill in the bases in between the primers, using the complementary bases on the extracted strand to guide them. When finished, the enzymes have synthesized a copy of the extracted DNA's gene.

By repeating this heating and repairing cycle several times, we can make many copies, or clones, of the original gene. (A clone, by the way, can be defined simply as 'exact copy', whether a gene, a sheep, a human, or a carrot.)

recipes, what PCR does is allow us to search for certain recipes, say those calling for 'four eggs' and make copies of the recipe. If we end up with several different recipes, we can repeat the search the next day, with greater specificity, perhaps combining 'four eggs and one cup of flour' until we end up with copies of the one recipe we want.

We usually let the PCR process cycle about twenty-five times, which conveniently takes overnight in a specially automated machine called a **thermocycler**. How many copies will we end up with? The first cycle gives one copy (plus the original), the second cycle makes a copy of the original and of the copy we just made, so that's four altogether. The third cycle makes a copy of each of those four, resulting in a total of eight, the fourth makes sixteen, the fifth thirty-two, the sixth sixty-four, and so on. Twenty-five cycles of the process yields zillions of copies of the gene. Having so many copies makes the gene easy to isolate, in a highly purified form, ready to be modified or transferred into other organisms.

Other gene banks and methods of obtaining genes

A third method of acquiring genes makes use of another type of gene bank, a depository, where scientists can deposit the physical DNA, cells lines, seeds, or whatever. A deposit made in this bank can often help satisfy proof of claim or patent disclosure requirements, as well as simply providing public access. The most widely used is the non-profit-making American Type Culture Collection (ATCC) in Virginia, USA.

Another method is the **reverse engineering** process. If we don't know anything about the DNA sequence of a particular gene, we might be able to isolate and purify the protein it produces. We can then determine the amino acid sequence from the purified protein. From the amino acid sequence we can synthesize a DNA sequence calling for those amino acids in the required sequence. If the sequence is not too long, we can synthesize the gene one base at a time. For long or more complex sequences, we can synthesize short simple sequences to serve as primers, one primer complementary to the sequence near one end of the gene, the other primer corresponding to the other end of the gene. Using these two DNA primers we can 'fish out' the natural gene using PCR as described in the previous section. This DNA for the gene is easily purified and ready for further investigation or manipulation.

Finally, the easiest and least expensive, but also least reliable method is called 'clone by phone'. You simply telephone a fellow scientist who has already isolated and cloned the gene you're interested in, and ask him or her to post it to you. Although this method is more unreliable than the others, it is one of the few techniques in which university and other public sector scientists enjoy a much greater success rate than private sector scientists.

Now that we have a conceptual grasp of molecular genetics, we can delve into the basis of genetic modification: how we actually transfer genes into an organism.

CHAPTER 3

Home cooking! DIY guide to genetic engineering

- How long has recombinant DNA technology been used?
- How do we actually perform gene transfer?
- Gene transfer is unnatural, isn't it?
- Don't bacterial genes cause disease?
- What's a 'marker gene'?

The last chapter gave us the tools, or perhaps the toys, to transfer genes from one organism to another. It is technically feasible to isolate a piece of DNA from any organism, for example a human, and insert it into a cell from any other, such as a fish or a tomato. Just as a woodworker eagerly tries out a new tool, and a child must play with a new toy, it seems human nature entices us to use and apply new knowledge. Let's see how we humans have applied our new molecular genetic tools.

Gathering the tools and ingredients

Before we can insert genes into an organism we need to have isolated and cloned one or more desired genes for transfer, a vehicle to deliver the genes, and a suitable recipient or host. In addition to these necessities, we'll almost certainly have other bits and pieces of DNA used to facilitate the overall process. Chief among these are the **marker genes**, so named because they are easy to detect in successfully transformed cells. Gene transfer, as we know it, is a very inefficient process. Millions of host cells are prepared as recipients for the transfer, but only a few of these target cells actually take up and express the introduced genes. A major step in the technical aspect of genetic engineering is identifying which of the few cells, if any, have been successfully transformed. In all likelihood, your important or desired genes are not apparent in the new host cells, so marker genes are used as indicators. Because the marker gene is attached to the genes of interest, expression of the marker in a host cell is a good indication that you have also successfully transferred the important genes. Some critics question using marker genes, so we'll discuss them in more detail later.

Transfer of the isolated gene is a fairly straightforward process if the intended host is a bacterium or other microbe. Microbiologists have been inserting foreign DNA into bacteria for many years and have the technical details pretty well sorted out.

However, if the recipient is a multicellular plant or animal, other obstacles arise. If the host is an animal, particularly a domestic food source animal, the technical process is much more difficult and still in its infancy. Each species of animal or plant has different requirements for successful genetic transformation. These requirements often have to be determined experimentally, even by trial and error. The individual requirements apply not only to inserting the foreign genes, but also to then recovering a whole organism from the genetically transformed cells.

The history of genetic engineering

Recombinant DNA, the physical linking of different pieces of DNA, started in earnest in the early 1970s, led by American scientists Paul Berg, Stan Cohen, and Herb Boyer. Microbiologists have long known that certain bacteria, treated appropriately, will take up pieces of DNA from their surrounding environment and insert the foreign DNA into their own genomes. The foreign DNA can even be recombinant DNA (rDNA) created in the lab. After this uptake of DNA, the host bacteria are said to be genetically transformed, engineered, or modified. The first products of this technology were bacteria, but the concept was universal, applicable to all organisms.

The successful engineering aroused considerable interest, particularly in the USA, as investors sought new improved medicines and foods, and scientists and activists expressed concern about the potential negative effects on the environment and health. As early as 1972, Paul Berg publicly called for a moratorium on molecular genetic research until the possible hazards of genetic engineering could be evaluated and discussed. The US National Academy of Sciences asked scientists to consider the various implications of rDNA. A group of prominent scientists met to discuss the potential hazards at Asilomar on the Monterey peninsula in 1975. As a result, the US National Institutes of Health (NIH) implemented a set of stringent guidelines (now largely relaxed owing to a complete lack of any 'untoward or unexpected' incidents).

Biotechnology became a buzzword, with start-up companies sprouting like weeds after a spring rain of venture capitalist cash. Genentech, Inc. became a household word as a leading biotechnology company and remains unusual in that it is still alive and productive, having made its fame in applying the new tools to human health objectives. Incorporated in 1976, within a year it had produced the first human protein in a bacterium, and by the second year had cloned human insulin. Genetically engineered human insulin has become the mainstay of diabetic treatment. In addition to the genetically modified forms of human insulin, Genentech and other companies developed a wide range of genetically modified products, including human growth hormone, factor VIII (a product to help blood clotting in haemophiliacs) and dornase alfa (Pulmozyme), an almost miraculous treatment for cystic fibrosis patients. More recently, Genentech developed recombinant products to fight certain forms of cancer. To get an idea of the extent of Genentech's genetically engineered products, check out their website (See Chapter 16).

Nowadays, Genentech and other companies develop human health products using genetic engineering with little fanfare and little public opposition. In contrast, agricultural applications of genetic technologies attract considerable attention—most of it unwanted. Of all the recombinant products developed by Genentech, most of which are highly intrusive into human bodies, the one receiving the most suspicion and negative publicity was one not intended for human application. Instead, it was developed for animals and licensed to Monsanto: bovine growth hormone (BST).

Getting into your genes

How do transferred genes get into the recipient host genome? The first step is to deliver DNA for a 'desired' gene into a cell and have it integrate in a stable manner into the cell's genome. For bacteria, that's it. All you need to do with the genetically transformed bacterial cells is then identify and separate them from the teeming masses of non-transformed ones. For higher organisms, we need the second step, whole organism regeneration.

Gene transfer is a cellular process. Delivery of DNA works one cell at a time. Despite the hype, successful DNA is still a very inefficient process, as only one in a zillion cells is successfully transformed in any attempt. Thankfully, providing several zillion host cells as potential recipients of the delivered genetic information is not usually a problem, so getting at least some cells transformed is, similarly, not usually a limiting factor.

The major obstacle facing successful genetic modification of almost all higher organisms—plants and animals—is usually the second step. After successfully delivering foreign DNA into the nucleus of a cell (the first step), we must induce that cell to grow into a complete organism. Because each cell has the genetic information to make a complete organism, all we need is to find what stimuli will push the cell on to and along that developmental course to regenerate into a complete organism. It may sound simple, but this is actually the hard part. For many species, we simply don't know what the 'right' stimuli are. There are several ways of successfully delivering foreign DNA into a given cell. Almost all tested species, plant and animal, have had cells genetically transformed with foreign DNA. Cells of relatively few species have successfully negotiated the second step. It always strikes me as ironic that the greatest technical obstacle to genetic engineering is not a genetic one, but a developmental and physiological one.

Depending on the objective, completing the second step is not always necessary. For some purposes, cellular transformation is all you need. Transgenic bacterial cells, happily churning out human insulin in a fermentation vat, need no more attention than a steady supply of food and other basic creature comforts. However, a wheat cell transformed to resist a nasty disease is of no use unless we can get it to regenerate into a whole plant, complete with fertile flowers from which we can obtain seeds. Farmers sow seeds, they cannot sow cells. Flour to make bread comes from seeds, not cells. In order to provide seeds, we need fertile transformed plants, so we must find whatever it takes to convince the transformed cell to grow into a whole, fertile plant.

The bad news is that every species responds to different regeneration stimuli, and some species are extremely reluctant to comply at all. Wheat is one of the most difficult. Getting foreign DNA into wheat cells was accomplished years ago. Obtaining a transgenic wheat plant is recent. (This is why we haven't seen transgenic wheat in the marketplace yet; GM wheat lines are currently in field trials *en route* to market.)

The good news is that you need only one transformed cell to regenerate to provide a transformed plant. The seeds from that one plant may be used to establish a transgenic crop. My own GM linseed variety can be traced back to a single Petri dish of cells. Of course, the transformed plant has to be carefully selected, as they all have somewhat different characteristics, and we, therefore, like to have as many as possible to choose from.

The plant species most easily transformed (meaning not only cellular transformation but with subsequent plant regeneration) is tobacco. For some reason, tobacco and its *Solanaceae* relatives, such as potato, tomato, and petunia seem to be the first to respond to cellular and genetic manipulations *in vitro* (in a Petri dish or test tube). The first experimental transgenic plants were tobacco. The first transgenic crop was tobacco, the first widespread consumer consumption of a transgenic product was GM tobacco (I'm not sure how it passed the health clearance, considering it was a GMO. GM tobacco probably causes cancer and a multitude of other nasty health conditions).

Other species required painstakingly cultivation and testing *in vitro* to determine the appropriate chemical and environmental conditions leading to full plant regeneration from cells. As fate would have it, some of the most important food crop species—cereals and grain legumes such as peas and beans—are the most difficult to regenerate. Only now are the *in vitro* culture conditions being elucidated to grow cells of these important crop plants into whole, fertile plants. Consequently, they are now amenable to recombinant DNA technology. Because of the technical difficulty in regeneration, that process is usually determined before an attempt is made to insert foreign genes; there's no point placing an important gene into a barley cell if that cell just languishes for a while and then dies.

A successful plant regeneration procedure isn't the end of it, however. Just because you have succeeded in introducing foreign DNA into a cell, and just because you have an efficient method for regenerating cells of that species into a plant, doesn't mean you can readily combine the two processes to start a production line of transgenic plants. Combining the two steps doesn't always work, unfortunately.

One of my research interests is to find how to generate transgenic lentils. Lentil is a new and valuable crop in western Canada. Conventional breeders have introduced great advances in lentil crop varieties, but there are a number of obstacles to efficient production. Diseases and weeds are at the top of most farmers' lists, and GM technology might be used to overcome those problems. However, because it's a minor species, few breeding institutions are applying biotechnology to lentil. My students and I developed a way to regenerate whole lentil plants from cells *in vitro*. That was in 1986 (sounds easy, but it took years). Next, we found a way to introduce foreign DNA into lentil cells. That was accomplished in 1990 (it took years, too). Then we tried combining the two procedures. We're still trying to put the two together to generate our first transgenic lentil. Apparently it's been done elsewhere (Australia), but we're still working at obtaining our first fertile transgenic lentil plant.

With this background, let's go back to the molecular lab where we prepare a gene for transfer.

The magic ingredient

Enzymes are to a genetic engineer what mirrors are to magicians, except the products are not illusions. Enzymes are proteins consisting of specific sequences of amino acids and synthesized by an organism according to DNA gene recipes. The enzymes facilitate a chemical reaction. Some enzymes help to build new chemicals, others help break down chemicals to nutrient parts.

Of particular interest to genetic engineers are smart **restriction endonuclease** enzymes. Restriction enzymes seek out specific base sequences on DNA and cause a cut, either a nick through one strand of the double-stranded DNA, or a cut through both strands. They're called 'smart' because they can recognize certain DNA base sequences, usually four or six bases long, in which to make their cut. The DNA base sequence GAATTC is recognized by the restriction endonuclease *EcoR*1. If this enzyme comes into contact with this particular base sequence on a piece of DNA, it will make a cut. Other base sequences are safe from destruction. Most of these restriction enzymes come from **pathogens** (disease-causing agents). During a hostile takeover, the infecting organism sends these enzymes into the cells to attack the target's DNA. Without intact DNA, the victim doesn't stand much of a chance, succumbing to the invader. Over 300 of these enzymes have been isolated and used by molecular geneticists, who carefully select which enzyme to use based on the DNA sequence of the pieces for cutting and splicing. With a judicious selection of restriction enzymes, one can cut a piece of DNA containing an intact gene from a whole DNA sample of an organism. Other enzymes can then be used to splice together series of DNA fragments from different sources. Finally, as long as one of the spliced pieces is a gene allowing replication in a bacterium, the artificial DNA can be made into a circle. This circle of DNA can be readily introduced into a bacterium where it will live happily as a plasmid (see Chapter 2), replicating along with the bacterium. Most artificial DNA segments are maintained in bacterial plasmids in this manner, as the bacterial 'carriers' can be frozen until the DNA is needed. When we acquire a new piece of DNA, whether from our own isolation or from a bank or other source, we put it into bacteria for safekeeping. When we need a stock of the DNA, we thaw the bacteria, let them grow overnight to create millions of copies, then use a DNA extraction procedure for plasmids. This yields a large quantity of identical DNA in about two days!

How do we insert genes into the plant cell?

There are several different methods of getting DNA into a cell. With bacteria, it's often simply a matter of giving the population of host bacteria a chemical or environmental treatment, then adding the DNA to the growth medium. Some of the bacterial cells will suck DNA up from the culture medium and insert it into its own genome. Even if the process is terribly inefficient, say only one in a million bacterial cells is so transformed, the process is feasible because it is easy to grow zillions of bacterial cells at one time. All it takes is one cell, one successful transformation event to grow a whole population of GM bacteria.

Higher organisms are more difficult, although again several methods have proved successful in different species. I will describe two of them, the two that my lab team uses to generate transgenic linseed.

Shooting your DNA load: a human-designed machine

The simplest method of introducing foreign DNA into cells is not nearly so elegant or biological as the more sophisticated method described in the following section. Instead, it has no subtlety whatever, is based on brute physical force and violence, and results in unnecessary cell death and dismemberment. Scientists colloquially refer to it as the 'shotgun method', an expression accurate both figuratively and literally. It exemplifies the human approach to the manipulation of life. But it works.

After acquiring a purified stock of the DNA to be transferred, the DNA is mixed with microscopic gold or tungsten pellets, like minuscule shotgun pellets, to which it adheres. The DNA-coated pellets are placed on a support in the line of fire from a gunpowder blast or, more recently and not nearly as dramatically, a blast of helium gas. The target cells are arrayed in the line of fire, such that the pellets enter the cells. The trick with this biolistic method is to find the appropriate conditions in which the pellets enter the cell but do not exit, causing injury but not killing the cell. What happens after the pellet enters the cell is a mystery, but we can assume the DNA, no longer stuck to the pellet, is transported or finds its way to the cell nucleus. Somehow, the foreign DNA is inserted into the cell DNA, perhaps through some sort of natural genetic repair mechanism. Exactly how this occurs is uncertain, but the end result is undeniable. The cell can acquire functional foreign genes. If the cell is then induced to regenerate into a whole plant, the plant and its ultimate progeny can carry and express the new genetic information.

This method is most commonly used in cereals such as wheat, rice, and maize, species unsuitable for the naturally occurring genetic engineer, *Agrobacterium*.

Agrobacterium: a naturally occurring genetic engineering agent

Agrobacterium tumefaciens is the Latin name of a naturally occurring genetic engineering agent. In the wild, it is a soil microbe, opportunistically waiting for a plant to suffer an injury close to the soil level where the bacterium can get at some exposed cells. The injury could be caused by anything from a grazing insect taking a nibble to local sandblasting from a windstorm.

If *Agrobacterium* happens to be nearby, it will attach itself to the injured plant cell. Acetosyringone (a wound healing chemical produced by some injured plants) serves not only the plant but also *Agrobacterium*, as a signal that this is a susceptible plant and to begin the pathogenic response. Thus begins the only known natural example of mating between different biological kingdoms: the infecting *Agrobacterium* insidiously subverts the plant cell for its own benefit. A series of chemical reactions (based on specialized enzyme activities) occurs in the bacterial cell to find and prepare a special piece of DNA (called T-DNA, for transfer-DNA) for introduction into the plant cell. The T-DNA is recognized by having particular short base sequences, left border (LB) and right border (RB), on either side of the T-DNA. Restriction endonuclease enzymes, encoded by *Agrobacterium* genes, recognize each border and cut one strand of the double-stranded DNA at each border site. The one strand of DNA running between the nicks in the LB and RB is removed and wrapped in protective proteins, while repair enzymes immediately work to resynthesize the excised strand of DNA, using the remaining strand as a template for the appropriate base sequence. The T-DNA, cocooned in its protective layer, is moved to a tunnel drilled between the bacterium cell and the plant cell to which it had earlier been attached. The T-DNA–protein complex is delivered to the plant cell through the connecting tunnel, where it eventually finds or is taken to the nucleus, home of the plant's own DNA. In a way that we do not yet understand, the T-DNA is inserted into the plant's DNA, where it becomes a fully functional part of the plant's genome. The location of insertion was once thought to be random, but it now appears not to be, although not entirely ordered, either. Each transformed cell will have the T-DNA inserted in a different part of the genome. These different loci of insertion give rise to different degrees of foreign gene activity in the modified cell, which may in turn affect the level of gene expression.

T-DNA in **wild strains** of *Agrobacterium* (i.e. those occurring in nature) contains several gene recipes, all relating to the genetic conquest of the plant cell. The insidious bacteria subvert the protein synthetic machinery of the plant cell to make proteins from these T-DNA genes. As one might expect, some of the newly introduced genes code for proteins that make nutrient compounds specifically for the *Agrobacterium*. The compounds, called **opines** (rare types of amino acid), are used preferentially for the nutritional benefit of the bacteria. Other genes, in a particularly clever twist, produce enzymes to make plant growth hormones. These genes, and their products, are of absolutely no use to the bacteria. But the plant cell responds to them by growing, reproducing over and over, dividing uncontrollably into a tumour-like mass of cells, each one continuously producing more growth hormones and more opines for the conquering *Agrobacterium*. Of course, with each division comes a new copy of the entire plant cell genome (the entire genetic blueprint of the cell nucleus), including now the insinuated T-DNA. More copies of the genes in the T-DNA result in yet more plant growth hormones, and yet more opines. The plant cell, by now having lost control of its own destiny, turns into a lumpy mass of cells. The result is the development of crown gall disease on the plant, the result of tumours forming from the plant cells at the site of the infection, usually close to the ground, the crown of the stem.

By studying *Agrobacterium* and its infection process, various scientists around the world reported that the bacterial ability to genetically transform the infected plant cell was separate from the functions of the genes transferred. That is, the genes on the T-DNA were just the cargo; they were not necessary for the actual gene transfer process other than providing something to deliver. Those genes controlling the natural transfer of DNA remained in the bacteria. The genes sent into the plant cell on the T-DNA were useful to the bacteria in that they subverted the plant cell into producing nutrients for the bacteria, but they did not directly affect the GM process itself. What this meant was that the genes carried on an artificial T-DNA could be almost anything. Strains of *Agrobacterium* could be found or developed totally lacking the disease-causing (**oncogenic**) genes, and genes of interest substituted.

Disarmed *Agrobacterium* strains

Scientists have developed different strains of *Agrobacteria*. Some strains have had their pathogenic T-DNA eliminated entirely, so they are incapable of causing crown gall disease. Yet they retain the mechanism to genetically transform a plant cell to which the bacterial cell is attached. In such circumstances, the *Agrobacterium* activates the various genes to initiate the T-DNA transfer. The proteins are made, because the genes regulating the transfer itself are not located on the T-DNA. They are elsewhere in the bacterial genome. However, the enzymes go searching for the LB and RB, and are frustrated. There is no T-DNA to transfer. It's like a courier wanting to make a delivery, but unable to find a package. The *Agrobacterium* in this case is expending energy, spinning its wheels, going nowhere. The plant cell survives with its genetic integrity intact.

Suppose now we provided this disarmed *Agrobacterium* strain with artificial T-DNA. We know the specific DNA base sequence of the LB and the RB. We synthesize a small piece of DNA containing an artificial LB and RB, and construct it so there is a functional gene between them. We give this small piece of DNA another couple of DNA sequences to allow it to replicate inside the *Agrobacterium*, make the artificial DNA into a circular ring, and then introduce this plasmid circle of DNA to the *Agrobacterium* in a Petri dish. We select an *Agrobacterium* that has taken up the circular DNA and let the colony grow, knowing that each time the bacterium replicates its own DNA, the artificial DNA also replicates. Each daughter cell in a growth division has a copy of the synthetic circular DNA, a portion of which is in between an LB and an RB. What then happens when we take this disarmed *Agrobacterium* and allow it to attach to a plant cell? As before, the bacterial machinery is set in motion, the enzymes to nick the LB and RB find the sequences, not on the bacterial DNA but in our artificial DNA. The rest of the transfer mechanism takes over, bundling the T-DNA strand between the artificial LB and RB, and conveys it to the plant cell. The courier of our analogy now happily delivers the package, not knowing the contents have been switched. This time, there is no tumour formation and there is no opine production, as there are no pathogenic genes in our artificial DNA. There is no pathology; no crown gall; no disease. There is a plant cell with a foreign piece of DNA in its genome. What then happens depends on the DNA base sequence we synthesized and had the *Agrobacterium* deliver. This time, the plant cell does not fall victim to the subversion of the bacterium; it is the *Agrobacterium* being exploited by us humans. We can now provide these *Agrobacterium* strains with whatever genetic package we have available, and the bacteria will faithfully look after the delivery into plant cells for us. They are naturally occurring genetic engineering agents.

Agrobacterium genes

Inserting *Agrobacterium* genes into a plant cell, as *Agrobacterium* does in the wild, has no commercial value, so it is curious that the first genes artificially inserted into plants using the subverted bacteria were simple *Agrobacterium* genes. When this work was being conducted, in the early 1980s, genes of interest were in short supply. One of the simplest was a gene from a different strain of *Agrobacterium*. The various *Agrobacterium* strains can be distinguished by the genes ordinarily carried on their T-DNA. A common class is the **nopaline** type. Nopaline is a particular opine, produced in plant cells infected with a nopaline strain of *Agrobacterium*. One of the genes on the bacterial T-DNA is a nopaline synthase gene (*nos*).* When this gene is transferred into a plant cell, the plant cell protein synthetic machinery reads and expresses the gene, resulting in the nopaline synthase enzyme (NOS). This enzyme, foreign to the plant, acts on common nutrients in the plant cell to make the opine nopaline. Nopaline is used preferentially by *Agrobacterium* as a food source, completing the subversion of the plant cell in a very clever manner. The conquering bacteria effectively genetically engineer the plant cell to make food for the invader using the plant's own energy and nutrient pool at essentially no cost to the bacteria. The fate of the vanquished seems to change little through human history or nature.

Other strains of *Agrobacterium* have genes for other but similar opines. **Octopine** is a related but distinct nutrient preferred by octopine strains. The octopine synthase gene (*ocs*) generates the enzyme octopine synthase (OCS) in a transformed plant cell, but nopaline is absent unless a nopaline strain is available to provide the *nos* gene. Nopaline and octopine are similar chemicals, but readily distinguished using a simple lab assay. The genes, present as they are on T-DNA of the respective bacterial strains, are readily available. It should come as no surprise that among the first genes transferred to plants as a human genetic modification was a nopaline gene, using a disarmed octopine *Agrobacterium* strain as a delivery system. Ordinarily, nopaline will not appear in plant cells infected with an octopine type *Agrobacterium*, and vice versa. When T-DNA containing a *nos* gene was provided to an octopine type *Agrobacterium*, and that bacterium then allowed to infect tobacco plants, the tobacco cells started producing nopaline. When those cells were grown into whole plants, nopaline was being produced throughout the plant. When the plants reached maturity, flowered, and set seed, nopaline was produced in progeny, exactly as predicted. Plant genetic engineering became reality.

Unfortunately, nopaline provided no practical benefit to anyone (except perhaps *Agrobacterium*), and tobacco, although a very useful experimental species, was losing favour as a commercial crop species.

Making money from GM technology

Two races began at once. One race was after 'useful' or commercially interesting genes. Marker genes were useful for experimentation, but had little commercial value. On the other hand, they are often necessary to be able to detect and isolate the few cells successfully transformed in an experiment. For most GMOs, the inserted DNA consists of at least one selectable marker gene plus the **gene of interest**, the gene conferring the commercial value to the organism. Often, other genes and

---

* See p. 30 for a note of the way genes and enzymes are named.

DNA sequences, helpful in the initial phases but irrelevant to the final organism, are also present.

The other race was to extend the disarmed *Agrobacterium* GM technology to crop species other than tobacco.

Going along for the ride: scorable and selectable marker genes

Marker genes have no value in a commercial GMO. Yet without them, the GMO probably wouldn't exist. Markers help scientists identify which, if any, of the zillions of cells in a transformation experiment have successfully taken up the introduced DNA. Without markers, the scientists have to painstakingly analyse each of those cells; the whole process becomes impracticable. Marker genes come in two categories, scorable and selectable:

1 **scorable** markers provide an indication of whether or not a cell or group of cells is transformed based on a quick and simple test
2 **selectable** markers provide not only the indication of transformation, but also allow a growth advantage to the transformed cells.

None of the marker genes is completely reliable, so most scientists, particularly in the early stages of technology development, use both a scorable and a selectable marker when attempting to develop a new GMO.

Scorable markers

Remember the discussion of how to obtain genes for transfer (p. 51). The first genes used in genetic modification experiments were simple markers, such as nopaline synthase (*nos*). These were easy to detect, enabling the scientists to tell when an experiment was successful in transferring functional DNA into a plant cell. In order for the scientists to know that an experimental method of inserting a gene worked, it was important to be able to quickly and easily identify not only that the DNA had been inserted, but also that it was functioning in the host cell. Nopaline can easily be detected in plant cells, using a simple inexpensive assay that takes about a day to run. Large numbers of experimental samples can be assayed and scored, directing the scientists to concentrate on the more successful parameters. However, *nos* is now obsolete, as it has several technical drawbacks. It is a scorable marker, not a selectable marker. That is, the presence of nopaline is an indicator of successful transformation in plant cells, but cannot be used to segregate or select transformed cells from non-transformed cells. Genetic transformation occurs on individual cells, and even the most efficient method is extremely low in efficiency—although a large number of cells are provided as potential hosts for gene insertion, very few are ever actually transformed. A selectable marker, one that would readily segregate the two populations of cells by giving a growth advantage to the transformed but not the non-transformed cells, would be more useful. What led to the demise of the *nos* gene as a useful marker, though, was that it was discovered to occur naturally in many plants, including crop species such as soya bean. The presence of natural nopaline in soya bean, a major target for genetic transformation, meant *nos* couldn't be used with any degree of confidence to indicate transformation because there was no simple way to distinguish natural soya bean nopaline from inserted *nos* nopaline.

Other simple scorable marker genes were sought and made available. The most common of these is beta-glucuronidase, technically *uid*-A but commonly and affectionately known as GUS. The GUS gene was developed from the bacterium *Escherichia coli* by Richard Jefferson at Cambridge in 1987 and, in an old-fashioned gesture rarely seen today, released into the public domain. Any *bona fide* scientist could request, and receive, the GUS gene from Richard. It immediately became the scorable marker of choice in plant genetic transformation experiments. Why? For one thing, it was freely available, without strings or obligations. For another, it had few of the disadvantages of nopaline while remaining simple, indeed easier, to score. Unlike nopaline, GUS could be scored using any of several different assays, each with its own advantages and disadvantages. Unfortunately, all kill the tested cells, so identifying a 'GUS-positive' cell precludes regenerating a whole organism. However, it is useful for verification after a putative transgenic plant is regenerated. A small tissue sample can be sacrificed for the GUS assay without jeopardizing the life of the entire plant.

The quickest and easiest method is unfortunately expensive and qualitative, giving only a yes or no answer to whether or not GUS was present in the cells. The test is simple because it is based on a chemical reaction with the gene product enzyme to make a striking bright blue pigment in the transformed cells. It was particularly attractive to a scientist trying to transform a difficult tissue or species. Seeing the distinctive blue pigment appear in the test tissue for the first time was usually a cause for celebration. The slower and more elaborate but less expensive method had the advantage of providing quantitative results. This assay would not only indicate the presence of GUS, but also measure how much was present, an indicator of how effectively, or 'strongly', the foreign gene was being expressed.

Both of these assays, and others, are still widely used in scoring plant transformation success. GUS has the decided advantage over nopaline in staying put, at least for a reasonable time. If one cell in a tissue of thousands of cells was successfully transformed with the GUS gene, the 'fast' assay could detect those transformed cells by their blue coloration, whereas the non-transformed cells remained green (from chlorophyll) or clear. GUS is only beginning to appear in GM crops in the market. It has no commercial value by itself, but was necessarily carried along with the gene of interest, because that gene, the one contributing the commercial value to the cultivar, could not be readily detected in the transformed cells. Although there were reports of 'GUS-like activity' in certain plant species, these false positives did not appear to confound results with the major crop species the way nopaline did with soya bean. Various regulatory bodies scrutinized both the GUS gene and the gene product for health and safety and environmental concerns. None was identified, probably because the gene is already widely distributed in the environment and in our bodies. The first GM products on the market carrying the GUS gene include soya beans and sugar beet.

Selectable markers

The scorable markers can be useful, but selectable markers are more popular because, with an efficient one, the scientist lets the marker do the work of segregating the few transformed cells from the many non-transformed cells. The most common selectable marker is the *npt*-II gene, conferring resistance to the antibiotic kanamycin. This gene was present in the Flavr-Savr™ tomato because when the Calgene scientists were developing their tomato, they needed a way to identify the tomato cells successfully transformed with the gene of interest, the inverted polygalacturonase gene. Since the commercially valuable gene was not functional in tomato cells in a Petri dish, the activity or expression of that gene could not be used directly to identify the desired transformed cells. It was also impracticable to regenerate hundreds of thousands of tomato plants, one from each cell, to try to find the few successfully transformed ones. So, the selectable marker gene was hooked up adjacent to the commercial gene of interest on the T-DNA as delivered by the *Agrobacterium*. Tomato cells growing in culture medium in Petri dishes were inoculated with the *Agrobacterium*, then transferred to another Petri dish containing fresh culture medium, but with added kanamycin. Ordinary tomato cells are inhibited by kanamycin, but tomato cells successfully transformed and expressing the *npt*-II gene are not. The activity of the *npt*-II gene product protected the tomato cell from the inhibitory effects of kanamycin. The few transformed tomato cells continued to grow in the medium and some were regenerated into whole plants. The whole plants were tested for fertility and the resulting tomato fruits were tested for the activity not of the *npt*-II gene but of the adjacent gene of interest. Usually, but not always, the successful transfer and activity of one gene indicates successful transfer and activity of the other genetic components in the T-DNA. In this case, the success of the *npt*-II gene in conferring kanamycin resistance to the tomato cells was a good indicator that the polygalacturonase gene would also be present.

The kanamycin resistance gene is also present in my GM linseed and was used to identify and select the successfully transformed linseed cells in those initial experiments back in 1988. Its only purpose to was to help identify the transformed cells. The gene is still present, and it still functions, but has no commercial use or value. In fact, the selectable marker gene is now a liability because some people have expressed concerns that it might jump on to bacteria and then confer antibiotic resistance to pathogenic organisms. More about this issue later, in Chapter 11.

Some selectable markers are themselves the gene of interest, greatly simplifying the whole process. For example, the *bar* or *pat* gene, conferring resistance to the herbicide glufosinate ammonium (the active chemical in AgrEvo's commercial formulations Liberty™ and Basta™), can be used as a selectable marker. The plant cells are inoculated with an *Agrobacterium* carrying the *bar* or *pat* gene in its T-DNA. They are then placed on a culture medium to which the glufosinate herbicide has been added. Non-transformed cells die from the herbicide; transformed cells live and grow. The scientist doesn't need to identify and then try to segregate the transformed from the non-transformed cells; the selection agent has done both steps in one. Whole plants can then be regenerated and immediately tested for herbicide resistance with Liberty™ or Basta™.

Other bits and pieces of DNA

What else is on the T-DNA transferred into GMOs and released to the environment? Are those extraneous bits and pieces really necessary?

From a commercial viewpoint, the most important component of the inserted DNA is the gene of interest. This is the gene that confers a commercially valuable trait, like the delayed ripening conferred by the inverted polygalacturonase gene in tomato, or the herbicide resistance genes in several GM crops. In addition, there is usually a selectable marker, often *npt*-II, to allow the initial transformed cells to be easily identified and segregated from the ordinary non-transformed cells in the original experiment. Sometimes there is a scorable marker gene, like GUS or *nos*, to assist with the identification. What else? What other foreign DNA might be lurking in our foods?

Prokaryotic markers are common, usually antibiotic resistance genes used in the original construction of the disarmed T-DNA. Prokaryotic genes do not function in plants or animals unless specifically modified to do so. The DNA base sequence doesn't usually require modification, but the promoter does. Promoters, remember, act as gene switches to activate or inactivate the expression of a gene. The prokaryotic promoters used in GM foods are not recognized by the host plant or animal cell, so the gene is not expressed in the transformed cells and the protein is not made. The gene remains non-functional. The *npt*-II gene discussed above was originally a prokaryotic gene, isolated from a bacterium, but the bacterial, prokaryotic promoter was replaced with a plant promoter to make it function in plant cells. Without substituting the promoter to one the plant cell would recognize, the *npt*-II gene would not be expressed in the plant cells, and therefore would be useless as a selectable marker there.

Prokaryotic markers were used when we needed to combine genes carried by two different bacteria. Like the marker genes discussed for GMOs above, we would have one bacterium carry one marker, and the second carry a different one. After mating or recombining the two bacterial sources, we would use the expression of both markers simultaneously to identify the bacteria successfully combining and expressing both markers. From there it's a simple matter to extract the relevant DNA from the identified bacterial colonies and test to ensure the genes, not only the marker genes but the associated genes of interest, were present and together, ready for transfer to the target plant or animal cell. Most GM foods on the market and coming to market have one or more of these prokaryotic genes, coming along like excess and now-unnecessary baggage, their purpose long fulfilled. Like the eukaryotic marker genes, the continued presence of prokaryotic markers in GM foods has raised concerns. We'll discuss these later also.

Finishing touches

Making a GMO is simple enough once the pieces of the technological puzzle are put in place. For microbes or cellular products, the pieces include DNA encoding a gene of interest and a vehicle to deliver the DNA into a suitable host microbe or cell. For higher organisms, such as crop plants, you not only need the gene of interest and a delivery system into suitable host cells, but you also need the ability to regenerate an entire organism from the transformed cell.

Once you have a suitable delivery system in place with a suitable regeneration protocol, you can insert virtually any DNA to obtain a GMO without having to modify the other aspects of the procedure. In my lab, for instance, we can take any isolated gene and deliver it into linseed cells, then regenerate whole plants from those cells to recover a GM linseed plant. From that one plant we can, through self-pollination, derive a new linseed GM variety. I am not able to offer this service in lentil yet, but we and others have done it to make GM oilseed rape and potato, and could probably do it in other species for which there is a published protocol. However, most scientists tend to specialize according to their main species of interest. In any case, the specific gene does not seem to make much difference to the GM process of inserting foreign DNA into a host cell. The gene seems to be simply the contents of a package. When we acquire a new gene of interest, we simply plug the DNA into our linseed protocol and start generating new GM linseed lines containing the new gene of interest. Most crop species are now at this stage.

CHAPTER 4

Salad days? Conventional and GM foods

- Real food, from ordinary crop varieties, is natural, wholesome, and pure, isn't it?
- What are some of the different methods used in 'conventional' plant breeding?
- How does a GM plant variety differ from a conventional plant variety?
- What are the different kinds of GM food?
- How are new varieties regulated and approved for marketing?
- How do farmers choose which variety to grow?
- Where do they get their seed?
- What happens to the harvested grain?
- Can we segregate GM from non-GM grain?
- Is it true that genes in nature are stable, conventionally produced foods are safe, and GM products are marketed with little or no regulatory scrutiny?

Popular misconceptions of how food gets to our table

For a person from an isolated farming community, a trip to a modern urban supermarket is a daunting experience. Especially alien is the predominance of highly processed packaged foods, designed for the modern cosmopolitan consumer whose purchasing pattern is based on convenience and price rather than nutrition and freshness. Food products are becoming many more steps removed from the farm. A common perception is that food nowadays is largely synthetic, produced in a factory from artificial ingredients. Although it is certainly true that many of our modern foodstuffs are highly processed, with more and more artificial ingredients, such as preservatives and colourants, the underlying, basic food product still comes from a farm, produced by a farmer.

Some misconceptions arise from traditional religious beliefs. Once in a while I will get a call from someone who begins 'I want to eat food the way God made it, and avoid genetically modified foods. Tell me what I can eat'. I can only tell them I don't know for sure how God made our foods and how each might have changed, whether by human or natural or divine intervention, in the meantime.

What is certain, though, is that almost all of our basic food sources, including microbes, crops, and animals, are substantially different, genetically and culturally, from what they were even 2000 years ago.

Traditional practice: 'acceptable' crop production methods

You may think I'm being obtuse: what those people want is to avoid foods produced from recombinant DNA technology, as opposed to foods from traditional/ordinary/conventional methods. I admit I am being obtuse. Obviously they want to avoid rDNA foods. But my intention is to help people to think clearly and define exactly their concerns and objections.

Before drawing a line between acceptable technology and unacceptable technology, let's see what classical or 'acceptable' breeding entails. We've seen what molecular genetic modification is, now we need to learn about conventional breeding. Only then can we properly define the boundary line.

Most food comes from plants. Plant breeding provides most crops. Most farmers grow modern varieties, technically called cultivars, of a given crop. In order to compare crops developed using genetic modification (GM) with those produced using 'classical', acceptable plant breeding, we need some background information.

What constitutes classical or, as some say, 'acceptable' plant breeding? What techniques do traditional plant breeders use to bring us the vast majority of foods and other useful crop plants? Do any of these involve genetic modification or other 'unnatural acts'? Most of us are not aware of what 'traditional' or 'conventional' breeding entails. Nor are most of us aware of how a new crop variety is evaluated and tested prior to being grown by farmers and put in the marketplace. In the next section we take a quick look at some 'conventional' crop breeding methods.

Standard plant breeding methods

I am not a plant breeder, although many people consider me one, as I have co-developed and released several new crop varieties and serve on the Canadian national crop variety registration committee. No, I have never been admitted into the plant breeder's cabal. Instead, I look on in awe as my more traditional colleagues stare at field trials of breeding lines, then pore over the resulting reams of computer-generated random numbers and identify, somehow, the breeding lines most likely to become the next commercial chartbuster. What amazes me most is that they are so often *correct*.

Selection

Modern conventional plant breeding seems an arcane combination of enlightened science and dark art. It must have started thousands of years ago, when some of our ancestors noticed certain of the wild-growing plants held more seeds, or bigger seeds, or had some other feature that made them different enough to avoid being consumed immediately. Perhaps the seeds were left behind by simple oversight, with no further thought given them. When the nomads returned (possibly many years later), they would have found a whole patch of 'superior' plants. By this time, they knew that plants came from seeds, and if they refrained from eating all the good seeds, they could use the remaining 'selected' good seeds to grow another, bigger patch of the crop in the next season. By exercising the first technique of plant breeding—selection—they became the first breeders.

Crossing

Over thousands of years, many other techniques have been added to the breeders' toolkit. Chief among these is crossing, in which the male pollen from one identified superior plant is collected and transferred on to the female part (stigma) of another superior plant, with the expectation that any resulting hybrid offspring will possess the superior traits of both parents.

Simple crossing developed the wheat variety Marquis, released for commercial production in 1909. Until recently, the statutory standard for breadmaking quality in Canadian wheat, Marquis was still a world standard. The breeders, A. P. Saunders and his son Charles, identified the benefits of Marquis by chewing on the kernels during the early field trials. Today their method would be illegal for any new variety deemed to be genetically modified, as it would not have passed food safety clearance at such an early stage in its development. Crossing is still the mainstay of plant breeding activities.

Emasculation

The breeders followed pollen-based crossing closely with emasculation. With this tool, the breeder unashamedly wields a scalpel to slice off the plant's male reproductive organs, properly called anthers. Most conventional breeders use this method to ensure that only the 'good' pollen (as chosen and provided by the breeder) succeeds in fertilizing the eggs in the tender young female ovary, producing seed for the next generation.

Intergeneric crossing

Sometimes a breeder forces the mating between two unrelated plants of different species; this is known as an intergeneric cross. The progeny of such couplings would rarely, if ever, occur in nature. On occasion, the breeder succeeds and produces 'man-made' crops. *Triticale* is an intergeneric hybrid between wheat and rye, fed mostly to animals but also to humans in multigrain breads. The goal was to develop a crop variety combining the breadmaking quality of wheat (*Triticum*) with the ability of rye (*Secale*) to grow in harsh environments. As with many such good ideas, the typical result carried the wrong combination—a tender wimpy plant with poor baking quality. However, some *Triticale* hybrids worked well enough to be grown with modest commercial success in various countries.

Ever-vigilant, the breeder controls the whole mating process like a puppeteer manipulating his charges. Yet the public has little idea how these 'conventional and acceptable' food products were developed. *Triticale* and other intergeneric foods are not labelled as such, nor do they require any additional regulatory scrutiny prior to commercialization.

Embryo rescue

Another 'conventional' breeding method developed in more recent years is embryo rescue, in which unrelated individual plants, sometimes even from different species, incapable of normal procreation together, are mated to produce a semi-formed aborted embryo. Taking a more direct hand now, the breeder steals the embryo from the ovary, placing it in a Petri dish or test tube, an artificial environment where it is deprived of its natural destiny. Instead, relying solely on synthetic nutrients, it grows into a sickly hybrid. Rarely do these pitiable creatures live very long, but a few manage to survive and some even reach reproductive maturity. The products of this technique are rarely robust enough to develop directly into a new variety. Instead, the technique is used to transfer a foreign gene first into an intermediary species, then into the crop species. That product might lead to commercial release. The crop varieties derived from this 'acceptable' technique are not labelled or scrutinized beyond the level required for ordinary new crop varieties.

Haploid breeding

One of the most intrusive plant breeding techniques is technically known as haploidy. Haploid breeding relies on the use of gametes, the sex cells of egg or pollen naturally carrying only a single set of chromosomes.

In nature, the pollen and egg combine to form an embryo with two sets of chromosomes, one from each parent. The normal embryo then grows into a complete organism, with each cell carrying the usual two sets of chromosomes. In haploidy, however, the natural process is perverted and undermined. Instead of a natural mating, the chosen gamete cells are forced to make a copy of their own single set of chromosomes to provide the second set. The resulting cell, and the plant subsequently derived from it, is called a double haploid. It contains the usual two sets of chromosomes, but instead of having one set from the father and one from the mother, it has two copies of one set of chromosomes. It is said to be homozygous, because it has two exact copies of every gene. Ordinary hybrids are heterozygous, as some genes from the father will differ from those from the mother.

Haploidy, usually combined with the crossing method, is employed because when it works (it doesn't work with all species, and is sporadic in others), it can reduce the overall breeding period by several years. It is most commonly used in breeding barley, rapeseed, and some other crops. Several methods are used are to induce haploidy, including chemical treatments such as colchicine, but the resulting varieties are not labelled or scrutinized beyond the level required for ordinary new cultivars.

Mutation breeding

The term mutation breeding is an honest but sometimes misunderstood representation of the breeders' activities. Technically, a mutation is any change to the DNA of an organism. This technique involves taking crop plants and exposing them to mutagenic agents—ionizing radiation or other radioactive compounds, or some of the most poisonous chemicals known to humanity. Given too high a dose, the plant dies from radiation poisoning or chemical toxicity. At lower doses, the plant grows normally, although portions of the DNA have been scrambled beyond all recognition. One gene may be destroyed, or a hundred, or a thousand—no one knows. The plant survives because it has two homologous copies of each gene. The second copy provides the genetic information when the first is annihilated, so the exposed plant lives a near normal life. A proportion of the progeny, however, pay the price when the scrambled genes are reunited in the embryo cell and both copies of the gene are defective. In most cases, the result of having both copies of the gene defective is lethal; the progeny dies. In those cases where the destroyed genes are not critical to survival, the progeny carries on as best it can while lacking at least some normal functions. Most of these, as one might expect, are sickly and infertile.

Occasionally, a mutant will display a feature previously unknown in the species; the breeder carefully inspects the mutant and the new trait. On extremely rare occasions, the breeder will take an interest in the novel trait and exploit it in the development of a new cultivar. An example of the type of improvement through induced mutation is reduced height of crop plants. This might not seem like much of an improvement to us as consumers. After all, who cares how tall a plant is? Surely in most cases we're concerned with the amount and quality of grain produced? In any case, it would seem that a taller, larger plant would have more stem and leaf area, more biomass, to produce more grain, so why would we want a shorter plant? Would a short plant with less biomass not generate less grain? Not always. Our most important cereal food crops, such as wheat and rice, produce their grain in ears or heads at the top of long stalks. If the grains are too heavy for the strength of the stem, the whole thing falls over, sometimes as far as the ground. If this happens, the grain is attacked by ground-dwelling bacteria, fungi, insects, and other organisms happy to get an easy meal so close to home. An added problem is that harvesting equipment has difficulty collecting the grain when it's too close to the ground. Substantial losses occur from excess grain production resulting in the stem falling over, or lodging.

As any child knows, a short stick of given diameter is harder to break than a long stick of the same material. Induced mutations can create 'dwarf' plants, of reduced stature without necessarily reduced grain yield capacity. The shorter stems are stronger, more able to keep the grain-heavy heads upright, out of the way of opportunistic feeders near the ground and within easy reach of harvesting equipment. With reduced loss from lodging, the total grain yield harvested is increased. European wheat cultivars are good examples of high yielding mutants, derived from one or more reduced height mutations.

Other mutations can similarly result in improved overall food production, not always by increasing the yield to the food product itself, but by decreasing the losses due to lodging, diseases, and so on.

Among the examples where mutation has directly affected the quality of the product is Linola™, the human food linseed oil from Australia that is consumed in the UK, the USA, Canada, and elsewhere. To generate Linola™, an extremely nasty chemical mutagenic agent, ethyl methane sulfonate (EMS), was applied to ordinary linseed. The breeder, Dr Allan Green, inspected thousands of progeny lines, choosing and crossing 'interesting' mutants until, eventually, he developed a line almost lacking a major constituent of ordinary linseed oil. Linseed oil, like all vegetable oils, is a mix of several constituent fatty acids, including, for example, the saturated fats palmitic acid and stearic acid, the monounsaturated oleic acid, and the polyunsaturated linoleic and linolenic acids. Traditional linseed oil is predominantly linolenic acid, which helps make linseed oil a premium industrial sealing oil because it dries quickly to a hard film. This feature is great for paints or sealants for concrete or cricket bats, but the same attribute makes it unsuitable as a commercial human food vegetable oil. The mutant linseed has almost eliminated linolenic acid in its oil. Linola™ fits nicely into human vegetable oil markets as it is quite similar to the premium oils produced by sunflower or safflower and actually has less linolenic acid than other major food oils.

We unwittingly consume intentionally mutated foods. Over 1400 cultivars of a wide range of species have been developed through mutation breeding in the past 50 years. Except in special cases, the mutant products are not labelled or scrutinized beyond the level required for ordinary new cultivars.

Somaclonal variation

Breeders induce mutations artificially, but on occasion nature provides spontaneous mutations. However, these natural mutations are usually too sporadic and unreliable to exploit in a breeding programme.

In the early 1980s, two Australian scientists, Phil Larkin and Bill Scowcroft, gave a name to a phenomenon that had been observed by various people over the years, although few wanted to admit was real. Numerous people working on plant cloning took cell or tissue samples in a Petri dish and altered the nutritional complement of the culture medium to induce plant regeneration. Academic physiologists or developmental biologists studying the process of regeneration conducted most such experiments, but some scientists had a commercial interest. For certain plant species, especially horticultural or rare species, a method of propagating the plants in culture, called micropropagation, could be worth a fair amount of money. Today, micropropagation is a big business, with many common houseplants having started life in the Petri dish or test tube. The critical objective of micropropagation, however, is to have clonal plants, genetically identical to the parent plant which was specifically chosen on the basis of its superior characteristics.

The developmental physiologists and others investigating whole plant regeneration from tissues in Petri dishes rarely looked too closely at the final product. Their interest was usually in the earlier stages, trying to understand the nature of early growth and development. Once the regenerating plantlets grew big enough to move from the Petri dish or test tube into soil, they were discarded. The few researchers who kept the plants long enough occasionally noted oddities in some of the test tube derived plants, but thought nothing of them. These unusual features were explained as resulting from the physiological stresses placed on plants growing in the unnatural environment and artificial culture medium of a Petri dish. It is not unusual for a plant regenerated in culture to be sickly, even after transfer to soil and placement in a healthy greenhouse, but then go on to produce perfectly normal seed-borne progeny.

The commercially minded micropropagationists, however, noticed these off-types but rarely spoke of them. Odd plantlets were usually destroyed as soon as they were discovered. In their business, it was important to have the plants all look absolutely identical to maintain the highest commercial value. Off-types jeopardized the value of the whole lot.

The off-types did occur, and sometimes their progeny also showed the strange trait, indicating a genetic as opposed to environmental (physiological) basis for the alteration. Most of us thought these off-types were mere curiosities, or like the micropropagationists, undesirables to be destroyed. The Australian scientists, however, suggested that these spontaneous genetic changes occurring in cells in Petri dishes might yield useful new traits, and named the phenomenon somo-clonal variation (SCV).

SCV is based on tissue culture and regeneration: the process of slicing a bit off a plant and putting it into a Petri dish, then forcing the injured cells not to die, or even to survive, but to grow into a whole new plant. Cells taken from a piece of leaf, or root, or even flower can be manipulated and tricked into 'regeneration' of shoots or embryos, ultimately grown into whole, fertile plants and capable of normal reproduction. The seed progeny from this individual are usually indistinguishable from 'normal' plants of the same cultivar, but, as with mutation breeding, on rare occasions a new feature appears. The breeder evaluates this new trait and, once again, on extremely rare occasions, he might exploit the novelty in a new cultivar. Several new cultivars developed from SCV are in commercial production. One of them is a linseed flax, described more fully below.

Cell selection

A modification of SCV is cell selection. Again, cells are grown in a Petri dish and stimulated to grow into a tumorous mass. As in human (or other) tumours, when cells grow in an uncontrolled manner, spontaneous genetic changes occur.

Instead of regenerating new plants from this mass and evaluating the plant progeny, as in SCV, the breeder takes a more direct approach by selecting the desired mutated cells while they are still in the Petri dish. These individual selected cells are then the only ones the breeder bothers to metamorphose into whole plants.

In order to select the desired cells, a chemical agent or poison that will kill any normal cells is added to the culture medium. Of the millions of cells in the Petri dish, the vast majority will perish. Any survivors are stimulated to regenerate into whole plants, as they are most likely to have undergone a mutation giving them the novel capacity to withstand the normally lethal selection agent. The limitation to this technique is that one can't select for 'higher seed yield', for example, because we don't have a chemical to add to the medium to identify such mutants. However, it has been used to select for herbicide resistance (just add the herbicide to the medium), salt tolerance (add a high concentration of salts), or even drought (add an agent to reduce accessibility of moisture in the medium). This technique offers major advantages over SCV, and even over mutation breeding.

- First, when employing SCV or mutation techniques, the breeder must evaluate hundreds, preferably thousands of whole plants and their progeny. This is expensive, time consuming, and, even for a plant breeder, boring. With cell selection, the breeder identifies 'interesting' types from among millions of cells while they are still in the Petri dish. The plant then developed from that 'interesting' or selected cell is more likely to be interesting in the same manner. Cellular selection is fast, inexpensive, and fascinating. It also provides the capacity to scan much larger numbers of potentially useful genetic mutants, as a single Petri dish can hold millions of cells, each potentially representing a different mutant.
- Second, as with cell selection, the breeder has a good idea of what advantageous trait the mutant plant cell (and subsequently plant) will carry, because it was selected and identified in the Petri dish. In mutation breeding and SCV, the breeder doesn't have a clue about what might pop up, or whether a novel feature might be of commercial value.

New crop cultivars have been developed from cell selection and are on the market. Pioneer Hi-Bred developed their herbicide-resistant Smart canolas using this technique. Most products are not labelled or scrutinized beyond the level required for ordinary new cultivars.

Existing technology

Humans have practised genetic technology (although often inadvertently) for thousands of years. Farmers routinely selected 'the best' of a crop or litter for continued propagation. Over time, this form of genetic engineering results in the population genetically shifting to reflect the selected traits. In the past hundred years, with our better understanding of genetics, the breeding process has become more orthodox and directed, with breeders intentionally choosing and mating parents to generate offspring with the right combination of genetic traits. However, conventional breeding involves taking the bad with the good. Often, a parent is chosen because it carries a single desired trait; the remaining 24 999 (or more) genes are either neutral or undesirable. Conventional crossing requires the combination of the entire genomes of the two parents, so in addition to the one desired gene, all the others come along for the ride. Most of the time and effort in traditional breeding is spent in eliminating as much of the undesirable genetic junk as feasible. Take, for example, a wheat-breeding programme, where the breeder crosses an elite commercial cultivar with a distant relative to introduce an important disease resistance gene from the foreigner. Unfortunately, the stranger delivers not only the disease-fighting gene, but a whole range of other, sometimes detrimental genes. One of these might make the resulting hybrid too tall, causing it to fall over before harvest. The breeder then has to analyse and cull all the too-tall progeny. At least the tall ones are easy to detect and remove. More commonly, the additional foreign genes interfere with the good breadmaking features of the domestic parent. Identifying those genes often takes considerable time and effort to eliminate.

Technological development in breeding now allows the single desired gene to be added to the complete genome of a single desirable parent. This process yields progeny almost identical to the parent, but with the addition of the one desired (transferred) trait and no undesirable genes. We call this process recombinant DNA (rDNA) technology. Then, through conventional propagation, the resulting progeny can produce a new, genetically elite, population lacking the undesirable genes.

Some opponents to GM object to 'those crosses that would not occur in nature', rejecting foods produced from such 'unnatural' breeding. However, many 'acceptable' crosses between plants of the same species involve plants grown so geographically dispersed they'd never mingle DNA without human intervention. Breeders in America often use plants found in Ethiopia or Nepal as parents. Under natural conditions these plants could not transfer pollen the required thousands of kilometres.

Consumers demanding only 'naturally occurring' food products might have to abandon most of their current foodstuffs. Even the potato, a basic staple in most diets, is very different today from its natural ancestors. Traditional farming methods in isolated parts of the Andes provide a glimpse of traditional potatoes. The crops display a diverse mix of potato landraces, primitive varieties consisting of genetically different colours, shapes, textures, and other attributes. In contrast, modern potato cultivars stand out for their uniformity and, generally, larger size.

Why have farmers abandoned the diversity of landraces in favour of modern cultivars? Historically, consumers prefer uniformity, farmers favour volume, and food processors demand both. Traditional varieties and landraces of most crops cannot compete in yield or quality. To be sanguine, modern cross-bred cultivars make more money for farmers and processors (the producers), and cost the consumers less.

The products of cross-breeding technology are not labelled or scrutinized beyond the level required for ordinary new cultivars. If 'unnatural' products are taboo, then a large number of consumers might be unwittingly eating self-proscribed foods.

Even before this recent technical development, however, almost none of the foods we now consume existed when human civilization arose some 40 thousand years ago. Indeed, civilization might be measured by the degree of selection, breeding, and intervention in our food supply. Those of us who demand only natural, unmodified food are necessarily limited to such a selection as wild berries, some fish, perhaps watercress, and whatever wild animals might be trapped and slaughtered. Even those would have undergone genetic alterations due to natural selection and evolution. They would also have been influenced by intentional or unintentional human-induced stresses on their populations and environment.

Why is conventional breeding acceptable?

Discussing the main techniques in crop breeding shows just how complex and intrusive 'acceptable' classical or conventional breeding can be. Usually the products require no special regulatory scrutiny or labelling. My objective is not to scare everyone into now demanding tighter regulatory scrutiny or labelling of these 'traditional' cultivars. On the contrary, it is to remind consumers that the current regulatory framework, largely invisible to the public eye, is extremely efficient in identifying and eliminating undesirable new foods. We do not need additional scrutiny for mutation-derived cultivars, for example, because the standard regulatory scrutiny is up to the task. No mutation-bred cultivar has ever caused harm, although some potentially hazardous ones were caught early, before any real damage was done. The same is true for other breeding methods, including recombinant DNA.

Yes, food scares continue. Contaminated feeds, dioxins, *E. coli*, benzene, *Salmonella*, and others warrant almost a daily column in our newspapers. Additional regulation of conventional breeding methods is unlikely to provide greater security and protection against food scares, because food hazards are almost invariably due to adulteration or contamination of foods, not to the actual cultivar or process by which they were developed.

Genetic engineering and rDNA
Into the traditional breeder's toolbox we've introduced several forms of rDNA to generate potential new crop varieties and food products. We looked at the genetic engineering technology in Chapter 3, so we have an idea how the technology compares with classical or traditional breeding technology. Later in this chapter we look at a real-life example of a genetically engineered crop variety in commercial production. Drawing a line between 'rDNA' and 'acceptable' breeding

methods seems more difficult because of the apparent continuum of different breeding technologies. Because of the many 'acceptable' or conventional breeding methods in common use, it is not a simple matter to dichotomize between rDNA technology and all others. Nor is it wise, if the distinction is based solely on safety concerns. GM varieties undergo far greater scrutiny for safety and environmental risks than, say, varieties developed from mutation breeding. In mutation breeding, we have no idea what genetic changes have been induced and little or no molecular characterization of even the evident novel trait. In rDNA breeding, we know exactly what genes have been introduced and have them fully characterized, right down to the molecules. Mutation breeding presents a minimal threat to environment or health safety. Genetic engineering is, if anything, even safer due to the more rigorous characterization and scrutiny.

This is not to suggest that mutation breeding presents an unregulated hazard that must be curtailed. Products of mutation breeding are properly regulated and fully safe. The history of safety in induced mutant varieties supports this assertion. My point is that if mutation breeding is acceptable and safe with the current level of regulatory scrutiny, then there is no logical basis to categorically 'draw the line' between rDNA and mutation breeding. An example is the herbicide-resistant canola varieties. The UK actively imports oil from Australian herbicide-tolerant canola, yet refuses oil from Canadian herbicide-tolerant canola. The stated rationale is that one was developed using conventional technology, the other by GM. Yet the potential adverse environmental and health effects are the same—virtually nil. If escape of a herbicide resistance gene from imported rapeseed is a legitimate environmental concern, why is oil from one herbicide-resistant canola prohibited altogether, and another admitted without additional scrutiny?

Similarly, Pioneer-HiBred used cell selection to develop their herbicide-resistant Smart canola and wish not only to import for processing but to cultivate the varieties as crops in the UK. They argue that they need no special scrutiny because the canola is not GM. Legally, they are correct, the Smart canola was not produced using rDNA. But if there is a concern over herbicide resistance genes escaping, does it matter if the source is GM or not?

These examples illustrate three salient problems characteristic of the whole GM debate.

1 We lack a precise, common definition of a GM product (see Chapter 1). Smart canola was regulated as GM in Canada because it presented a novel trait (herbicide resistance). It is exempted from GM regulation in the UK because it is not a product of rDNA. It is the same product. If it poses a health risk to Canadians, it poses an identical risk to Britons. Yet in one country, it came under extraordinary regulatory scrutiny, in the other, almost none. A proper scientific review would entail the similar health scrutiny in both jurisdictions.

2 We confuse and coalesce different classes of GM products requiring different kinds and degrees of regulatory scrutiny. Earlier we discussed three different types of GM product:

– a whole living GM organism containing functional DNA (e.g. a GM tomato, a GM soya bean)
– a processed product of the GMO containing degraded, non-functional DNA (e.g. paste from a GM tomato, tofu from GM soya bean)
– an extract from a GMO, containing neither GM DNA nor protein (e.g. oil or lecithin from GM soya bean).

Each of these types of product elicits different scientific concerns. We need not be too worried about pollen escape from tofu, for example. But in regulatory review, and in the public mind, all three are seen as 'products of rDNA' and equally suspect.

3 We need to keep the question of safety in context. Nothing is absolutely risk-free. In establishing regulatory procedures, we need to ask 'How does the GM product differ from the closest conventional version?' The canola oil from Australia and the canola oil from Canada are both squeezed out of seeds of herbicide-resistant plants. Neither oil carries more than trace amounts of DNA or protein. Yet one is welcomed into the UK market with minimal regulation, the other denied access altogether.

So just what regulation is in place for products of ordinary breeding? Now that we know how various breeding methods work, let's investigate how we get the conventional products on to the market.

From the breeder to your plate: cultivar registration and commercial release

The goal of plant breeding is to provide 'improved' crop varieties, technically called cultivars. The improvements can be anything from increased seed yield to enhanced disease resistance to improved quality. Regardless of the 'improved' trait, all new crop varieties must, by international law, meet three criteria.

1 First, a new variety must be genetically modified and different from all other varieties and organisms. It must be genetically distinct.
2 Second, the new variety must produce a uniform appearance. A field of the crop cannot be populated with varied plants, with some tall, others short, light green with darker green and so on. All of the plants in a variety must look like each other.
3 Third, the new variety must be genetically stable. If, for some reason, a candidate variety breeding line seems to be unstable, it will be eliminated.

By the time the breeder is ready to seek registered variety status for a candidate breeding line, sufficient observations will have been made to enable a determination on all three criteria: distinct, uniform and stable, or DUS in industry parlance. Without all three criteria being met, the candidate line, no matter how positive it might be in other respects, cannot be registered and therefore cannot be commercialized in international trade.

Plant breeders each have a particular favourite method of deriving the 'improved' cultivar. Even within a basic technique there are sub-techniques. Crossing, introgression, backcrossing, the pedigreed method, single seed descent are all sub-techniques of ordinary breeding practised by 'conventional' plant breeders in bringing us new improved cultivars. One thing they all have in common, though, is that it takes a long time to develop a new crop variety. For most crops, about 8 to 13 years pass between the time the breeder starts the process, until the resulting new and successful variety is registered for sale to farmers. Then it usually takes another couple of years to increase seed supply to have enough to sell to commercial farmers. By the time it ends up on your plate, the new variety is probably obsolete in the mind of the breeder, who has a much-improved version under development. The average new cultivar has a life of only a few years before it is superseded by a superior new cultivar.

Some countries, the UK and Australia, for example, have a system where formal variety registration is a fairly easy process, but seed sales to farmers are heavily influenced by independent organizations who conduct their own evaluations of registered cultivars and make specific recommendations or 'lists' for local or regional farmers. In either case, by the time a farmer chooses which cultivar to grow, the election is based on those cultivars independently evaluated and placed on a recommended list. The final result in either system provides farmers, and ultimately consumers, with products evaluated by independent experts and judged to be of the highest quality.

In the UK, new crop varieties are evaluated by the National Institute for Agricultural Botany (NIAB). NIAB publishes brochures with brief descriptions of the recommended varieties of each crop species and data tables providing performance data for important agronomic parameters. Figure 4 provides an example.

The 1998 recommended list for linseed includes about two dozen registered varieties. The data comparisons include relative seed yield, oil content, standing power, earliness of ripening, and other parameters of great interest to farmers but of little concern to final consumers. Similar lists are available for other crop types. Farmers choose varieties by studying the list, comparing the performance of each variety, and evaluating the data and the text notation of any special features for each variety. Before farmers can obtain seed of a new variety, however, they must await multiplication of seed stocks for that variety. Breeders ordinarily have a small amount of genetically pure breeder seed of their new lines. This seed must be used as a parental population, grown to provide sufficient seed to satisfy commercial farmers' demands.

The first farmers to get a new cultivar are called seed growers, having been judged as outstanding in their ability to multiply seed of a new cultivar in the highest possible quality. The breeder provides genetically pure seed of the new cultivar. The seed grower takes this seed and grows it, not to make a commercial

UK DESCRIPTIVE LIST OF SPRING LINSEED 1998

Based on trials from 1993–97. The control for yield comparisons is the mean of Antares, Barbara, Mikael and Zoltan. Differences of less than 8% in yield or 0.5% in oil content should be treated with reserve.

	Industrial oil varieties																				Edible oil varieties		
	Geria	Agristar	Jupiter	Flechette	Zoltan	Barbara	Peak	Mikael	Danube	Crystal	Antares	Moonraker	Flanders	Abby	Royale	Bolas	McGregor	Pacific	Gold Merchant	Norlin	Windermere	989	Coniston
Yield as % control (1.74 t/ha) 5 year mean	106	105	105	103	102	102	100	100	99	98	96	96	95	95	94	(92)	92	91	87	87	100	99	94
Agronomic characters																							
Standing power	5	6	6	7	7	7	7	7	5	6	7	6	6	7	6	8	7	8	7	7	6	7	6
Shortness of stem	6	7	6	6	7	7	6	8	7	7	6	8	6	8	6	8	5	5	6	5	5	5	5
Earliness of flowering	6	8	8	5	7	7	4	8	6	7	7	9	5	9	6	7	2	5	4	3	2	4	2
Earliness of ripening	5	4	5	3	5	5	5	6	5	5	5	6	6	5	4	5	5	5	5	7	5	5	4
Thousand seed weight (g)	7.0	8.5	8.6	7.9	8.0	8.9	5.7	9.1	7.1	8.5	8.1	8.5	6.0	8.5	8.2	8.5	5.6	8.2	6.6	6.5	5.6	5.9	5.7
Seed quality at 9% moisture Oil content of seed	39.7	39.6	39.2	39.5	40.0	39.1	39.6	39.4	41.4	39.4	38.7	38.7	40.3	40.1	38.9	39.1	38.8	39.6	41.6	37.4	41.9	40.1	41.7
Year first listed	1998	1998	1997	1998	1995	1992	1995	1993	1996	1993	1990	1998	1994	1997	1995	1993	1991	1995	1996	1990	1996	1997	1995

A high figure indicates the variety shows that character to a high degree.
() Limited data

Figure 4   Sample of NIAB recommended list of linseed cultivars for the UK from 1998. Reproduced with permission of NIAB.

Variety registration: the merit system

The long development period for a new cultivar includes several years of field trials. Many countries have a system to evaluate the plant breeder's best candidate cultivars and either accept them into the marketplace or reject them. The Canadian system for most field crops, including wheat, canola, barley, and linseed is typical of the 'merit' approach, so will serve as an example here. Other jurisdictions registering new varieties based on merit will differ in detail, but are substantively similar.

A breeder spends several years in developing a new candidate cultivar, each year selecting the best plants from a particular cross, of which there may be several thousand. The early years are spent backcrossing to eliminate as many undesirable traits as possible, and discarding any unstable or undesirable types. Early field trials involve short rows of plants grown from seeds from a single chosen plant. If that row performed well, seed will be collected from it at maturity and used to grow a larger row or small plot (several short rows) next season. If the short row contains undesirable plants, they are discarded. Often, the whole row is discarded. After a few years of continued evaluation, the majority of lines have been discarded. The remaining lines are analysed in greater detail, looking at seed yield, time from seeding to harvest maturity, and a whole range of mundane parameters, such as height and flower colour. In addition, the harvested seeds are all measured in every imaginable manner, weight, density, and chemical analyses to give indications of grain quality.

After harvest each year, all the information on the performance of each line is collated and computerized, allowing full comparison with all other entries for every parameter. The breeder spends days poring over these data sheets. Any lines showing any degree of instability in any aspect are eliminated from further testing. Those clearly inferior in major parameters, such as seed yield or time to mature, or a disease susceptibility are likewise eliminated from further testing. Only those with excellent performance across the board are advanced to another year of testing. The breeder might start with 2000 breeding lines in any given year, ending up after a few years with only one or two from the initial batch. Or perhaps none.

When the breeder has what appears to be a good performing line, and a population of genetically stable seed, the line is entered (by providing a sample of the seed) into the national crop testing system which, in Canada, we call the Co-op trials. An independent coordinator, usually a federal government employee, organizes the field trials. The field trials consist of several standard cultivars of the crop type in commercial production, plus all the candidate lines from the various breeders, public and private, in the jurisdiction for which registration and commercial release is sought.

Each prospective new line directly competes not only with the current standard or commercial cultivars, but also with its competitors' best new lines. The trial is conducted at several locations, to ensure that any geographical advantage or disadvantage is noted, and also to ensure data is collected even if one or two locations must be discounted due to adverse weather during the growing season. The breeder at this stage has little or no influence over the process, and all candidates in the test are treated equally—for example, no special treatments are given to herbicide-resistant lines. Data are collected on each line throughout the growing season, including such agronomic traits as height, time to flower, maturity date, and seed yield. An independent public assessor also collects disease data to measure how the new candidate stands up to important plant diseases in the area, and finally a more comprehensive grain quality analysis is conducted, measuring the important chemical constituents of the grain. For example, a candidate cultivar of bread wheat will undergo a series of tests to measure its breadmaking ability. Any line not measuring up to the standards is rejected, regardless of how well it does in other tests. The coordinator collects and collates all the data from each location. Each year, the coordinator meets the contributing breeders to analyse the data and eliminate all but the best lines. By the time a candidate cultivar breeding line is considered for registration, necessary for commercial release, it has been analysed by the breeder and by independent experts for several years.

Finally, a 'competent authority' committee of experts evaluates those lines performing over at least two and usually three years in the national field trials. The expert committee evaluates the reams of data and votes on the merit, relative to the standard cultivars and also to the other candidate cultivars. On the basis of that vote, the candidate is registered or rejected.

The main expert committee for field crops in western Canada (the Prairie Registration Recommending Committee for Grain, PRRCG) meets each February to deliberate and vote on candidate varieties. February is the earliest the data from the previous field season can be collated and distributed to each member of the committee. The committee members are drawn from national as well as local breeding institutions, universities, and private companies. Each member has to be intimately involved in the plant breeding process and carry expertise on at least one aspect of breeding, agronomy, and pathology or grain chemistry.

This system is quite rigorous. By the time a line is presented for the final vote, it has survived several years of scrutiny. Depending on the crop type and the breeder's specific methods, perhaps only one line in 4000 initial candidate lines makes it to the vote. It is not unusual for a plant breeder to release only one or two new cultivars in a lifetime and still be considered a successful breeder. The benefit of this 'merit' system is that farmers know they are getting a high quality product when they buy certified seed of a registered cultivar.

crop, but to provide more seed to sell to regular farmers, who in turn grow the commercial crop. With the breeder providing only a small amount of the breeder seed, the seed growers often require two or three years of seed multiplication to provide sufficient seed stock to supply the demand from farmers for the new cultivar. This adds to the total time from initiation of breeding to actual commercial production.

Seed growers sell certified seed to commercial farmers. The selling price includes costs of production, handling, advertising, overheads, and so on as

---

Where do farmers get their seeds?

Many farmers get their seeds from their own stocks. Others buy seeds from a grain company or from neighbours.

Some farmers grow the same seed year after year. 'If it was good enough for Grandpa, it's good enough for me' is their attitude. Every time they grow a crop, they save enough seed for the subsequent crop. The seed is fresh, because it has just been rejuvenated. Seed loses viability over time; farmers don't sow seed from the same batch that Grandpa grew.

'The grass is always greener on the other side' surely originated with a farmer. They are the archetypal nosy neighbours, always curious and envious of the crop across the road. It's little wonder many farmers supplement their income by saving some of their harvest and selling 'brown bag' seed across the fence.

Then there is certified seed. Unlike the earlier examples of saved seed or brown bag seed, certified seed is sold by registered variety name. In fact, it is an offence to sell brown bag or 'grown from' saved seed by cultivar or variety name. Depending on the region and crop type, a farmer has a choice from six to fifty or more cultivars. Although all cultivars must be genetically distinct, certain quality characteristics must be similar. The quality standards allow the ultimate blending of the commodity without regard to the particular cultivar. After harvest, when the farmer sells the harvested seed, it gets mixed with seed of up to fifty other cultivars of the same quality grown in that area.

Most successful farmers buy seed every year, but this practice varies widely according to national and local custom, crop type, and price. Seed of hybrid cultivars always has to be purchased fresh every year, because hybrid plants do not breed true. When a farmer saves seed from hybrids for replanting—and believe me most have tried it once, but only once—the resulting crop looks like an awful, non-uniform collection of apparently unrelated plants.

For 'open pollinated' crops, seed can be saved from one year to the next, but the quality diminishes quickly. I recommend farmers buy certified seed each year. The premium product almost always covers the cost of the initial outlay. Many farmers either don't want to or can't afford to. So they continue to grow saved seed. That's their privilege.

The farmer's privilege (sometimes called the farmer's exemption) is more than an expression. Internationally recognized laws and treaties protect it. It can be overridden only by an explicit contract between the farmer and the seed vendor.

usual, and also a royalty payment to the breeding institution. Most public breeding institutions use royalties from the sale of certified seed of their registered cultivars to defray costs of continued plant breeding programmes, but these amounts alone are usually insufficient to maintain a plant breeding programme. Royalty moneys from my varieties support research programmes, most often as student stipends.

The new cultivars now coming into farmers' hands were, for the most part, initially generated fifteen years ago or more. The first GM plant was produced in 1983. It was an experimental tobacco carrying a simple marker gene. In only two or three years, the fledgling technology was extended to agronomically useful genes in crop species. The first GM crops, those now in the marketplace, really are 'first generation' technology.

Like conventional varieties, a GM crop variety must undergo the standard evaluation process. Unlike standard varieties, however, it must also pass the various environmental and food safety assessments specific to GM products. Also, unlike conventional varieties, in which approval in one jurisdiction provides access to worldwide markets, the GM variety must undergo the separate GM scrutiny of each market to which it may be exported.

Delivering the goods: the grain handling system

Each farmer grows the crop, harvests the grain, and takes it to a local storage facility, a grain elevator, as a delivery. So do other farmers in the region. The grain storage facility usually keeps the grain in cavernous bins until it can be transported to processors or to overseas markets. Having these giant grain bins means the elevator company can only keep separate as many different grains as there are bins. So, when a North American farmer delivers a load of standard grade 2 wheat, it gets dumped in the bin labelled 'standard grade 2 wheat' along with all the other standard grade 2 wheat loads dropped off by all the other farmers in the region. There is no provision for storing separate cultivars or even recording them.

Although the ultimate consumer is generally blind to the entire breeding and commercialization process, most are confident from experience that the products they buy—bread, vegetable oil, or whatever—are safe and nutritious. Few have any idea what particular cultivar of wheat went into the bread they buy or bake, or what cultivar of sunflower provided the oil in the bottle of sunflower oil. In most cases, it is a blend of many different cultivars, but each one will have the same high quality of breadmaking characteristics or oil composition, respectively.

Trying to identify specific cultivars in a blend of grain seed is extremely difficult. Identification from a loaf of bread or a bottle of oil is virtually impossible. Furthermore, each batch of oil or bread will contain a different blend of contributing cultivars. Typically, a shipload of soy, maize, or wheat seeds contains blends of dozens, if not hundreds, of different cultivars. They all pass the same quality controls before being loaded, and often have to pass inspection before being unloaded. The cultivars in each shipload will vary according to the shipment's origin and the source of the bulk commodity within a growing region, as different geographical regions will have different cultivar proportions and local farmer preferences. The next shipload will have a different proportion of cultivars in the blend.

Segregation of GM and non-GM grain

Segregating GM from non-GM grain would require at least doubling the current grain handling industry, as there would have to be counterpart GM storage bins for every non-GM storage bin. For every 'grade 2 hard red spring wheat' bin there would have to be a 'grade 2 GM hard red spring wheat' bin. In addition, the grain must continue to be segregated throughout its entire journey, in road tankers, rail freight wagons, or ships, and through processing facilities until its ultimate destiny on the grocery shelf. Obviously, the cost of this infrastructure for segregation of GM grain would be substantial, but if we are willing to pay, it could be done. Monsanto has been accused of refusing to segregate their GM soy and maize from regular soy and maize. Monsanto faces its share of legitimate criticism, but this is not their fault. It's not Monsanto's decision to segregate or blend, that decision is up to the grain handling companies.

Segregation already occurs for certain commodity products. Grade 1 wheat is segregated from grade 2 wheat. The grading takes place at the elevator at the time of delivery. Every farmer argues for the highest grade, as that provides the highest price. Grading is based on relatively simple categories: presence and amount of weed or other seeds, dirt, broken kernels, and 'foreign matter' (which we discuss in Chapter 5) in a given load. Some have argued that if segregation can be so easily done with different grades of wheat, it can also be done with GM and non-GM crops. However, segregating GM crops would not be so simple, as the receiving elevator agent has no practical way to verify whether a particular load of grain is GM or not. Asking the farmer if the grain is GM or not is one way to base a determination, but depending on the differential in price benefits, it might not be very reliable. If there's no price differential, the farmer may have blended the grain harvested from two or more fields, some of which might have been sown to GM and others to conventional varieties. So, although it is theoretically possible to segregate GM from non-GM varieties, there's no inexpensive way to do it reliably or with the apparently low level of tolerance demanded. GM crops growing in agricultural communities will become co-mingled with non-GM varieties. Pollen blows around cross-pollinating plants of the same species without regard for GM designation. Seeds get spilled. Farm machinery traps seeds inside, to be blended with the next load of grain or to drop out on the next field. Seed bags get mislabelled. All of these things happen far more often than we like to admit.

Nevertheless, if we demand segregation of GM from non-GM varieties, and

A tale of two varieties

An example of conventional breeding technology

Shortly after Larkin and Scowcroft published their views on somoclonal variation (SCV) using wheat as an example, my students and I initiated a similar programme with linseed. After generating some 12 000 linseed regenerants, we noted only a few off-types or possible somaclonal variants. Seed from those that seemed interesting for any reason were provided to my colleague, Dr Gordon Rowland, our 'traditional' linseed breeder. Gordon field tested the somaclonal lines in his trials, comparing their performance with current registered cultivars as well as his breeding lines undergoing evaluation for possible registration as new cultivars. Within a year or two, most of the SCV lines were eliminated as being either inferior or essentially no different from breeding lines already in the trials. A few lines were maintained for a few years, but the number of SCV lines gradually diminished to one.

I was pleased that Gordon retained one, at least. But when I looked at the data, I could see no reason to keep the line. It was not deficient in any aspect, but it had no outstanding or positive features. When I asked Gordon about this, he said 'Well, let's keep it in and see how it performs next year'. Not noticing any apparent advantage of this line, I would have thrown it out, but Gordon was the breeder, he knew better than I did how to interpret the numbers. Each year for the next several, the SCV line was one of those uncertain borderline cases—should we discard it or not? It always performed well, but not outstandingly. It had no apparent deficiencies, but no particular selling features, either. Its seed yield, probably the most important parameter, was close to the top, but never the actual leader. Its maturity was similarly close to the best, but never reached that pinnacle either. We tested the line over several years, in dozens of trials all over the country. I was still unsure we had a worthwhile cultivar. It was a good performer, but many cultivars already in the market were also good performers. Without an outstanding feature somewhere, such as the highest seed yield or earliest maturity, people weren't going to buy it in preference to what they already had available.

When the time came to make a final decision, Gordon showed me the computer printout, comprising all the performance data and comparisons with all other commercial cultivars and breeding lines over the years of testing. The SCV line was the top performing linseed in Canada. How could this be? I was stunned. Then I realized, when we were looking at good years or good regions, the line was near but not at the top of the performers. When we looked at poor years, it was also near but not at the top. The ones at the top in the good years, edging out the SCV line, were nowhere near the top in the poor years, and vice versa. Similarly with time to maturity. The other lines maturing earlier than the SCV line were generally lower in seed yield. Overall, the SCV line combined the best seed yield with the earliest maturity across the range of farm environments in western Canada and promised solid performance in all sea-sons, good and bad. We presented the candidate for consideration to the PRRCG, who approved the recommendation for registration. We called it CDC Normandy. You might have seen it growing or even eaten it, as it's in commercial production and worldwide distribution. It and other cultivars from somaclonal variation are not labelled or scrutinized beyond that required for ordinary new cultivars.

An example of applied rDNA: GM linseed

Sulfonylureas (SUs) are one of the more popular groups of herbicide. Several commercial formulations exist, dominated by DuPont, makers of such herbi-cides as Glean™, Ally™, and Refine™. These herbicides are popular with cereal farmers because they very effectively control common and nasty broadleaf weeds at extremely low doses (a teaspoon or two per acre) at reasonable cost. They also control many of the broadleaf crop plants that inadvertently grow in a wheatfield. An unfortunate side effect of some SUs is their tendency to remain active in the soil for extended periods. Depending on the nature of the soil and the environment, that extended period could be many years.

Wheat farmers in Saskatchewan learned to their chagrin that Glean™, for one, would take many years to decompose naturally in the soil, precluding farmers from growing broadleafed crops. Partly because of this problem with the residue, Glean™ is no longer available on the market in Canada or the US. Although none of the other SUs is as persistent, and some have virtually no residue problem, some do have residual activity in certain soil types and regions.

Farmers were in a bind. They wanted to continue to use the SU in their cereal crops, but the residue meant they couldn't grow another non-cereal crop in the subsequent years. Continuous cropping to cereals was one answer, but it is not a sustainable option. Continuous cropping leads to a soil imbal-ance from nutrient depletion and build-up of pathogens. The only other option, summer fallowing until the residue had degraded naturally, is also not a sustainable practice, as it results in soil erosion and non-productivity of the land. It's also not economically sustainable, as land taken out of production doesn't generate much income. Some farmers are still waiting, after twelve years or more, to put fields back into useful production. Farmers had no choice but to employ non-sustainable farming practices.

I thought it would be worthwhile developing a GM linseed cultivar capable of being grown in such contaminated land. It would provide a rotational option to farmers. They could avoid the non-sustainable practice of continu-ally growing cereals year after year. They could avoid the alternative non-sustainable practice of summer fallow, with its negative environmental consequences of soil erosion and non-productivity. With a linseed cultivar tol-erant to SU residues in the soil, farmers with this soil contaminant problem could employ proper and sustainable rotations with cereals and a broadleaf crop—the GM linseed. This could be an environmentally, agronomically and economically sustainable GM crop cultivar. Unfortunately, it would have to wait for the technology to develop, as no gene conferring resistance to SU had been isolated and no one had yet generated a GM linseed.

The first few transgenic plants, mostly experimental species, such as tobacco and *Arabidopsis*, had been genetically transformed with marker genes, and the race was on to extend this success to crop species with the ultimate aim of inserting genes of agronomic value. Although the basic concepts of genetic transformation using *Agrobacterium* (and later, the particle gun) were common across many plants, each species has its own particular nuances. The technical methods successful with tobacco did not work on wheat, rapeseed, or most other crop species. With several postgraduate students, undergraduate students, a lab manager, and various part-time technicians, I'd been working with disarmed *Agrobacterium* for a couple of years before finally enjoying some success in transferring marker genes into linseed. While we continued developing and improving the linseed transformation technique, we were anxious to try something beyond marker genes, something useful. We were like kids given a new computer, but only basic software, no exciting games. I recalled my interest in helping farmers overcome their problems with SU herbicides. A gene conferring resistance to SUs would be a nice bit of software.

Shortly afterwards, my colleague George Haughn isolated such a gene and gave it to me. My students used our linseed transformation method to insert it into major commercial linseed cultivars, eventually developing thirty GM lines to test. Over several years, all but two were eliminated—some performed poorly for ordinary agronomic traits like yield, other did not express the new gene strongly enough to be useful to farmers. Two lines, both derived from the excellent linseed variety Norlin, were excellent performers and also showed full SU herbicide resistance. They were entered into the national registration trials.

The results from the national variety registration trials were encouraging for both lines as well. In all measured parameters, there was high correlation between each of the GM lines and the parent variety Norlin. Each year, when the national coordinator released the data from the season's trials, each contributing breeder studies the performance of the candidate lines. Those performing well would be tested again in next year's test. Those lines showing a weakness would be eliminated from further testing and, with that, their chance of ever being released for commercial production. New candidate cultivars are usually considered for registration after three years in the national trials. Both GM lines made the grade each year, as neither had exposed any weaknesses and always performed well. After three years of these national trials, in addition to all the other field trials conducted over five years, in soil containing herbicide residue and without, we had no basis for eliminating either line from consideration for variety registration. But we also had no basis for choosing one GM line over the other. Both conferred an excellent degree of soil herbicide tolerance, and both provided excellent agronomic and quality performance.

Because of costs of regulatory compliance and possible confusion in the marketplace, we didn't want to register two virtually identical GM varieties. Gordon and I ended up flipping a coin to determine which line would be put forward at the next annual variety registration meeting. The toss gave the choice to designated GM line 12115, also known as FP967.

FP967 was put to the PRRCG recommending committee in February 1994 and accepted. We named it CDC Triffid. A year later, the first GM canolas were also accepted, to be followed by an ever-increasing number of GM candidate cultivars seeking variety registration status.

are prepared to pay the price, it will be done. What, though, if we consumers also decide to segregate other cultivars based on breeding methods? Segregation for mutation bred cultivars? Cultivars from intergeneric crossing? Where does it end? To be realistic, it ends when consumers decide they don't wish to pay the additional costs for segregation they see as unnecessary. The higher the price, the sooner they'll see it as unnecessary.

Drawing the line

How can we draw a line between acceptable and unacceptable breeding methods? Unfortunately, the existing breeding methods are not isolated and discrete: they are instead continuous, shading gradually into one another. There is no logical dichotomy on which to base a linear distinction. Why draw a line between rDNA and 'everything else' when the result would have rDNA on one side and the potentially more hazardous mutation breeding, or irradiation, on the other, 'safe' side? The same line would identify as impermissible those products of rDNA technology in wide and largely acceptable use, such as insulin, vitamin C, and vegetarian cheeses. There is no scientific justification for such a distinction. Also, people express different concerns. Some would draw the line between selection and crossing, for example, whereas others might accept haploid breeding but not mutation breeding. Some, of course, would attempt to excise rDNA from 'everything else', but cannot scientifically justify that line.

Popular misconceptions

There is a popular but nevertheless incorrect assumption that current crop cultivars, animal breeds, and food products are natural (as found in nature). As we've seen, almost all current cultivars of crops are very different, genetically, from their ancestral relatives. Animal breeds have all been carefully bred and selected for attributes desirable for domestication, meat production, and human consumption. Microbes used in various food production processes—for making beer, bread, wine, and cheese, for example—are all very different now from what they were. Evolution, driven by genetic instability, occurs even without human intervention. Nature demands gene instability and devised means to ensure it.

Another popular misconception is that current crop varieties are 'safe' (i.e. that there is no risk involved). I agree that current cultivars are, in general, safe. But it's not the technique that produced them that's safe; it's the products that are safe, because they have been scrutinized using current, routine regulations. The current cultivars are safe, not because the breeding method is inherently safe but because any unsafe candidate varieties have been identified and eliminated during the rigorous breeding development and evaluation process.

Planting ideas

Is genetic engineering just an extension of conventional breeding technologies, as claimed by many of the developers? Or is it so novel and revolutionary that it cannot be compared with existing technology, as demanded by various activist groups? As with most controversial issues, the real answer lies somewhere between the extreme views. After learning about the technical process of genetic engineering as well as some of those used in conventional breeding, we can begin to see for ourselves where genetic modification fits.

In many technical ways, rDNA is indeed revolutionary. Never before have breeders been able to isolate single useful genes and transfer only them to develop superior varieties. In many other ways, the products of GM are not so different from what could be generated using conventional methods. For example, much of the non-GM canola crop in Australia is grown using varieties carrying a herbicide-resistant mutation, despite lower seed yields of 15% associated with that mutation. A GM version might be able to provide the same trait, but without the yield penalty accompanying the 'natural' mutation. Similarly, genetic engineering provides crop varieties capable of growing in polluted, contaminated soils. Functionally identical varieties can be, and have been, identified from spontaneous mutation or induced mutation. One of the hypothetical risks associated with mutation breeding is that, although we can identify the new and useful trait, we have no idea what other genes might have been mutated at the same time. It is entirely possible that, in the course of mutating a gene to result in shorter stature a less obvious mutation affected toxin production in the grain. What is the logical basis for intense scrutiny and regulation of the GM version, but not the 'conventional' version, which conceivably could well carry substantially greater risk?

CHAPTER 5

Food: the offal truth

- Will banning GM foods eliminate food scares?
- Does ordinary food contain DNA?
- What else is in our 'pure' food?
- How do we measure toxins?
- Are there toxins in other commonly ingested products, such as tobacco?
- What do tolerances and allowances mean?
- What else is in 'pure' food?
- Are we eating GM DNA and protein? How much?
- What about other things in food, like pesticides?
- What is genetic homology?
- Why can't we just go back to the way it was in the 'good old days'

Food safety: what's your gut reaction ?

We all eat something every day. It's no wonder food safety and security are top priorities for everyone. It's difficult to overcome the emotional impact, but threats to food safety and security, more than any other issue in the GM debate, are fraught with the most egregious misunderstanding and misinformation. To some, regular food is pure, natural, and wholesome whereas GM seems impure, unnatural, and unwholesome. This chapter explodes this myth, as we consider food and food production issues—GM and otherwise.

We need to evaluate the food safety risks of GM food in the global context of ordinary food production systems. Consider the stories of food contamination and adulteration of the past few years:

- benzene in Perrier™ water
- antifreeze in wine
- *Listeria* bacteria in French dairy products
- dioxins in chicken, eggs, and meat
- and of course, BSE from infected beef.

On top of these we are presented with scary stories of GM foods,

'Frankenfoods' to some. GM is not immune to safety and security lapses, but it might be used to relieve some of our ongoing food problems.

Poisoned by a mutant tomato?

One of the major and potentially valid concerns about GM foods is that they might inadvertently poison us. Some people say GM products are not scrutinized rigorously enough, that we don't know the long-term effects of ingestion. They claim that our regulators, in their safety evaluations, depend almost entirely on the analyses and test results conducted by the biotechnology companies, some of which are not known for a deep sense of openness and disclosure, especially of non-flattering data.

No one, not even the avaricious multinational, wants to be responsible (i.e. legally liable) for poisoning unsuspecting consumers (i.e. prospective litigants). So just what is the appropriate amount of testing required before a product is considered 'safe' for human consumption?

New crops, regardless of breeding technique (and including GMOs), must pass a series of chemical composition analyses and meet minimum standards before being allowed commercial release. GMOs, in addition, undergo more exacting tests to provide greater 'comfort' and security that the product is at least as safe as conventional food crop cultivars.

What, then, is the likelihood of being poisoned by a GMO? To address this question, we need to consider the risk associated with ordinary food poisoning, then compare that with the additional risk, if any, imposed by GM foods.

What's in store?

When I travel, I like to spend an hour or so at my destination going through a local food market, just to see what the people are eating. In the UK, I notice a wide selection and plenty of nutritious food. I see heaps of fresh fruit and vegetables, but notice the supposedly fresh peas looking dull and listless compared to my recollections from past years. (Later I learned that British pea processors used to apply artificial colorant to make the peas look nice, but ceased the practice several years ago). I also see fewer brands but more variety in prepared and processed foods than I see in a supermarket at home. UK foods seem even further removed from the farm than North American foods, in that a greater proportion pass through more processing steps. What is in all these foodstuffs? Various public opinion surveys show most people don't realize what they're putting into their mouths. Or, more precisely, they don't know what's in what they're putting into their mouths.

What is in our food? Do any foods contain DNA? Of course they do! As we learned in Chapter 2, all plants, animals, and microbes use DNA to carry their genetic information. Every cell carries some DNA, along with other cell components—proteins, oils, carbohydrates, fibre, and so on. The only foods not carrying DNA are highly processed food products, such as oil, starch, or sugar, where DNA and other components of the originating organism are destroyed or removed during processing.

Are there any bacterial or fungal components? Yes, indeed. Food often carries bacterial or fungal contaminants. The microscopic organisms themselves might be dead from pasteurization, sterilization, cooking, or whatever, but they leave their remains, including their DNA, for you to enjoy.

Thomas Hoban, a Professor of Sociology and Anthropology at North Carolina State University in the USA, is interested in people's opinions on GMOs, particularly GM food. He and his collaborators conduct public opinion surveys on the subject, compiling data from around the world. One of the findings was the frighteningly high proportion of people who believe that ordinary tomatoes do not contain genes, but GM tomatoes do. In fact, both GM and regular tomatoes carry enough DNA to encode over 25 thousand proteins.

Poisoned by DNA?

Keith Downey is an 'old-fashioned' plant breeder. Now retired, he spent his entire career working for the Canadian government developing new varieties of rapeseed using 'traditional' plant breeding methods. In fact, Keith is considered the 'father of canola' for leading a team of scientists in developing a non-toxic form of rapeseed called canola in most of the world. Britain, one of the few hold-outs, refers to both the toxic and non-toxic types as 'rapeseed' or 'oilseed rape', causing untold and unnecessary confusion to consumers in the UK.

A few years ago, Keith was asked to join a peace conference summit in Belgium. Plant Genetic Systems (PGS), a small but aggressive biotechnology company based in Ghent, had genetically modified canola and was eager to field test the modified plants. Local activists didn't like the tests and destroyed the plants in the field. The summit was called to discuss how to resolve the issue: activists were demanding a moratorium on field tests until the modified plants were proven 'safe', PGS officials claimed they needed to conduct the field trials to acquire the data on which to establish safety. Keith was invited as an external expert resource person because he was not on the payroll of either the company or the activist side. According to Keith, the meeting between the leaders of the activists and PGS began guarded and tense but then deteriorated rapidly with participants readily and intimately sharing their innermost emotions. It terminated when the activist camp stormed out, their leader shaking his fist, shouting from the door 'You'll never convince me to eat DNA!'

None of the 'new' genes is truly new to our diet, because we have eaten them (albeit sometimes inadvertently, as in the case of bacteria). If we have no hesitation in eating a tomato and bean salad, why do we question eating a tomato with a bean gene? Foods that we can safely eat separately (like tomatoes and beans) can be safely eaten together (like tomatoes plus beans). Ultimately, all those genes and proteins are mixed up together in our gut anyway. What a GM tomato carrying a bean gene does is add them together earlier.

Ingredient, additive, contaminant, or adulterant?

We like to think of food as being wholesome, natural, and pure. Most food is, at least within reasonable standards of tolerance. We become understandably upset when we hear of various contaminants or adulterants in our food supply. But when does a common additive, say a vitamin enrichment, become an adulterant? And what about natural impurities—are they healthy?

Let's look at one of our most wholesome foods, milk. What's in natural milk straight out of a cow? Milk is a 'nurse product', jammed full of many nutrients. Unfortunately, because those same nutrients are attractive to other organisms, including nasty bacteria, we have to pasteurize milk to kill the bacteria. People who consider pasteurized milk adulterated, and therefore prefer 'organic, unpasteurized' milk, run a big risk. The rest of us consume the corpses and remnants of the bacteria.

Consider other popular historic and wholesome foods. Bread, cheese, beer, and wine are all processed to at least some degree. What happens in the processing? These foods depend on 'friendly' microbes and microbial action to conduct much of the processing. But it's not always a 'natural' process, as modern techniques—many of which are newer than GM—are used to maximize and optimize food production. And they commonly use 'unnatural' microbes, not always from rDNA, but modified through 'conventional' biotechnology. What are the 'long-term' effects of these microbes and processes? We don't know, because some of them haven't been in existence very long. Food processing is one of the most innovative, fastest changing industries on earth. A substantial portion of new patents relate to new food processing methods and products. Yet these new products appear on market shelves without too many questions or concerns about their safety or effect on the environment. It seems illogical to subject GMOs to intense suspicion, yet virtually ignore these other new technologies.

Ordinarily wholesome foods, such as eggs or chicken, can be inadvertently contaminated. A food fight, not related to GM this time, broke out in 1999 when trace amounts of carcinogenic dioxins were discovered in Belgian animal feed. The cost of the ensuing recall and clean up was enormous. However, the scandal was just one example of the contamination of our conventional food supply. In this case, the toxins were noticed and the results publicized, but what about all the other contamination events that are not noticed or reported? No day goes by without our consuming some unwanted component of food, because all non-processed food contains at least some bacteria and other potentially unpleasant substances.

Before this starts to sound like a testimonial for vegetarianism, let's look at the natural composition of some common plant foods. Some of the most toxic substances known to humanity comes from plants. Aflatoxins from microbes growing on nuts, oilseeds, and other food plants are one example. Aflatoxins cause high fever, jaundice, pain, vomiting, and even death. Over a hundred people died in one outbreak in 1974, before GM foods were released, from eating 'natural' maize. You might argue that these are contaminants, not a natural component of the plant. OK, let's consider only 'natural' components. Plants, even food plants, have evolved a wide range of mechanisms to deter browsing microbes, insects, worms, and other animals. Many of these strategies involve toxins. **Cyanogenic glycosides**, substances that generate cyanide under certain conditions, are naturally produced in many food plants, from apples and apricots to beans and cassava. Soya beans, potatoes, and other common foods produce toxic **lectins** (naturally-occurring pesticides). Other nasty but naturally occurring chemicals include **alkaloids**, tomatine in tomato and solanine in potato. Plant breeding has reduced the amounts of these chemicals in the edible parts of the plants, but this is not always 100% effective. Sometimes we see potatoes improperly covered by earth; parts of the tuber exposed to sunlight turn green, an indicator of solanine. Don't eat them, even if they come from an organic producer. These are a few examples of many, many natural chemicals in our foods: toxins, carcinogens, teratogens and other distasteful categorizations. Perhaps we might use GM technology to remove these anti-nutritional substances from our foods.

What about the simplest and most widely consumed and basic item, water? Not content to simply drink water from the domestic or city water supply (who knows what 'they' might have contaminated it with—perhaps even fluoride!), many people buy bottled water. An analysis by the Natural Resources Defense Council (one of the more credible and responsible activist organizations) showed most bottled water in the USA to be no different from ordinary tap water. In fact, some brands of bottled water, even those proclaiming to be from pristine springs or glacial lakes, came out of a domestic supply pipe. In almost a quarter of the brands tested, contaminants, including arsenic and bacteria, exceeded statutory limits.

No food, even pure water, is 'pure' in the scientific sense. All foods carry additional substances, either naturally or as contaminants. In practice, when you buy a food item described as 'pure', it means the contaminants are present within a certain limit of tolerance, and the presence of the contaminants will not cause harm to most consumers. The lesson for us is to consider GM foods in the context of conventional foods. If we assume ordinary foods are pure and devoid of contaminants, then any argument we build on that premise will be faulty. When a scary story claims a GM food carries some amount of bacteria, toxin, or other unpleasant component, compare that with the undesirable composition of the non-GM version.

Dietary exposure

Conventional food safety evaluations make much of not only the presence of various substances—natural or contaminant—in the food, but also the amounts of these substances actually consumed. This concept is called **dietary exposure.**

Traditionally, dietary exposure to poisons was based on their being 'present' or 'not present'; if a pool of water contained arsenic, for example, it was signposted 'Arsenic' or 'Poison—do not drink'. Humans, at least literate ones, did not consume the water and did not allow their animals near it either. Otherwise, ponds and lakes were considered 'safe', the implication being that there was no arsenic (or other poison) present in the water. Nowadays, arsenic (along with other things) can be detected in virtually all sources of water. Has some process, natural or otherwise, poisoned our wells? A more likely explanation is that technology has developed more sensitive assays for all substances. A sample of water measured today might contain 10 micrograms of arsenic per litre (a microgram is 0.000 001 of a gram). If we measured the same sample using the technology of 100 years ago, we would not detect arsenic at all; it would register 'no arsenic'. 'Safe' is not an absolute. There is no 'zero risk', there is rarely 'zero content', unless you consider our ability to measure simply hasn't advanced to the point to measure that substance to the next degree of magnitude. We drink arsenic every day. Despite this, few people die of arsenic poisoning from drinking water.

Similarly, cigarettes have been shown to contain many nasty poisons, including cyanide. But few smokers die of cyanide poisoning. In addition to cyanide, cigarettes contain a broad array of over three dozen chemicals, from acrylonitrile to styrene. This does not include residues of the 130-plus registered pesticides used to treat tobacco growing as a crop, including endosulfan, a killer of insects and, at high doses, humans. The Government of British Columbia, along with the Canadian Council for Tobacco Control, posted the actual constituents of cigarette tobacco on their web site. If you're a smoker and want to quit, or if you're a non-smoker and are thinking of starting, get on the internet and take a look (*http://www.cctc.ca/bcreports/*).

Some people consider smoking a voluntary, chronic form of suicide. What's the difference between suicide by ingesting a large dose of cyanide for immediate effect, or ingesting smaller doses over a longer period for a lingering death? I don't place much credibility in someone telling me he doesn't want to see GMOs on the market until we can be certain there's no long term ill-health effect, meanwhile smoking a cigarette, apparently oblivious to the contradiction.

Most foods contain anti-nutritional components, ranging from natural poisons (such as cyanide in lima beans or apricots) to substances that mildly interfere with nutrient uptake, such as trypsin inhibitors (more naturally-occurring pesticides) in soya beans. Also, all foods contain contaminants, ranging from simple inorganic soil particles and more complex organic soil particles to biological contaminants such as faecal matter and microbes and their products, including the most toxic substances known to humanity.

Here again we also have to consider the communication problem. When a scientist conducts an assay for a substance, and fails to find any, we say it is **below the level of detection** (BLD). This is not the same as saying 'no' or 'zero', because different assays might show some level of the substance. We cannot say there is no substance present, because we cannot prove a negative. Perhaps next week someone will devise a more sensitive assay or testing machine and show there is some of the substance present. Similarly, scientists often use several assays to measure the same substance. Rarely do the quantitative results correlate exactly, so scientists choose which assay to use based on any of a number of factors. Some work better with different sample types, for example, if the sample is fresh and moist, or older and dried. Often the choice is made by practicalities: the equipment is available and there are people who know how to use it. The alternative assay might require different expertise or equipment, or more expensive materials.

So the issue is no longer a simple dichotomy ('safe' vs. 'not safe'); it is a question of 'how much'. How much arsenic is 'safe'? Unfortunately, quantitative answers are, obviously, more complicated than the simple dichotomous, qualitative, 'safe' vs. 'not safe'. How much arsenic is 'safe' depends on your definition of 'safe'. In absolute terms, if 'safe' means zero risk, then only zero amount of arsenic will satisfy you that you won't die from arsenic poisoning. However, setting a lifestyle and diet to ensure zero ingestion of arsenic would necessarily lead to other problems. The obvious one is imminent death from other causes, such as suffocation (arsenic particles are in almost every breath you take), starvation (arsenic can be detected in virtually every foodstuff; we eat about 25–50 micrograms per day), or dehydration (as noted, arsenic is a natural component of 'pure' water). These problems will present a more pressing and legitimate cause of anxiety than chronic intake of tiny amounts of arsenic.

For those of us wanting to continue living for more than a few days, what is 'safe'? Unfortunately, and as usual, it depends (life is so much more complicated that it used to be) on several factors.

- The chemical form of the toxin, for example, is it pure or is it compounded with other things?
- What are the 'other things'?
- Is it ingested, inhaled, or topically applied?
- Is it taken all at once, or spread over a long time?
- Are you more or less sensitive to this substance than other people?
- How does the toxin work? Does it kill you outright, or make you prone to cancer? Or does it cause a non-lethal but debilitating condition?
- Does a sub-lethal amount cause no or only short term effects?
- Is there a treatment to overcome this poison?

- Is there a weight effect, that is, can a large person sustain more than a light person?
- Is there an age effect? Can an adult take more than a child, even accounting for differences in body mass?

After considering all these complications, perhaps it's easier to return to the simple definition of 'safe', and not worry about the minuscule amount of arsenic or cyanide or whatever in our water and foodstuffs. Just because we can measure cyanide in parts per billion or per trillion, should we, even without the need to evaluate the results?

Food and water are not the only sources of toxic substances. How about mercury? Mercury is also highly toxic, causing kidney and brain damage. How much mercury do you have in your mouth? It depends on how many fillings you have, as mercury is a common component of dental fillings. Mercury is also found in many food products, as well as (of course) in cigarettes. The risk level for mercury starts at 0.3 micrograms per kilogram of body weight each day.

Measuring toxicity

According to toxicologists, everything is potentially toxic. When it becomes poisonous is simply a matter of dosage. Toxicologists use measurements to determine relative toxicity of compounds, as not every chemical is equally hazardous. Some are so toxic only a tiny amount is enough to kill; other chemicals are less hazardous. Pesticides are an example. Some are nasty chemicals designed to kill agricultural pests but don't readily discriminate; humans are also susceptible. Other chemical pesticides, such as the toxin from the bacterium *Bacillus thuringiensis* (usually just called *B.t.*), are very specific in the species they affect and thus have low toxicity to humans or other animals.

Toxicity is not the only component of hazard or risk. Substances can be hazardous without being toxic. The chemical implicated in more human deaths than all other chemicals combined has a very low toxicity: it's H_2O (better known as water).

Toxicologists developed the LD_{50} to indicate degree of hazard of a particular substance (see Box). The LD_{50} of arsenic in rats is about 60.5 milligrams per kilogram of body weight. The LD_{50} of another common food contaminant, aflatoxin, is 0.5–10 milligrams per kilogram of body weight. At lower doses it causes cancer and other unpleasant conditions. As you can see, the naturally occurring aflatoxin (produced from food fungi) is even more hazardous than the naturally occurring food component, arsenic.

According to the US Food and Drug Administration (FDA), the 'action level' for aflatoxin is substantially less than arsenic, at 20 parts per billion. That is, if 20 or more parts per billion of aflatoxin is found in a particular food lot (except milk, where the action level is 0.5 parts per billion), then remedial action must be taken. This could mean dumping the whole shipload, or treatment, for exam-

---

What is LD$_{50}$?

The LD$_{50}$ is simply the amount of the poison required to kill (lethal dose) half (50%) of the subjects in a test. Scientists interested in toxicity often refer to the LD$_{50}$ as a measure of just how poisonous something is. Each person (or other animal) will tolerate a different amount of a poison before succumbing, based on their weight, or age, or other physiological or genetic make-up.

To overcome this variation across individuals, they devised a measure of the effect of a given dose on a group or population. One difficulty in using LD$_{50}$, despite it sounding like such a simple and precise figure, is that biological organisms are highly variable. There might be substantial difference according to method of ingestion (inhaling vs. eating, for example), or whether the exposure to the poison is acute, all at once, or chronic, over a period of time. Also, the LD$_{50}$ is calculated according to each compound, as toxins are rarely pure. The LD$_{50}$ of mercury, for example, varies by what it's compounded with: when ingested by a population of rats, the LD$_{50}$ for mercury(II) oxide is 18 milligrams per kilogram of body weight; for mercury(II) sulfate it is 57 milligrams per kilogram.

---

ple, by heat inactivation or irradiation; but usually it means blending with other, less contaminated loads to dilute the levels to below the action threshold. Although aflatoxin is far more toxic than arsenic, it hasn't caught on in the public imagination. 'Aflatoxin and old lace' just doesn't have the same ring to it.

Tolerances and allowances

In recognizing all foods carry substances we'd rather not eat but are not harmful in small amounts (in fact, some are positively required in small amounts), regulators set limits on acceptable quantities in our foods. These limits, known as **tolerances** and **allowances**, are calculated according to the nature of the extraneous material, how toxic or dangerous it is, and how easy it is to manage, both politically and functionally.

In the USA, a major grain-exporting nation, US Sample grade of mixed grain can contain, according to the USDA handbook, up to

. . .8 or more stones that have an aggregate weight in excess of 0.2 percent of the sample weight; 2 or more pieces of glass; 3 or more Crotalaria (*Crotalaria* spp.); 2 or more castor beans (*Ricinus communis* L.); 8 or more cockleburs (*Xanthium* spp.) or similar seeds singly or in combination; 4 or more pieces of an unknown foreign substance(s) or a recognized harmful or toxic substance(s); 10 or more rodent pellets, bird droppings, or an equivalent quantity of other animal filth per 1,000 grams of mixed grain. . .'

This means roughly 0.2% of the weight of the grain, or 2 grams of extraneous matter per kilogram, can be accepted for human consumption. Notice also that the extraneous material might include 'recognized harmful or toxic substances', along with faecal matter.

In Canada, another grain-exporting nation, the Canadian Grain Commission (CGC) is responsible for inspecting shipments to ensure the grain doesn't exceed tolerances and allowance limits. Unfortunately, the CGC doesn't publicly publish the tolerances because they don't want to alert international customers to the fact that they're eating Canadian rat shit. However, in private conversations with a CGC inspector, I learned the tolerance is about the same as in the US (0.2%). The inspector emphasized that the CGC is very concerned about foreign matter in grain shipments and they take every effort to ensure a shipment is as clean as possible, even to the point of requiring apparently dirty loads to be stopped and cleaned. Nevertheless, you can be assured you get a daily intake of rat shit and insect parts with every mouthful. Furthermore, the screenings (i.e. all the bits and pieces removed during the cleaning process) end up being fed to animals, so any impurities are recycled that way.

Consumers in the UK also get their share of inadvertent nutrients. Ministry of Agriculture, Fisheries and Food (MAFF) scientists at the Central Science Lab in York analysed cereal-based foods and found 21% of 567 samples contained mites, up to 20 000 of these tiny organisms per kilogram in one sample. In all likelihood, every time you open your mouth, you're allowing entry to all manner of undesirable organisms and substances. In the vast majority of cases, we experience no harm from these supplementary nutrients. I've learned to accept it and not think too much about it.

Are we eating GM DNA?

We have all ingested products of recombinant DNA, either intentionally, through such approved and labelled products as GM tomato paste, or unintentionally. The inadvertent consumption is not always malicious adulteration by the companies blending GM with non-GM foodstuffs, then refusing to admit their activities. More often it is through ordinary mistakes, where a small amount of GM gets mixed with non-GM. Such admixtures are typical in the food handling business. Various reports of analyses of foodstuffs show a small amount of such GM admixtures appearing even in 'organic' products. Since it is impracticable to guarantee that a food product has zero GM composition, the EU is considering a tolerance of 1% for GM material in foods. That is, a food containing less than 1% GM may be considered 'GM-free'. Other values being suggested range from 5% (the standard tolerance for organic systems) to the unworkable absolute of zero.

Another inadvertent mechanism by which you might have consumed GM product relates to the recent fashion for embellishing salads with flower petals to add some colour. In 1997, the EU approved the first GM plant for European-wide commercialization, a modified carnation from Florigene. This product was developed as an ornamental flower, so was not scrutinized for food use. However, consumers might unwittingly decide to liven up a salad with the lovely blue petals, thus inadvertently consuming rDNA.

Consumers in North America have been eating GM DNA and proteins for years, most often without knowing about it because labelling laws require a label only when the modified product is substantially altered from the base product. Europeans, similarly, are exposed to some GM ingredients from approved products, notably maize and soy. These are the main sources cited when we are presented with the statistic that over 60% of processed foods contain GM ingredients.

Calculating the amount of rDNA in a given GM food is complicated by a number of factors. One is the amount of actual consumption of the GM food product, often hidden behind a façade of 'confidential business information'. The companies are often reluctant to release actual sales figures for their product lines, especially GMOs, to the competition.

Another complicating factor is the presentation of GMO material in foods. We have to be sure what we're measuring. A whole fresh soya bean is one thing, complete with intact DNA. Soya paste from GM soya beans is another, as the DNA has been degraded during processing and the remnants are virtually indistinguishable from native DNA. Soya oil from GM soya beans is a third category, as it ordinarily contains no measurable DNA whatever, native or GM.

Then we get into blends involving GM products, say GM soya beans and non-GM soya beans, and blends of several different ingredients in many processed foods, some of which may be GM or may not be. Even more removed is meat from animals fed GM grain.

Finally, how do we account for the dietary intake of rDNA, when the novel gene is a normal and natural component of another common food? Suppose, for example, a tomato gene is inserted into a soya bean. In a given day, you might well eat foods containing both soya and tomato. If we conduct an analysis and detect a tomato gene, how do we know whether it came from a GM soya product, or simply from an ordinary tomato? How do we accurately calculate how much rDNA is likely to be consumed by an ordinary human in the course of the day? We can't.

What we can do is take each GMO and estimate rDNA dietary exposure from human consumption patterns (see Box for calculations). We can work out that the GM increased the amount of DNA in linseed by about 0.000 000 7%. Overall, it is a minuscule amount, probably measurable only hypothetically or indirectly, as in our estimated calculations. In any case, the body doesn't know the difference between ordinary DNA and rDNA. It doesn't care if you've consumed a GM soya bean with an inserted tomato gene or an ordinary tomato along with an ordinary soya product. Furthermore, regulatory agencies do not consider DNA in food to be a health hazard. What might pose a health hazard is the associated novel protein.

Calculating dietary exposure

Let's take our GM linseed CDC Triffid as an example. Triffid is a niche market variety, expected to account for no more than about 10–15% of the total linseed acreage in Canada. Let's assume it becomes very popular and captures 25% of the total acreage.

Most linseed is sold for crushing as an industrial product, going into the manufacture of paints, varnishes, inks, and so on. However, a small portion of the seed ends up being consumed by humans. Whole linseed is used in humans as a natural and, when consumed in moderate quantities, gentle laxative. Consumption estimates vary up to the 10% mark; let's be very generous, and suggest 25% of the linseed destined for industrial crushing ends up consumed without standard processing or cooking (which itself denatures the DNA and proteins). That is, let's assume that 25% of the industrial linseed shipped from Canada to crushing plants in the UK is diverted before processing and fed directly to humans as fresh seed, not baked or otherwise cooked.

One component for which we do have reasonable figures is the amount of linseed exported in a given year. About 70 000 metric tonnes goes from Canada to the UK in a typical year. So, roughly

70 000 000 kilos × 0.25 (percentage GM linseed) × 0.25 (percentage consumed fresh)
= 4 375 000 kilos

of GM linseed might be expected to be consumed in the UK in one year. If the population of the UK is approximately 60 million, then the average consumption of linseed there is

4 375 000/60 000 000 people = 0.073 kilograms or 73 grams per person per year;
73 grams/365 (days in a year)
= 0.02 grams per day.

Now, we need to figure how much of that 0.2 grams per day is DNA. This is a difficult measurement because of the tiny amount of DNA in a linseed. The DNA in one linseed cell weighs about half a picogram, or about 0.000 000 000 5 grams.

Then we have to figure how much of the total DNA is rDNA. Linseed carries about 300 000 000 DNA bases in the normal genome. The genetic modification added about 20 000 DNA bases. This means the GM increased the amount of DNA in linseed by about 0.000 000 7%.

Are GM foods a good source of (novel) protein?

A more meaningful calculation might be the dietary exposure to a novel protein generated by the rDNA. Again, see the Box for the detailed calculations. Using the same assumptions as before, the dietary exposure works out to 9.4 micrograms of novel protein per person per year. To put this in perspective, the amount of arsenic that most people ordinarily ingest in food or water—around 50 micrograms per day, or about 18.25 milligrams per year, is not considered to be of health concern. The expected average dietary exposure to this novel protein from the GM linseed is, therefore, about 200 times *less* than the average dietary exposure to the 'safe' and general accepted level of exposure to arsenic.

Dietary exposure to (novel) proteins

The GM linseed is 32.3% protein, so multiplying the total weight of consumed GM linseed by the proportion protein gives

4 375 000 kilograms × 0.323 = 1 413 125 kilograms

of total protein from the GM linseed consumed in the UK in one year.

The GM linseed contains three eukaryotic genes, but only two are expressed in the seed. Of these two, one, *als*, is ubiquitous among plants and its protein product, ALS, cannot be distinguished from the endogenous linseed ALS. This leaves only one true and detectable novel protein in the seed, NPT-II. What is the dietary exposure to NPT-II protein from human consumption of the GM linseed? NPT-II protein accounts for 432 nanograms per gram (or 0.432 milligrams per kilogram) of total protein. Put another way, about 0.00004% of total protein is the novel product, NPT-II.

When we multiply by the total amount of protein consumed, we have

0.432 milligrams × 1 413 125 kilograms = 565 250 mg, or 565 g

of NPT-II protein consumed in the UK in one year from consumption of this GM linseed. Spread over 60 000 000 people, this makes the dietary exposure 0.000 009 4 grams (9.4 micrograms) of novel protein per person per year.

As noted earlier, many foods naturally contain anti-nutritional substances in small quantities. The amounts of these substances are monitored during the normal course of development of new strains. Lines showing higher than usual concentrations of anti-nutritional compounds are eliminated early in the breeding process. Many foods, including soya bean and linseed, naturally produce cyanogenic glycosides in small amounts. These substances can, in certain conditions, generate the nasty toxin cyanide. The cyanide (HCN) content of fresh ground flaxseed is about 8 micrograms per 100 grams, produced from enzymatic reactions with the various cyanogenic glycosides present in greater, but highly variable, quantities in all linseed varieties. Triffid was monitored and the amount of this anti-nutritional substance was about the same as ordinary linseed; the GM linseed is no different from other cultivars in cyanogenic glycoside content. Is cyanide content something we should be concerned about? Let's check the calculations (see Box). I don't like the idea of consuming any amount of cyanide, but, for the sake of argument, how does 5.8 micrograms of cyanide from GM linseed compare with other sources of cyanide?

•   The US Environmental Protection Agency (EPA) (see Ch. 16, 266) has set a maximum contaminant level of cyanide in drinking water of 0.2 milligrams of cyanide per litre of water (200 micrograms per litre).
•   One cigarette contains 138 micrograms of cyanide.

In order to ingest the same amount of cyanide from linseed as from one cigarette, you would have to consume 1.725 kilograms of seed in one sitting. Considering the laxative properties of linseed, this would be a very long sitting indeed.

Cyanide content of seeds

Under the scenario above, 4 375 000 kilograms of whole flaxseed are consumed in the UK in one year, or about 73 grams per person. In 73 grams of flaxseed are 5.8 micrograms of cyanide. The average person in the UK would then consume about 5.8 micrograms of cyanide from the GM linseed over the course of one year.

Arsenic, cyanide, and NPT-II protein are all naturally occurring substances we consume in small quantities every day, but we probably don't want to know and certainly don't want to be reminded that we're consuming them. When Edwina Currie, then Tory health minister in the UK, informed people *Salmonella* bacteria was present in chicken and eggs, the common interpretation was that the *Salmonella* problem was new. It wasn't. *Salmonella* has been in our foods for ages, and will probably continue with us, along with arsenic, cyanide, aflatoxin, and a multitude of other 'natural' toxins. The mere presence of a potentially hazardous substance ought not be a cause for undue concern. A high concentration ought to be, regardless of whether the presenting foodstuff is GM or conventional.

Have you ever discovered an old jar of jam at the back of the fridge and carefully spooned out the furry stuff on the surface before consuming the remainder of the jam? Many people do this, unaware that moulds secrete chemicals into their surroundings well beyond the borders of their mycelia (the visible growth on the surface). If the mould is a toxic one, the toxin could well have infiltrated throughout the jam. Consumers eat far greater quantities of contaminants from such inadvertent but nevertheless voluntary actions than from food they buy in the shops. If we are sincerely concerned about the amount of potentially hazardous substances we consume with GM foods, or even with conventional foods, why are we still spooning the moulds from jam, or carefully cutting the furry ends off cheese, or the soft spot from the peaches? Can we claim credibility for our concern over 'contaminant' rDNA and novel protein in GM foods when we continue to voluntarily consume far greater quantities of known health hazards?

What about all these pesticides in our foods? Won't GMOs increase chemical residues in our foods?

The chemical pesticide industry has a code of ethics. Unlike most such codes of ethics, established with the best of intentions, this code may actually work against consumers. The code prohibits members of the industry discussing relative safety of chemical products, as in 'Our chemical is safer than our competitors' product!' Because of this, we tend to think that all chemicals have similar health and safety risks and, because no one in the industry talks about it, they must all be bad, and so they're all equally bad.

I'm not a member of the industry, so I can disclose without fear of breaking the code. Here it is: not all chemicals are equally nasty. In general, newer products are safer than older ones, and some on the market now are quite benign. That doesn't mean you should drink the stuff. All pesticides have labels with safety instructions, yet too many people ignore them. All chemicals, including H_2O, should be treated with respect.

Endosulfan is an agricultural chemical used in cotton crops. As Australia expands its cotton-growing area, more endosulfan is sprayed to control insects. A problem arises because the endosulfan sprayed in the cotton-growing environment gets into cattle sharing the neighbourhood. When the meat from the exposed cattle is exported to Japan, the authorities there analyse the meat, find residues of endosulfan and reject the shipment.

Endosulfan residues affect Australians the same way they do Japanese. If there is any human health hazard, Australians will suffer. Australian authorities have an excellent record of food safety regulation and are unlikely to allow human consumption of a potentially hazardous food product. However, the Japanese authorities have a notorious reputation internationally for using any means available to negotiate a better price. Is the detectable presence of endosulfan in beef a real health and safety issue or is it political mischief? In either case, Australian meat rejected by Japanese officials is often simply re-routed to domestic Australian markets.

It seems contradictory that people are consuming endosulfan, *B.t.*, and other pesticides from conventional and organic farming systems, yet seem reluctant to approve products designed to reduce the use of such pesticides. GM *B.t.* cotton would be one such product. The GM cotton is insect-resistant, so it doesn't need endosulfan treatment. Using such a GM variety, cattle and cotton could share agricultural environments without jeopardizing international markets, and consumers would be exposed to less pesticide residue in their food.

The Prince of Wales and others fear that pesticide-resistant GM crops will lead to an increase in pesticide usage and therefore to an increase in pesticide residue on foods. Many of the first GM products are indeed designed for pesticide application, so it seems a reasonable line of thought. However, early US federal Department of Agriculture (USDA) studies note decreases in pesticide usage in seven of twelve regions growing pesticide-resistant GM crops in 1997 (the remaining five were unchanged). More recently, US soya bean farmers have reported a decrease in pesticide usage of between 10% and 30% on GM crops, which make up 55% of the soya crop in 1999. If these GM crops are designed for pesticide application, why is there no change or even a decrease in pesticide usage?

The companies say the GM crops are intended not to increase pesticide use but to shift market share from one brand to another. Monsanto's Roundup-Ready™ crops, for example, are designed to get farmers to use Monsanto's glyphosate-based herbicide Roundup™ to control weeds in the crop instead of a collection of herbicides from other manufacturers. Monsanto thus attracts customers away from their competitors and, of greater interest to us, they allow use of a single product (in our example, Roundup™) instead of using up to several different herbicides to control the range of weed species present in the crop, as is the usual practice.

Another advantage to us is that modern pesticides, the ones for which resistance genes are being developed, are generally safer, used in lower doses, and more environmentally benign than older pesticides. No matter how careful we are, we will always encounter at least some pesticide residue on foods. My preference is to go with the newer pesticides.

When is a bacon sandwich not a bacon sandwich?

Society not only tolerates but respects religious and ethical food prohibitions, ranging from different forms of vegetarianism to restrictions on specific foods. GM food producers must grapple with legitimate concern from these various consumers. But first the dietary observer must determine exactly what is proscribed.

Consider, for example, the Jewish and Muslim prohibition of pork. What is the status of a GM vegetable containing a gene isolated from a pig? If someone is restricted from eating pork, what do we do about a veggie burger containing soya beans with a pig gene? I called a local rabbi and asked him this question. He emphasized that each Jew must confer with his or her own rabbi on this question. He explained the Jewish prohibition against pork was based on the 'essence' of the beast, manifest certainly in the flesh but potentially in other aspects as well. As far as he was concerned, though, a gene isolated from a pig no longer carried the 'essence' of the pig, and was therefore exempt from the prohibition. From other discussions, I learned that no Jewish leader has condemned the presence of a pig gene in otherwise acceptable food. I advise Jews to consult with their rabbi before consuming veggie burgers carrying pig genes. No need to panic, no such products exist yet. Even here, though, GM does not present a totally new problem. Jews (and others with a pork prohibition) grappled with the same fundamental problem years ago, when insulin from pigs was first developed for treatment of diabetics. Porcine insulin presents no problem for Jewish diabetics.

Many vegetarians lack the counsel of a spiritual and cultural leader and so must decide for themselves what constitutes an acceptable vegetarian diet. No doubt, some vegetarians will decide that a single pig gene in a soya burger is sufficient to prohibit consumption. Others—perhaps even vegans—will decide, like the rabbi, that the single pig gene lacks the 'essence' of the animal and so the burger is therefore suitable for consumption.

Even here, though, drawing a line is difficult. Consider what happens if scientists wanted to improve the nutrient balance in legumes. We might use a gene from a Brazil nut, producing a protein rich in cysteine and methionine, amino acids which are deficient in soya bean and other legumes. We have to reject this gene, though, because the resulting protein is allergenic. As an alternative, we find a more suitable, non-allergenic protein from a tomato gene, although this gene provides a protein not quite as rich in the two amino acids. So then we modify the DNA to provide a protein enriched in the two amino acids. Our soya bean with the modified tomato gene would seem perfect for vegetarian consumption, having better nutritional balance, not being allergenic, and lacking animal genes or products. It would seem acceptable to vegetarians. We later discover the modified tomato protein is identical to a pig protein. Is it still suitable for vegetarian consumers? If not, at what point does it or did it become prohibited?

Let's throw in another question. We just discussed a genetically modified tomato gene. Now assume we find a natural unmodified tomato gene is identical to a pig gene. If ordinary tomatoes (and, in all likelihood, other fruits and vegetables) are suddenly blacklisted because they share a gene with a pig, what do people then eat? If ordinary fruits and vegetables sharing pig genes are not prohibited, there'd be no scientific basis to prohibit GM plants carrying a gene similar or identical to those in pigs.

Molecular genetics research incites far more ethical debate than do simple GM foods. For example, do plants contain genes homologous to animal genes? Yes. We've known about DNA and microbes for years, but homology between human genes and plant genes is a concept new to the general public. We're not surprised that wheat and barley share many genes, but—remember from Chapter 2—even humans share some 7000 genes with the *C. elegans* worms.

Many life processes, from the metabolism of common nutrients to the efficient use of energy to the synthesis and maintenance of DNA, are common across species. It is not surprising, then, that many of the genes controlling these functions are likewise similar. This homology among common genes raises interesting ethical questions, suitable for dinner table discussions. For example, we've already considered the ethical issue of a pig gene in a veggie burger. Assuming we reject the pig–veggie burger, how do we consider consuming a watercress sprout carrying genes homologous to those in pigs? Logic would dictate we eliminate all foods carrying pig genes, or those substantially similar to pig genes. However, such prohibition is unlikely to be supported by adherents because it is not life-sustainable. If we decide to accept the cress despite the presence of the pig-like genetic material, can we return to the rejected pig gene–veggie burger, modify the inserted porcine gene to make it less similar to the pig and more similar to, say, wheat? What if we just use the homologous gene from the wheat in the first place? It's still homologous to the gene found in pigs. In this respect, vegetarians, Jews, Muslims and others, consume, perhaps unwittingly, genes homologous to those in pigs, beef, and other animals every day.

Last bites

Everyone is concerned about food safety and security. A fundamental problem in the public debate over GMOs as food is the frequency with which issues are discussed out of context and without proper perspective. Consider the cases of food scares in recent years, some of which were listed at the opening of this chapter. Is food production becoming more sloppy, leading to the apparent increase in cases of food adulteration and contamination? Alternatively, perhaps technology has advanced to the point where such incidents are only now being detected? All foods, whether from GM, conventional, or organic farming systems, carry contaminants and other undesirable components. Regulatory agencies and consumers need to evaluate the nature of the substances and the degree of hazard presented in relation to currently accepted products. Surely, if a food product presents a health hazard, it ought to be regulated regardless of the method by which it was produced.

'The good old days'

One of the commonly stated arguments against GM technology, indeed all modern technology, is that life is getting too complicated. Perhaps you want to return to life as it was 100 years ago or more, because you think living was so much happier and fulfilling, food was fresher and healthier?

Let's take a moment to cast our memories back to those idyllic days. Certainly, there was no GM food production, and no one worried about cholesterol or food-borne carcinogens. Of course, most people didn't live long enough to get heart disease or cancer; those who managed to avoid infant mortality or war-related deaths at a young age usually succumbed to typhus, cholera, diphtheria, galloping consumption, influenza, or any of a multitude of other traditional diseases first. Then there were the occupational hazards; military service took its toll of course, but also coal miner's disease (black lung or pneumoconiosis), wool sorter's disease (anthrax), and the various venereal diseases were disabling, if not lethal. If anyone did contract heart disease or cancer, it was all too often undiagnosed and in any case, untreated. Non-lethal afflictions might have been treated with impure but highly toxic mercury salts or, if you were lucky, leeches, in many cases mercifully converting the lesser condition to a terminal one. Of course, anyone born with a congenital condition such as cystic fibrosis or muscular dystrophy didn't have a chance to begin with, and anyone developing diabetes was doomed. Then, as now, food production was said to be adequate to feed the population, but politics seemed to get in the way. It wasn't a problem with production, they said, but distribution. There was no mass transport system and only rudimentary means of food preservation. The range of diet was extremely limited, even when there was enough food to go round. Nutritional deficiencies abounded—rickets, scurvy, and ordinary malnourishment. Famines were a regular event, with mass food riots a standard feature of seventeenth- and eighteenth-century British life. But it wasn't all bad. Families were closer in the old days because there was little travel or migration, although most people never knew their grandparents or grandchildren. And regular ergot infections in cereal crops allowed people to get naturally stoned on Nature's LSD.

Life expectancy didn't start to rise until the late nineteenth century; infant mortality didn't decline until the early twentieth. I'm not suggesting that life isn't more complicated now, and I certainly agree that some aspects of life from an earlier age are preferable. No doubt there are beneficial aspects of simpler lifestyles we ought to revisit. My point is that we sometimes have an unrealistic and excessively romantic perspective of history. In our nostalgia we tend to concentrate on the perceived positive conditions and minimize the brutal realities. But technology has not introduced all of the evils of modern society, and genetic technology is not the original and exclusive source of threats to our food supply. As we evaluate the health risks associated with GMOs, let's ensure we're taking a proper perspective.

CHAPTER 6

The issues—where's the beef?

- Are you concerned with the process of GM or with GM products?
- Why is the public attitude toward GM in America so different from that in the UK?
- What are the contentious issues?
- Didn't GM L-tryptophan kill people in the early 1980s?
- A respected scientist showed GM potatoes were toxic, didn't he?
- Can't GM foods cause new allergic reactions?
- Why are pesticide-resistant crops the first products?
- Are we creating superweeds?
- What are artificial hybrids?

What's the problem?

The debate over genetic engineering often confuses process and product. On a recent visit to the UK, I had dinner with two friends who are both very concerned over GM foods. Knowing I was involved in GM research, they asked my opinion. I replied that I usually ask people the basis for their concern—was it the entire process of genetic engineering, or did specific GM products drive their anxiety. One of my hosts stated emphatically that it was the entire technology, that we humans had no business meddling with nature. The other disagreed, saying 'No, humans have been meddling with nature for ages, GM is simply one more example'. She was concerned, instead, that particular GM products might damage the environment. The ensuing lively discussion illustrates one common problem in the public GM debate. There is a widespread concern, but the underlying anxiety can vary considerably. Often, concerned people haven't identified the basis for their anxiety. Let's identify the differences.

Concern may be advanced on an ethical or religious basis, covering the entire process or technology. If, however, we are concerned with GM as a health or environmental hazard, we need to evaluate the results of the application of the technology. A tomato with an inverted tomato gene is a product. A bacterium containing a human insulin gene is a product. People opposed to the *process* of GM will be concerned with both of these examples, while those anxious about hazards of specific GM *products* might happily accept both.

Cutting the cheese: concern with the safety of GM technology

It's difficult to evaluate the safety or risks associated with a process or method without looking at the resulting products as a collection.

The complications arise because evaluation of a technology is usually based on an analysis of the products of using the technology. Scrutinizing the health and safety of a technique is like trying to determine the risks associated with a body of information. If the technology itself introduces hazards to the resulting product, then every product of that technology is a potential time bomb. For instance, every building constructed on a poorly engineered foundation will be unstable, regardless of the structure erected on top. This doesn't necessarily mean each and every GMO is equally suspect, but it does suggest inherent problems will arise across a wide range of GM species and traits.

On the basis of public opinion surveys and popular press articles, it seems that many people in Europe are concerned about genetic technology in general. In North America, anxiety over GMOs, when it arises, is largely concentrated on specific GM products, less on the technology itself.

Why does there seem to be so much more public resistance to GM technology in Europe than in North America?

During my recent visit to the UK (I hadn't been back for several years) I was anxious to see how the European influence had changed the lifestyle. While *en route* I thought about a point a colleague had made to me during a discussion of why people in Europe, including the British, were more apt to disapprove of GM in general. The point made was that now in the EU people are more concerned with health than in past years; they enjoy a higher standard of living, are more aware of health issues, and are seeking healthier lifestyles than in North America. Superficial perhaps, but it seemed to make sense. I wanted to see for myself. On arrival at Heathrow, I immediately noticed the large proportion of people smoking. It struck me as unusual, because so few people smoke any more in Canada, whether because of the rising costs of tobacco products or the health issue, I don't know. But the difference was remarkable. So much for the concern over the healthy lifestyle in the UK.

I made my way to the courtesy coach/bus/taxi tunnel behind the terminal to await transport to my hotel. This cast concrete rectangular tunnel, several hundred metres long, offered three lanes for vehicular traffic, but only a narrow pavement for people waiting for their conveyance. The diesel fumes were not as strong as they used to be, but in that confined space were still far stronger than I wanted to endure. I wondered about the impact of those fumes on my health. Unfortunately, the only pedestrian exit from the tunnel was the main concourse; taking refuge in there meant possibly missing the irregular and unscheduled bus. About a dozen other people, spread along the pavement, waited patiently and without apparent discomfort. Perhaps they're used to it. Or perhaps they're oblivious to the hazard.

Education vs. ignorance?

Scientists often assume the more the public knows the facts about genetic technology, the more comfortable they are with it. To a casual observer this certainly seems to be the case, in that most people familiar with the technologies are at least moderate supporters. When I started dealing with government regulators in the mid-1980s, most, having no formal training in molecular genetics, were either openly hostile or guardedly suspicious of the technology. Now, with regulators having had such training, most, at least on a personal level, support the orderly and properly regulated introduction of GMOs into the marketplace. Some regulators remain openly hostile. On the other hand, the majority of rabid anti-technology activists appear to have little scientific knowledge of genetics, whereas the scientifically trained activists tend to be more focused in their opposition, concentrating on explicit concerns with specific GM products.

This comfortable and widely held assumption was blown to bits in 1998, when Dr Julian Kinderlerer from Sheffield University reported on a survey of people's attitudes toward GM foods in the UK. When people were asked about GM in general, many were negative. But they also admitted they didn't know much about it. They were given a condensed training course on GM technology, then re-took the survey. Everyone, including the organizers, expected the increased knowledge of genetic technologies would result in an increase in positive responses. It didn't. The number of negative responses increased. It appeared the more a person knew of the technology, the more likely they were to reject it. This is anathema to scientists, who always held that the problem in the UK was ignorance of the technology. It also tells something of the innate arrogance of many scientists.

I doubt the basic problem is that people in the UK are opposed to the underlying technology in general. Witness, for example, the wide acceptance of the same technology when used for pharmaceutical production, such as GM insulin for diabetics or GM dornase alfa (Pulmozyme) for cystic fibrosis patients. If there was a fundamental opposition to the act of taking a gene from one organism and placing it another, then the opposition to these products would be similar to the opposition to GM foods.

If the differential between attitudes in the UK and North America is not one of 'educated vs. ignorant', and if people in the UK are not fundamentally opposed to the process, why such a large discrepancy? Let's consider the major issues.

The major issues in the GM food fight

Food production

Europeans already produce too much food. They already pay farmers huge subsidies for their production, so more food means even higher subsidies and higher taxes. There's no need for more food in Europe. This explanation might explain the 'shocking' result of the Sheffield survey, that after the 'education in GM' people realized this technique really could produce substantially more food!

I agree the technology will result in increased food production capability. If GM can provide say, an increase in maize seed yield of 10%, then 10% more grain might be generated. In many parts of the world, an increase in food production is desired, and such products welcomed. In other parts, perhaps including the UK and Europe as suggested above, an increase in food production is undesirable. However, the same GM product delivering a 10% yield increase need not be used for increased grain production. Instead, that GM crop cultivar enables a 10% reduction in land used for agricultural production while maintaining the same amount of grain production as earlier cultivars. That is, a 100 acre plot of farmland in the UK might be divided into a 90 acre plot—used to grow the new GM cultivar and yield the same amount of grain as previously was produced on the entire 100 acres—and a 10 acre area that could be set aside for other purposes, perhaps as wildlife refuges. In an area where food is not limited, productive land often is. Additional food production may not always be necessary, but additional land is always in demand.

Environmental effects

The European countryside is being devastated by intensive agriculture. The reduction in the number of birds, both the number and diversity of species and within species, is being attributed to these practices. GM appears to exacerbate the intensification of agricultural production, with the predicted result being a further diminution of birds, insects, and other wildlife.

In casual conversations with non-scientific friends in the UK, I hear them express great concern over the intensification of agriculture. GM technology is seen as an adjunct to agricultural intensification, hence the source of additional anxiety. The underlying problem is not GM. It is agricultural intensification. Some of the environmental groups seem to have recognized this concern, English Nature being one. If the problems associated with intense agriculture can be satisfactorily addressed, there would be a concomitant reduction in anxiety over GM crops. Unfortunately, the intensity of agriculture in the EU is such a massive problem, political and social as well as agricultural, it is unlikely to be rectified in the short term. In any case, it is not GM technology *per se* that reduces wildlife numbers; those numbers were dropping long before GM technology existed. It is, however, easy to see that GM might exacerbate agricultural intensity in the EU. Is there a way to exploit GM technology to attenuate instead of accelerate the problems of agricultural intensity? One way, noted above, was to allow GM crops to take some portion of current cropland out of production and set it aside as wildlife refugia.

This is a topic where GM management comes to the fore. It is not necessary to ban potentially beneficial products, GM or other, if the risks can be properly managed. One of the stated risks with a real GM product is the *Bacillus thuringiensis (B.t.)* toxin gene in various crop species. This bacterial gene makes a chemical toxic to insects, so the plants expressing this gene acquire insect resistance. The legitimate concern is that widespread use of crops containing their own *B.t.* toxin will lead more quickly to *B.t.*-resistant insect populations. Another concern is that *B.t.* might kill non-pest insects, such as lacewings and Monarch butterflies, as well as the target pest species, thus contributing to reduced biodiversity in the environment. Both of these concerns, legitimate as they may be, are management issues.

To address the first issue of rapid resistance being developed, regulations, based on expert recommendations, stipulate some proportion (usually around 20%) of the field be planted to non-*B.t.* crops to enable the target insect pests to survive without the selection pressure to develop resistance. We all recognize that insect resistance to *B.t.* will develop eventually, GM or no GM, because *B.t.* is used extensively by organic farmers. The arguments are over how long it will take, and what is the suitable size of the refugia to delay the appearance of resistant pests for as long as possible.

For the second point, concerning impact on non-target species, one management solution is to ban the *B.t.* crop cultivar from regions indicated as a potential problem. GM *B.t.* rapeseed need not be grown in the UK. This does not mean GM rapeseed oil shouldn't be consumed in the UK, only that there may be areas where *B.t.* should not be cultivated in the environment. The regulatory system should be established to allow GM *B.t.* rapeseed oil for food use (presuming it passes other legitimate regulatory requirements, of course), but not necessarily to allow GM rapeseed for cultivation. Other places in the world may be able to cultivate and provide the GM rapeseed to the UK market without damage to non-target species in its local environment. The *B.t.* issue generates considerable controversy. Much of it is unnecessary, based as it is on misinformation and misinterpretation. We'll investigate this aspect in more detail later.

Agricultural intensity in the EU is a major environmental problem. A blanket ban on GMOs will not reduce current levels of environmental destruction caused by intense agriculture in Europe. Judiciously selected, GMOs might be used to reduce the intensity of agriculture and assist in the reclamation of a healthy wild environment in Europe. North American agricultural practices are not nearly as intense as in the EU, yet GM crops are widely grown.

The American view is somewhat different. Whereas in the UK, farms and wildlife for the most part must share the same land, in North America, farms are often separate from wildlife areas. For example, Saskatchewan has half the farmland in Canada, yet only about one-third of the land is farmed—the remainder is essentially wilderness with little effect of agriculture on the natural populations.

Big multinational companies develop all the products

Many people are concerned that big corporate farms controlled by big multinational companies are supplanting the traditional family farm and way of life. Food production is becoming further and further removed from urban society. Food is too highly processed and changes hands too many times between the farm and the dinner plate. Also, the UK public has traditionally had a more socialistic view of profit-seeking business than the public in America.

Yes, the majority of GMOs have been developed and placed on the market by Monsanto, DuPont, AgrEvo, Zeneca, Pioneer, Novartis, and other large companies. The products now available were developed, for the most part, in the 1980s when the technology was still in its infancy. Few institutions had the skilled expertise as well as the investment capital to develop GMOs. Public institutions, a major source of crop and animal breeding 'in the public interest' around the globe were squeezed by budget cuts throughout the 1980s. The world-renowned Plant Breeding Institute (PBI) in Cambridge was dismantled and sold in 1987. At that time the PBI was responsible for having developed almost all the wheat varieties grown in the UK. Other public breeding establishments were also pared down or sold. Public institutions were drained of many of their best scientists by companies offering up to double salaries and other incentives. The big multinationals were, for the most part, the only remaining institutions capable of putting up the ante to play the game.

The big companies do have the majority of GM products, and the big companies will continue to derive the greatest benefits from those GM products. But they're not alone. Small companies and public institutions have always been in the game, albeit with fewer resources and a lower profile. Some of the small company and public institution GM products are described in more detail in Chapter 11. A virus-resistant GM papaya was developed for Hawaiian papaya growers facing devastation. The GM fruit came from the scientists at the University of Hawaii and Cornell University in the USA. A small company,

Florigene, developed the first GM plant approved for marketing across the European Union—a blue carnation. The GM tomato paste on sale in UK supermarkets was initially developed at the University of Nottingham. And, of course, CDC Triffid linseed.

Contempt for the regulatory process

Many people in Europe describe their regulatory agencies as, to be charitable, incompetent, or, more candidly, corrupt. In any case, the agencies are seen as incapable of properly assessing and approving new products, especially complex ones that might carry some environmental health or safety risk. Scientific advisers and committees are often political patronage appointments, as witnessed by the scandal of EU corruption. In the UK, many people blame MAFF for the BSE fiasco and now simply don't believe assurances provided by the Ministry. In North America, people are more confident in their regulators and are more generally prepared to defer to the regulatory process to evaluate the risks of new products.

European bureaucracy is indeed huge and apparently unapproachable. There's no question of the examples of incompetence and corruption in the EU system. But North American bureaucracy cannot be devoid of incompetence or corruption. Perhaps it simply isn't as evident. Perhaps part of the problem is that the bureaucracy in the EU is so dominated by political issues. Whatever the reason, regulators in North America enjoy the luxury of public confidence to a degree beyond the realm of comprehension by their European counterparts.

Eugenics

Fear of genetic meddling to create a 'master race' of humans is much closer to the hearts of Europeans than of North Americans. The attempted genetic manipulation, albeit at a social rather than technical molecular level, to create a master race, was closer to reality in Europe than elsewhere. It's not so much that North Americans are not horrified at the thought of such social engineering, but rather that Europeans, within living memory, had to deal with the reality, whereas in other parts of the world the issue may be seen as a more distant, even hypothetical one.

Information sources

People on both sides of the ocean like to have access to the facts and credible information before deciding their position on a controversial issue. But they prefer different information sources.

People in the UK are astonished at how Americans seem indifferent to the GM controversy. Don't they know how hazardous GMOs might be? Americans, in contrast, are fascinated by the hysteria in the UK. People stake their opinions and positions on the basis of the credible information they acquire. Various public opinion surveys show that UK residents place a high degree of credibility in scientific information coming from activist groups. Not surprisingly, considering the source, the position is often one of considerable suspicion and scepticism. In North America, similar surveys consistently state the most credible sources of scientific information to be the family physician, followed closely by public scientists at universities and governments. Activist groups are well down the list. According to a recent survey by sociologist Tom Hoban at North Carolina State University, only 5% of Americans place much trust in activist group sources. Over half say they place 'none' of their trust in activist group literature. The medical community and public scientists tend to be less opposed to GM technology than activists.

Urgency of the public debate

For many Europeans, the first encounter with GM technology was being told they were already eating GMOs. It was, literally and figuratively, being 'shoved down their throats' by the companies with little or no regulation or public consultation. No wonder people are frantic. The less intense emotions displayed by the American public might be due to the more vague uneasy sense of, in the words of the American icon philosopher Yogi Berra, 'déjà vu all over again'.

If I'd been told the food I've been eating recently was treated in a new, potentially hazardous manner, I'd vigorously and emotionally demand a time-out to investigate the matter, too, as many Europeans have. Why, then, do most Americans not respond in what would appear to be a common and natural reaction? It isn't that the American public isn't aware of GM, or that they aren't shocked by potential threats to the food supply, or even that they don't care to engage in a public debate. It could simply be that they feel they had conducted the public debate some years ago and don't feel the need to replay it now.

The underlying technology of GM, rDNA or 'genetic engineering', is not as new as many Europeans believe. Early gene-splicing methods were developed by American scientists Paul Berg, Stan Cohen, and Herb Boyer, and expanded rapidly by others in the early 1970s. The applications of the technology were then mainly health and medical products, but the 'gene-splicing' technology, GM, is the same as that applied today to food. The US public did engage in a spirited and comprehensive debate from that time. The opposition was well represented by, among others, such USA media notables as Jeremy Rifkin. GM technology has been with us since the early 1970s. GM products have been on the market since the early 1980s. There have been no environmental disasters and no mass poisonings attributable to GM technology. The underlying technology is now widely, if not completely, accepted in the USA. So perhaps the American public believes they've already conducted the relevant debate and feel no need to revive it just because the same technology is now being applied to agriculture instead of health.

A common concern

Despite these apparent differences between consumers in North America and the UK, there is at least one common concern. There's no public demand for GM food. What consumers are lined up pounding at Zeneca's door demanding food that produces its own pesticides? All the high-profile GM products so far are of benefit only to the farmer and the company (especially the company), with little advantage, if any, for the consumer. Many GM proponents are anxiously awaiting the day when a GM product evokes substantial public demand. At present, most GM products are being pushed on to the markets and met by consumers with, at best, indifference or, at worst, outright hostility. 'Attitudes will change' say the companies, 'when consumers "pull" a desired novel GM product through the marketplace. Then we'll see the opposition activists and regulations dissipate as hungry consumers demand access to the product'. I'm not sure it will be that easy, but having real consumer interest will certainly make a difference.

We already have an example of a GMO purported to benefit the consumer: the Flavr-Savr™ tomato. This was placed on the US market several years ago, touted as providing vine-ripe, fresh picked flavour, even in the middle of winter. At first, consumers bought both the hype and the tomato. Then they didn't buy either; the GM tomatoes beat a hasty retreat from the marketplace. We'll explore why later, but for now we can use it as the example to negate the assertion that a GM product designed to benefit consumers will be not only accepted in the market but embraced.

Each of these issues shows an underlying concern based not on genetic technology *per se*, but rather with an intimately connected issue, whether a perceived unnecessary increase in food production, or intensity of agricultural production, domination by multinationals, distrust of regulatory officials, or non-necessity of products. Concerned consumers might recognize their own anxieties as being within one or more of these camps. If so, ask yourself if you are really concerned with genetic technology, or with one of the associated issues or specific products of the technology.

We've seen why the first generation GM products in crops are so heavily based on pesticide resistance. We're seeing on the market the first rudimentary results of experiments conducted in the 1980s—it takes that long to get a product out. The first wave of products was of necessarily simple traits, as that was the state of the technology at the time. But that first wave is passing. Fewer and fewer pesticide-resistant GMOs are being developed. Instead, the second wave of GM products, just coming on to the market now, carries features more relevant to general consumers. These include low calorie sugar beets (which convert sucrose to lower calorie fructans), starch-modified potatoes designed to fry in less oil, oilseed crops with healthier oils (less saturated fats), and various crops with improved nutritional composition—either reduction of undesirable components or supplementation with desirable ones. The third wave, still in experimental labs, will look quite different again when they are eventually released in ten or twelve years' time. These GMOs include plants making pharmaceutical or neutraceutical products or other high value chemicals. Such plants are not designed for widespread environmental release or commodity food markets.

There will always be legitimate concerns over health and environment necessitating regulatory scrutiny of GMOs over and above that currently imposed on 'conventional' new products. But conventionally produced new products generate health and environmental concerns, too.

Specific products require additional regulatory management

Every time some bright scientist takes a recently isolated gene from one organism and sticks it into another, a unique risk situation arises. Each GMO needs to be assessed on its own merits. The majority of GMOs, though, probably present a manageable degree of risk, such that commercialization might be appropriate under certain conditions.

These include crops with GM insect resistance, such as the *B.t.* maize and soya. The crops require management to minimize the threat of populations becoming resistant to the *B.t.* toxin, which has been used widely to control pests by farmers, including organic producers, since the 1950s. GM plants with genes conferring resistance to stresses such as diseases or freezing temperatures need additional assessment, not for their own sake, but to investigate the consequences of transfer of the genes to wild species in the cultivated region. If, for example, a wild plant acquires resistance to cold or fungal diseases, how will that affect its ecological niche? Will the gene suddenly provide an evolutionary advantage to that plant over other species growing in the neighbourhood?

In each case, however, we must keep the question in perspective. If the concern over gene spread is valid, the method of initial production is irrelevant. We are concerned over GM rapeseed passing its herbicide resistance gene via pollen into related but wild species growing in the UK. The same concern demands scrutiny of conventional herbicide-resistant rapeseed in the UK. If the acquisition of a trait is going to cause a problem, why does the source of the trait, whether GM or conventional, make a difference?

Another perspective concerns GMOs tolerant of environmental stress. Crops modified to withstand unseasonable frost are not yet on the market, but are in development. We'll need to determine how to manage any gene escape from these crop plants into wild relatives. Herbicide resistance genes don't give any advantage to plants in the wild (because herbicides aren't sprayed in the wild). But a wild plant with recently acquired frost tolerance might have an advantage over other species and come to dominate the population, upsetting the natural balance and biodiversity in regions prone to unseasonable frosts— the very areas most likely to cultivate a GM frost-tolerant crop.

We need to ensure the safety of our food supply. Some plants are being modified to produce pharmaceutical chemicals. We need to ensure these modified plants do not end up in the food chain. Apart from liability issues, the developers have no desire to see any such mix-up between, say, a food-type rapeseed and a pharmaceutical-producing rapeseed, as the pharmaceutical product is far more valuable to the company than the gross commodity oil, so it's in everyone's best interest to keep them well separated. But, knowing rapeseed's proclivity for distributing its pollen far and wide, how is that accomplished? One way might be to establish huge isolation distances and segregated seed handling systems. We needn't be concerned with the latter; the company will ensure their valuable pharmaceutical seed is nowhere near the vulgar gross commodity. Isolation distances are already in place and used in current, non-GM crops. Canola, the food oil crop, is derived from and remains closely related to rapeseed, which produces an industrial oil unsuitable for human consumption (some say the same for canola oil). Depending on the exact species (*Brassica napus, B. rapa,* or *B. juncea*), the fields must be several hundreds of metres apart to minimize cross-pollination. It should be feasible, then to establish isolation distances for higher value products to minimize cross-contamination. An alternative might be to put the valuable gene into a plant species with less outcrossing from released pollen, or into a species not used primarily as a food crop.

These are only examples of the legitimate environmental and food safety concerns that need to be addressed in evaluating specific modified organisms, whether generated via GM or conventional. Unfortunately, they are sometimes obscured by the hysteria surrounding the process.

The stories behind some scary GM stories

I heard GM L-tryptophan harmed people in the USA:— isn't that an example of GM gone wrong?

It is a common mistake, even for seasoned scientists, to equate a potentially hazardous product with the technique used to develop it.

A popular health food supplement, L-tryptophan, is one of the essential amino acid building blocks of proteins. It is sometimes consumed by people

who believe it helpful in any number of ways, supposedly alleviating everything from insomnia to stress to premenstrual syndrome. All organisms need
L-tryptophan to make proteins requiring that particular amino acid. In addition, some organisms, including humans, further process or metabolize
L-tryptophan into other chemicals such as neurotransmitters.

A Japanese health food and pharmaceutical company, Showa Denko, made
some changes to its production line of L-tryptophan. Commercial L-tryptophan is ordinarily produced through bacterial fermentation: specially selected
and conventionally genetically modified strains of *Bacillus amyloliquefaciens* in
huge vats synthesize and pump out large quantities of the amino acid, along
with other cell products. The company extracts the L-tryptophan from the fermentation slush, cleans it up, and sells it in large quantities to other companies.
The receiving company bottles it with their own name on the label and sells it
to distributors, who in turn place it in the shops where it's sold at grossly
inflated prices. Showa Denko was a major producer, manufacturing most of
the L-tryptophan on the US market, even though it was sold under many
different brand names.

In 1989, attempting to increase production and decrease manufacturing
costs, the company made a couple of changes:

- They switched bacteria from a conventionally modified strain to another
  strain—the same species, but modified by rDNA techniques. The new
  strain, called Strain V, had twice as many genes for tryptophan synthesis as
  older strains, as well as genetic enhancements from other bacteria to
  stimulate increased tryptophan synthesis.
- They changed the activated carbon filtration system used to clean out the
  various impurities from the tryptophan in the fermentation sludge.
  Tryptophan was the major constituent, but dozens of other chemicals were
  also present, mostly in tiny quantities. The purification process was supposed to remove these contaminants. Showa Denko decided they could cut
  the filtration in half.

Shortly after these changes were introduced, some consumers in the USA
came down with a new disease, eventually named eosinophilia–myalgia syndrome (EMS). Depending on whose figures you believe, anywhere from 1500
people to 'ten thousand' became seriously ill, with 27 to 38 or more dying from
the disease.

The statistical connection between the victims and Showa Denko came
quickly. The US Food and Drug Administration (FDA) pulled the supplement
from the shelves and have not returned it, although it is available with a pre-
scription in the USA, and over the counter as a food supplement in some other
countries, including Canada and the UK. The respected Centers for Disease
Control in Atlanta and the Mayo Clinic began investigations, as did Showa
Denko.

Almost as rapid was the indictment of genetic engineering technology as the

cause of the tragedy, an indictment that continues today in literature emanating from activist camps. The argument is that the use of GM technology results
in unexpected, unpredictable, and sometimes tragic consequences. Although
the argument had been put forward in the past, until Showa Denko and EMS
came along there were no examples of GM technology having any unexpected,
unpredicted, and certainly not tragic consequences.

There is no question, no debate, that several batches of tryptophan originating in Showa Denko fermentation vats caused harm to individuals. But was
it a problem with the GM process that gave rise to the GM bacteria, or was it a
problem with the purification of the tryptophan product?

Subsequent analyses found some of the contaminants, present in parts per
million, were not adequately removed during the purification process. Initially,
a contaminant compound identified as 1,1′-ethylidenebis[tryptophan] (EBT),
more familiarly known as 'peak E' or 'peak 97', was implicated as a causal agent
in EMS. EBT results from two molecules of tryptophan hybridizing to form
what chemists call a dimeric form. Although other molecular contaminants
have since been additionally suggested, EBT remains a primary culprit.

However, several contaminants remain unidentified. Furthermore, there is
concern that the problem was one not of contamination, but of purity. The
Showa Denko product was 99.6% pure L-tryptophan, somewhat higher than
the required purity, leading some to suggest that the intense purity itself might
be responsible for the problems, arguing that humans are simply not used to
chemicals of such purity.

How EBT and the other contaminants failed to be removed during the
purification is a matter of speculation, as Showa Denko has not released their
internal investigation on the matter. The FDA and the CDC are convinced that
the genetic modification was not at fault.

So, how do we know the genetic modification didn't inadvertently transfer
genes for the contaminants to the bacteria? We can't analyse the actual DNA
in the GM bacteria because Showa Denko hasn't provided samples. We can't
say for certain that the bacteria didn't carry genes to synthesize the contaminant toxins. We also don't know if the contaminants are from unusual
chemical reactions occurring in such high concentrations of tryptophan. We
do know, however, that contaminant chemicals, including EBT, are present in
minute quantities in batches of L-tryptophan and the related product 5-
hydroxytryptophan (5-HT) from other manufacturers using non-GM
bacteria. The problem is not unique to the GM bacteria. EMS and related
conditions have been reported in users of L-tryptophan and 5-HT after the
GM bacteria and its products were removed from the market, so the GM
process cannot be at fault. Also, batches of L-tryptophan from conventional
bacterial strains had been implicated in EMS dating back to before the Showa
Denko tragedy.

We can speculate on the exact mechanism, but it is clear that the process
used to modify the bacteria is not responsible for EMS. The best way to

minimize such tragedies to is to enforce better quality control of the product throughout the manufacturing process.

Toxic contaminant problems are well known to the industry and to consumers who frequently have to deal with product recalls. The original order from the FDA recalling L-tryptophan was carried in a routine notice of various other recalls, ranging from prepared sandwiches contaminated with bacteria to 'extra-strength' condoms prone to breakage. On a recent trip to the supermarket I saw two product recall notices. One was for a confection with sultanas as a major ingredient. Somehow, the recalled batch carried peanuts instead of sultanas. Considering the allergic effect peanuts have on some people, this could have been a major disaster if we didn't have the regulatory structure to deal with it calmly and effectively. There was a small notice in the newspaper and a larger notice at the grocery, and the product was removed from the shelves. In some ways, the L-tryptophan incident shows that GM products are more like conventional products in some respects—they are still subject to batch faults in the quality control, contamination, and the other bugs in the machine haunting commercial production of food products.

Our interest in this case is to draw a distinction between the product and the process. If a bad batch of a product resulted in the ban of the process, we would have few products on our shelves, as there are several product recalls every week based on inadvertent contaminants or mistaken labels on consumer goods. An isolated bad batch of a product does not indict the process used to make the batch.

Incidentally, Showa Denko is no longer producing L-tryptophan, and no manufacturer is using GM bacteria to manufacture L-tryptophan. And the FDA still has not found L-tryptophan to be 'safe' at *any* dosage.

A respected scientist showed GM potatoes to be toxic, didn't he?

The second example of misunderstanding and confusion between product and process concerns the imbroglio centred on Dr Arpad Pusztai, formerly of the Rowett Institute in Scotland. Dr Pusztai was investigating health safety concerns of GM potatoes when he noted what he thought were some dramatic results, which he felt he had to share with the world immediately. We'll discuss the specifics of this unfortunate situation later; at the moment, our interest is in the difficulty in distinction between process and product.

Dr Pusztai started out investigating food safety questions concerning GM potatoes, a noble enough objective. But his experimental design focused on the product, lectins (natural pesticides produced by plants), not on the process, GM. The experiments might have generated some useful information on lectins (they didn't, as we'll see later), but not about GM, because they failed to properly account or control for the process. Proper scientific design to investigate the GM process demands testing, with appropriate controls, a broad range of GM products, not just one. On this basis alone, the entire foundation of the research project was faulty, the interpretations meaningless. Unfortunately, Dr Pusztai tarnished his own reputation by interpreting his results on the basis of the process instead of on the product.

In any case, his exposé of the toxic effects of GM potatoes on rats was premature; no one else had previously reviewed his results. Peer review points out simple and embarrassing mistakes we all make from time to time, such as misreading the results of the positive control for the results of the experimental batch. Clearly, we expect the positive control, the poison-spiked potato group, to show ill effects. Dr Pusztai later admitted his error on not seeking peer review prior to 'going public'. If he had, he might have saved his hard-earned reputation and saved considerable, and continuing, public anxiety.

Why the attention to the false accounts of poisonous transgenic potato? This was seen as a great victory, first by those opposed to transgenic technology, because it appeared that a transgenic potato caused poisoning in rats. Then, when it became apparent that it was a mistake, that the procedure was flawed, the proponents saw it as a victory. This is an unfortunate event focused on two opposing camps. The real issue is, why is it newsworthy that poison fed to rats, whether added to their potato feed through transgenic technology or as a simple additive sprinkled on their food, results in poisoning of the animals?

Many people are calling for a full repeat of his experiments. Perhaps Dr Pusztai was correct, and GM potatoes are toxic. There is enough doubt, they say, to warrant proper investigation. I disagree. We have the answer already. Why spend all that additional money and subject innocent rats to the unnecessary experiments? Millions of Americans have been eating GM potatoes for several years, without adverse effect. In addition to providing larger sample numbers, over a longer time, it costs us nothing. A repeat of Dr Pusztai's experiments will tell us nothing we don't already know from the human experiment on American consumers.

A butterfly brouhaha

A third example of confusion between process and product is the Monarch butterfly incident, in which Monarch larvae fed on GM maize pollen containing *B.t.* toxin. The larvae did not fare as well as larvae fed on ordinary maize pollen; many observers concluded the GM was responsible. However, the scientists conducting the research, John Losey and his team at Cornell, did not make this mistake. In their short letter to *Nature* describing the experiment, they explicitly stated the problem was due to the presence of the *B.t.* toxin. Unfortunately, they did not include a treatment consisting of ordinary pollen spiked with ordinary *B.t.* powder. They omitted a crucial control. We'll discuss this *B.t.* toxin problem again.

These examples show how it is often difficult to separate a problem with a technique and a problem with the product of the technique. Would there have been as much media attention to the L-tryptophan problem had it been from a conventional bacterium? Would Dr Pusztai have received as much attention if he had conducted a study of rats fed ordinary potatoes spiked with a poison? What would happen if the Monarchs suffered from being fed pollen spiked with 'organic' *B.t.* powder? In each case, the 'hook' that attracted attention was the supposed GM aspect. The media doesn't often give much coverage to a story of harm coming to people who eat a contaminated food supplement. Even esoteric scientific journals are reluctant to publish results from routine experiments involving toxins added to feed making test animals ill.

Going nuts: the Brazil nut gene story

There has been much press coverage of the Brazil nut gene causing new, severe allergic reactions in people who had not previously been allergic to soya. Depending on where you heard or read the story, the allergenic GM soya was caught either just prior to commercial release, or only after several people had unexpectedly reacted to some soya-containing food product. With the knowledge that soya is a component of over 60% of our processed foods, people (rightfully) demanded to know which foods to avoid. 'How dare the Americans force their allergenic soya beans on us? How dare they refuse to tell us which shipments contained these soya beans? Thank goodness for the activists who alerted us to this danger before it was too late.'

My daughter Stephanie is allergic to Brazil nuts. She goes into anaphylactic shock from eating even a tiny portion of a Brazil nut and then has 15–20 minutes to be treated with an injection or face a likely untimely death.

Stephanie's grandmother Ann, who lives in the UK, was horrified to learn of the Brazil nut gene in soya, as Stephanie was scheduled to visit within a few months. 'How will I find food that doesn't contain these soya beans?' she cried 'If most processed foods contain soy products, she'll have to starve while she's here!' Ann, a bright and intelligent person, became quite emotional on this point. During a momentary lucid hiatus I managed to ask her what she thought Stephanie ate at home in Canada, where Stephanie has been eating unlabelled GM soya-containing foods for some time without going into anaphylactic shock. Why hasn't she been adversely affected? Because there is no Brazil nut protein, no Brazil nut gene, in soya beans.

The history of this popular misconception is interesting as well as illuminating. We are all aware of the massive problem of world hunger from general lack of food, but we are less aware of large populations who, although they may have enough to eat, suffer serious dietary deficiencies due to nutritional imbalance. Despite being able to generate satisfactory quantities of certain crops, these people do not enjoy a balanced diet. A primary example is sub-Saharan and West Africa, where people consume a diet high in grain legumes, mostly pulses. Although these peas and beans are generally nutritious, they are deficient in a couple of critical nutrients, so a diet predominantly or exclusively of the beans leads to health problems. The nutrients are the amino acids, methionine and cysteine, two of the amino acid building blocks of proteins. The beans get by without using much of these amino acids, so they don't synthesize large quantities or stockpile them. Humans usually balance their bean diet with cereals or other foodstuffs, ones that do contain more of these amino acids (most other foods contain at least some satisfactory quantities). However, in fringe or subsistence agricultural areas, alternative foods or supplements are not always available.

The Brazil nut (any nut or seed, for that matter) is a 'nurse' tissue—it contains a ready source of nutrients and energy so when the nut germinates and begins life, it doesn't have to work too hard getting established and then looking out for itself. This is why nuts are so nutritious (and fattening). It so happens that the Brazil nut stores a high concentration of the nutrient amino acids, cysteine and methionine, in a nutrient storage protein. By isolating the gene responsible we acquire the recipe for a protein rich in these amino acids.

If we could take this gene and place it into grain legumes, such as faba or soya bean, we could eradicate the nutritional deficiency, and also improve the general nutrient balance in grain legumes overall, at virtually no cost.

This was probably the most noble objective of agricultural biotechnology yet. It was promulgated by a small biotech firm in California in the mid-1980s. However, before any GM bean was generated, scientists themselves pointed out the folly of transferring a gene for an allergenic protein into a food crop. The work was later revived by Pioneer Hi-Bred, another major player in the game. This time, the project objective was intended to balance animal feed rather than human foodstuffs. Much of the soya crop is fed to animals; they would also benefit from nutritionally balanced foods. During the course of the work, Pioneer themselves conducted allergenicity studies with the Brazil nut protein, as it hadn't previously been conclusively shown that this particular protein was the one responsible for the allergic response. It was. Pioneer killed the project and, to their credit, published the results. The activists learned of the results linking the Brazil nut protein with the allergic response and sounded the alarm, ten years after the scientific community attended the project's funeral. No bean was ever produced with the Brazil nut gene.

Such a product as the Brazil nut storage protein gene in a food product (such as soya or faba bean) must never be allowed on the market, regardless of the proposed management strategy to minimize risk. There are acceptable alternatives to achieve the same end, and the risks involved in a mistake are too high. Even the company acknowledges they would be liable for any damages. This particular product was simply not worth the risks.

The objective remains noble, and others are looking at alternative means to achieve the goal. Just because the best source of these amino acids is unsuitable doesn't mean other rich sources are similarly unsuitable.

Two ways to skin a cat

Most people accept genetic manipulation when we use cross-breeding or for medical treatments. Most diabetics on insulin now are shooting genetically engineered insulin into their bodies. What's the philosophical difference between inserting a human gene into a bacterium and selling the product, and inserting a bacterial gene into a plant and selling the product? The genetic technology is the same in each case. Perhaps the concern is not the technology *per se*, but the applications of the technology. Is it that medical treatments are good, while increased food production is unnecessary? If so, then why are companies continuing to develop crops using old technology?

I can understand why, if we develop a crop that carries, say, a new toxin, we would need to carefully scrutinize that aspect in the GM line before releasing it. But should another plant, genetically modified by the transfer of a gene from the same species come under the same scrutiny and assessment?

Fungal disease—conventional vs. GM

We can use an example to illustrate the questionable differential in our attitude toward specific GM products and their conventional alternatives. Suppose a pathogenic fungus sometimes invades rapeseed-growing regions causing substantial damage. Plant breeders in that area have a choice:

A Do nothing and let the infestation destroy the crops and industry.
B Breed conventionally from a distant foreign rapeseed cultivar with a disease resistance gene.
C Breed from that same foreign rapeseed gene using GM.

If breeders wish to help farmers and consumers, choice A is not an option, leaving us with B or C.

Unfortunately, this hypothetical foreign rapeseed does not perform very well as a crop (almost invariably the case in real life, too). But by cross-pollinating this exotic rapeseed with the domestic crop plant, we might develop new lines, ones that are good crop types and also carry the fungal disease resistance. Unfortunately again, this process takes about twelve years; too long to help farmers facing bankruptcy from the current infestation.

Alternatively, genetic engineering might be used to isolate the disease resistance gene from the foreign line and transfer it directly into the domestic variety. This process takes about six to eight years. Not only does it almost halve the time to start helping farmers (and stabilizing markets), it ensures the undesirable features of the foreign rapeseed are left behind.

What's the scientifically valid rationale to give additional regulatory attention to a particular method of genetic modification of a plant? Conventional procedures require analysis of the candidate cultivar, including such parameters as seed yield and productivity, length of growing season, response to diseases, and a chemical analysis of the seed grain, among others. These are required regardless of method of breeding.

From a purely scientific viewpoint, the GM rapeseed in the example above should require less scrutiny than a product of ordinary breeding, because the GM variety is composed almost entirely of the known, conventional variety, plus one other gene from another rapeseed variety. The product of conventional breeding contains many genes from the foreign source; other than the one providing disease resistance, these cannot even be identified in most cases. Any 'unexpected or unintended' effects in the GM lines would almost certainly be noted during the regular evaluations. Undesirable genes from the foreign variety carried along in the conventional lines may not be noted or eliminated, ending up on the market.

The debate on the merits and demerits of GM and GMOs needs to be placed in perspective. Before we condemn a technology or product, we need to evaluate and compare the currently available and acceptable alternative. L-Tryptophan from bacterial fermentation vats carries a risk of contamination, regardless of the method used to generate the special strains of bacteria. By basing regulations on process, contaminants in a batch from the conventional bacteria might end up on the market. By scrutinizing products, bad batches from *any* process are more likely to be caught and eliminated before they can cause harm.

Why are pesticide-resistant crops the first products?

Once the technique was developed to use the ability of disarmed strains of *Agrobacterium* to transfer functional genes into plants (see Chapter 3), the race was on to find, and transfer, commercially useful genes.

Few genes had been isolated in the mid-1980s. Isolating a gene, even a simple one from simple bacteria, took plenty of time and plenty of money. The genes that had been isolated were generally either marker genes like *nos* or genes massively expressed in certain tissues, like ovalbumin in eggs. None of these had much expected value in crop plants.

The most pressing issues for crops were production-oriented objectives, overall grain yield, and other agronomic traits such as earlier crop maturity or enhanced weed control. In those early days, the technology allowed us to transfer one or a few genes at best, and, as noted above, we didn't actually have many genes anyway, useful or otherwise. Seed yield was known to be a complex trait, regulated by many different genes acting in concert. Similarly, maturity was a complex, multigene trait. It was not feasible to try to reduce time to maturity using molecular approaches. Disease resistance was a possibility, as we already knew that at least some disease resistance genes are fairly simple. Stress tolerance, such as resistance to frost or salty soils, was another possibility. Although we knew from conventional breeding research that such traits could be quite complex and beyond our capability at that time, there were also some relatively simple genetic mechanisms known to provide stress tolerance. This was probably when someone pointed out the ability of the Arctic flounder to live in the liquid but sub-freezing (about −2° C) temperatures in the Arctic, and pondered the possibility of isolating whatever gene the fish used for transfer to tomatoes and other cold-sensitive plants. Although this gene is probably unsuitable for making crops frost tolerant, it might have other applications. For example, it might be used in wheat designed especially to make frozen dough—the gene might give the dough better storage capability, longer 'freezer-life'.

To provide a novel trait to a crop using molecular techniques, you need to have an isolated gene, a piece of DNA coding for a particular protein providing the function of the trait in question. To isolate the piece of DNA from all the other genes in the donor organism, you need to know either something about the DNA sequence or more about the function of the trait. Few DNA sequences were known then; DNA sequencing was in its infancy and still very expensive and time consuming. To approach the gene from the trait side, you needed to know as much as possible about the trait at a molecular and biochemical level. Again, not much was known at a molecular level about 'seed yield' or 'maturity'. We also had to be cautious not to be confused by a particular mechanism of a trait. There are many different ways a plant could appear salt-tolerant, for example. Some ways might be genetically or physiologically simple, others more complex. Some plants use a single gene, producing a single protein, to exclude salt from the inside of the cells and thus preclude damage. Others have complex anatomical structures called hydathodes to protect from the ravages of excess salt. Such structures probably require dozens of genes working in concert to function properly. If we don't know which mechanism we're after, we're unlikely to succeed.

Because of all these complications, many of which still exist, we could not simply introduce the useful traits we wanted. Salt tolerance remains a top priority in many parts of the world, yet is still poorly understood at a molecular genetic level. Another excellent example is nitrogen fixation. A major expenditure for farmers is nitrogen-based fertilizer. Nitrogen is plentiful: it's even in the air, in fact about 78% of air is nitrogen, but most plants can't make use of it in that form. Instead, plants need a form of nitrogen found in fertilizers— organic or conventional—and these are expensive. In a process called **nitrogen fixation**, some bacteria (*Rhizobia*) are able to take the nitrogen from the air and convert it to a form plants can use as fertilizer. Certain plants, notably legumes, struck a deal with *Rhizobia* aeons ago: the plants would house the bacteria if the bacteria would make fertilizer for the plants. Thus began one of the most successful symbiotic relationships in the history of nature.

One of the first 'big science' ideas for genetic engineering was to take the genes responsible for nitrogen fixation from *Rhizobia* and transfer them to other crops. Farmers would save a fortune on fertilizer costs if they could grow plants that make their own. Nitrogen fixation, especially in wheat, was a major selling point of crop genetic engineering for venture capitalists and granting agencies right back to the 1970s, long before any transgenic plants had been revealed. A huge amount of funding went into research on providing plants capable of harnessing nitrogen from the air. We still don't have nitrogen-fixing wheat, or any other plant other than those, such as legumes, that could do it anyway. It turned out that nitrogen fixation is an extremely complex relationship between the plant and bacteria, involving many genes from both species. It's still beyond our ability to manipulate and transfer into other plants. Because of their fixation on nitrogen fixation, many investors became disillusioned at the failure to produce the self-fertilizing wheat within a few years, and withdrew funding, killing many small start-up biotechnology companies in the process.

This left the big chemical companies, along with a few residual small companies and public labs, to do their own thing. In the world of plant genetic engineering, Monsanto was already a major player, as was Swiss-based giant Ciba-Geigy (later, after merging with Sandoz, known as Novartis) and the public Max Planck Institut für Züchtungsforschung in Cologne, Germany.

Meanwhile, other companies were developing similar genes conferring tolerance to their own products. DuPont was developing genes conferring resistance to their sulfonylurea group of herbicides. Hoechst (which later, after merging with Schering, became AgrEvo) were trying to find resistance to their non-selective herbicide glufosinate ammonium, the active ingredient in Basta™, Liberty™, and other commercial herbicide formulations.

One of the small biotechnology companies, Plant Genetic Systems, was based in Belgium. PGS had a very talented staff of scientists aggressively working on a number of creative projects. One was to develop an artificial way to make hybrid plants in those species where hybridization was not feasible using conventional methods. Such a development would enable farmers to benefit from hybrid vigour in those crops the same way they currently enjoy the substantially higher yields afforded by hybrids in maize. Another PGS project was to beat Hoechst to finding a gene conferring resistance to Basta™, the major non-selective herbicide produced by that chemical giant. Unlike Calgene, PGS managed their scientific discoveries so skilfully such that, when Hoechst (by this time AgrEvo) came to buy out the upstarts at PGS, they ended up not in an acquisition but in a merger. AgrEvo acquired PGS financially, but PGS personnel were placed in a number of key scientific managerial positions, far beyond what Calgene was able to accomplish within Monsanto.

The most common trait in GM crops is herbicide resistance, followed by insect resistance. Insect resistance was developed simultaneously with the herbicide resistance because the most commonly used gene conferring resistance to insects was a simple bacterial gene with a substantial scientific history and database. *Bacillus thuringiensis (B.t.)* is a naturally occurring bacterium, used widely since the late 1950s in insecticidal powder formulations to control mainly caterpillar pests in domestic gardens and commercial and organic farm operations. Because it was a prokaryotic gene in a natural bacterial species, the gene was quickly isolated, characterized, and cloned. Many companies tried to improve the insecticidal activity or alter the insect species target range of the gene by modifying the DNA sequence, adding different promoters, and finding different natural versions in related strains of the bacteria. Of course, any such improvements due to the company's modifications enabled the opportunity for patent protection as well. Several companies developed *B.t.*. gene variations and inserted them into various crops, some observing very efficient insecticidal properties. This trait also marked a legal watershed. Unlike the herbicide resistance situation where the big companies developed genes conferring resistance to their own herbicide, the original *B.t.* patents had expired. Many companies had an interest, not just emotional, in *B.t.* Major legal action involving charges of patent infringement was initiated involving many companies, big and small, each claiming an intellectual property position on various forms of *B.t.*-based insect resistance genes. The lawyers are still counting the money.

The first GM crop products on the market were pesticide-resistant because they were the first commercially valuable products out of the research labs. The big companies had the capital as well as the background biochemical knowledge of their own products to devote to developing resistance genes. Genes conferring resistance to a simple chemical such as a pesticide were themselves relatively simple and so more easily isolated and cloned. Almost all of these current GM products are the result of research into the first isolated genes and were developed in the 1980s. They were all generated only a few years after the first transgenic plants were produced in 1983. My GM linseed was 'born' as a single transgenic plant in 1988. The foreign genes in it are now obsolete, having been superseded by superior versions, as are the genes in the GM products on the market and under regulatory review. The generation of genes and genetic constructs under development in the research labs now will not hit the market for several years. However, it takes up to fifteen years to bring a crop, transgenic or conventional, to market, so we're experiencing the lag time between the scientific development and the market release.

I'm not as concerned as some people are about the dominance of pesticide-resistant GM crops. Although they will continue with us, they are already fading as the first wave of transgenic technology gives way to the second. Soon, pesticide resistance will constitute a minor proportion of GM crop traits.

Are we creating superweeds?

One of the greatest fears in the public mind is the release of herbicide-resistant GM crops escaping to become uncontrollable superweeds devastating the countryside. It's unfortunate that 'herbicide-resistant' implies the plant is resistant to (or tolerant* of) *all* herbicides. All plants are naturally resistant to some herbicides. At best, it means a GM plant is resistant to one additional herbicide, or, at worst, a class of similar herbicides. Monsanto's Roundup-Ready™ cotton will survive a dose of glyphosate (the active ingredient in Roundup™), but is still susceptible to all the other herbicides to which cotton is ordinarily sensitive. AgrEvo's Liberty™-Link canola will withstand a dose of Liberty™, but will die from a dose of Roundup™.

The escape of the herbicide resistant plant (or pollen) from cultivated farmland to the wild is a legitimate concern that needs to be addressed. Are escaped plants of the same species ordinarily controlled with this herbicide? If so, can the plant be controlled otherwise? If there's another common herbicide capable of controlling the GM plant, then its unlikely to become a pest either in the natural environment or the managed (farm) environment. Do the GM plants have any environmental advantage over non-GM plants in the wild? Herbicide resistance is not an advantage in the absence of the herbicide, so if that herbicide is not ordinarily used to control that species, the escape of routine numbers of GM plants should not present a problem. In the absence of the selection pressure (in this case, the herbicide), the plant and gene will not overtake other plants of the same species. Ordinarily, the direct escape of a herbicide-resistant plant into either the natural or managed environment is not problematic. In the managed environment of a farm, the wayward plants can be controlled with either tillage (not even GM plants can withstand being sliced up by cold steel) or with other herbicides to which the plant is still sensitive. In the wild, the GM plant has no particular advantage over other plants, as the herbicide is not usually sprayed over a natural unmanaged environment. Without such a selective advantage, the population will almost certainly dissipate to zero within a few years, as more aggressive species out-compete the GM plant for space and nutrients. Crop plants don't usually survive well without the tender loving care of human intervention to protect them from the harsh realities of life in the jungle.

In the managed environment, a different situation arises if the GM crop is a close-enough relative of a local weed to permit interbreeding. If the herbicide is used to control the weedy species, then the herbicide resistance gene might compromise the utility of the herbicide in controlling that weed. What is needed here is an assurance that other herbicides are still available to

---

*   Some authorities prefer this milder term, but most non-weed scientists use 'tolerant' and 'resistant' interchangeably.

control the weed, even if it does acquire a herbicide resistance gene from the GM plant.

A real problem might arise if several different varieties of GM crops are grown in close proximity, such as Roundup-Ready™ canola and Liberty™-Link canola. There are already reports of canola plants displaying resistance to both Roundup™ and Liberty™ in farmers' fields in Alberta. Fortunately, other herbicide products are available to control such hybrids, but this example serves to illustrate what might happen if we allow genes conferring different herbicide resistance to 'pyramid', resulting in a plant difficult to eradicate. Interestingly, this is not widely seen as a natural environment problem because herbicide resistance is not an issue in unmanaged, natural environments. It is instead a farm management problem. A farmer growing Roundup-Ready™ canola expects to be able to enjoy complete weed control by spraying Roundup™ on the crop. If Roundup™-resistant plants other than the crop are present in the field, they will not be controlled by the Roundup™ herbicide application and the crop may be downgraded because of the Roundup™-resistant weeds.

In any case, GM herbicide-resistant plants are not superweeds immune to all herbicides. All plants are susceptible to some herbicides, and all have natural resistance to other herbicides. Wheat, for example, has a natural genetic mechanism to break down sulfonylurea (SU) herbicides before the herbicide can adversely affect the wheat plant. This is why SU herbicides can be sprayed on the wheat crop; the herbicide kills weeds but not the wheat. All plants, including all GM plants, are susceptible to at least some herbicides. No herbicide resistance gene offers an advantage to plants in the wild, because herbicides are not usually found in the wild. Certainly, there are management issues to be resolved before releasing GM herbicide-resistant crop varieties, and there are likely places where certain GM crops should not be cultivated due to the environmental risks.

What are artificial hybrids?

Maize and some other crops have achieved major agronomic advances owing to the development of hybrid technology using conventional breeding methods. Hybrid systems, in which usually the pollen from one line of plants aborts, necessitates cross-pollination, or hybridization, from other plants. The seed yield resulting from the cross-pollination can be substantially higher. This is called **hybrid vigour**, and is an important objective for those species not readily hybridized using conventional technology.

Plant Genetic Systems (PGS) found a gene promoter active only in cells lining the pollen-holding structures in the stamens of the flower. As the pollen matures in the normal plant, this promoter becomes active in these cells and the gene activity helps the pollen grains mature. PGS isolated the gene and its promoter, but discarded the gene part, keeping the promoter. Then they hooked the promoter to a gene coding for an enzyme designed to attack and degrade nucleic acids in the cell. Then they inserted the synthetic gene and promoter into tobacco, and waited for the GM plants to regenerate and mature. As the flowers developed, they kept close watch over the stamens. The GM tobacco plants seemed entirely normal. But when they started to form flowers, the stamens, particularly the anthers where the pollen is stored, aborted. The synthetic gene acted as expected. The flower development proceeded normally, with pollen cells developing in the anthers. But when they reached maturity, the inserted promoter activated the suicide gene only in the cells lining the pollen sacs. The enzyme destroyed all the nucleic acid in the cells and the pollen, resulting in dead pollen. The rest of the plant was unaffected. The only apparent result was a pollenless, male-sterile tobacco plant. The only way these plants could form seeds is if the ovaries were pollinated from other, non-GM tobacco plants. This was an artificial hybrid system.

PGS quickly adapted the technology to other, more important crop species. Among the first was oilseed rape, where the system seemed to work very well. PGS received one of the first UK approvals for commercial GMO cultivation, albeit limited to seed production, not consumption, with an artificial rapeseed hybrid. Several commercial canola varieties in Canada are now hybrids, including some of the PGS/AgrEvo varieties. The hybrids are gaining popularity with farmers, indicating the hybridization is functioning and providing the farmers with the promised increased productivity.

Of course, there's a price to pay. With hybrid seed, farmers need to buy fresh seed each year. Because the pollen comes from philandering males unknown, the progeny can exhibit all sort of uncertain traits if they are grown out as plants instead of processed as grain or consumed. Farmers accustomed to saving part of their harvested seed for next year's planting are disappointed at the poor stand and non-uniformity of the crop. They may try this once, then return to buying fresh seed year after year. Some farmers don't like the idea of buying fresh seed each year, so they return to whatever variety they had been growing before trying the hybrid. What has happened with hybrid maize is that most farmers, once they try hybrid technology, stay with it. It's likely they'll do the same with GM hybrids. Farmers recognize that the additional cost of buying seed every year is more than offset by the increase in income from the hybrid productivity. This GM technology is here to stay and will probably be extended to other crop species currently lacking hybrid technology.

CHAPTER 7

Figure it out

- What do all the numbers mean?
- Is risk assessment just a numbers racket?
- How reliable is DNA fingerprinting?
- How do we measure 'infinity'?

Life is a risk

All new products carry some degree of risk. For that matter, all products and activities, not just new ones, carry some risk. According to James Walsh, author of *True odds* (see Chapter 16), your chance of dying from flesh-eating bacteria is 1 in a million; from being hit by lightning, 1 in 30 000; from cancer due to eating peanut butter sandwiches every day, 1 in 5000. If you smoke a pack of cigarettes each day, your risk of dying from a smoking-related disease is a whopping 1 in 6. Some of these events are accidental and can't be easily avoided, while others are easily avoided—no one needs to smoke or eat peanut butter sandwiches every day (and who would want to?). The degree to which we can avoid risk is an important consideration overall. You can't escape risk of personal injury in modern life, even by staying in bed. An unusually reliable source, Bill Bryson, in *Notes from a big country*, see Chapter 16 (quoting from official statistics) says 400 000 Americans are injured by their bedding (bed, pillow, or mattress) each year.

Opponents of GM technology point out, correctly, that 'No developer of GMOs has assured us the GMO is risk-free!' They neglect to indicate that developers of conventional products similarly decline to provide the same assurance for their non-GM products. Taken in isolation and out of context, it appears that accepting GMOs means we're accepting unknown additional risks. The only way we can determine if we are being asked to accept these risks is to compare the calculated risks of the GMO with those of a comparable but conventional version of the same type of product. For example, a GM *B.t.* maize plant can be evaluated properly and fully only in relation to an ordinary maize plant (the same variety, grown in the same locations) combined with the conventional means to control insect pests in that conventional maize crop, preferably an ordinary, non-GM *B.t.* formulation. Failure to consider all of the relevant comparisons leads to erroneous conclusions, inviting potentially disastrous consequences.

Risk assessment and the numbers racket

Evaluating the risks associated with GMOs, or anything else, for that matter, involves analysing and comparing numbers. Often, the figures are either astronomically large or infinitesimally small. Unfortunately, the way many scientists and other experts present numerical values and calculations inadvertently befuddles the general public. Although such complicated mathematical presentation might be essential in an academic forum, it is not necessary here. What we might lose in statistical precision in this chapter we gain in conceptual understanding.

A major concept in risk assessment is chance. For example, what is the chance, or likelihood, of gene escape from GM rapeseed? How does that chance compare with other risks? Before we delve more deeply into these risks, we need a quick primer on chance, small numbers, big numbers, and infinity.

Chances are. . .

Nowadays there's always at least one article on genetic technology in the morning paper; I'm always anxious to see how they presented it. In the newsagent's I found myself in the queue behind a customer carrying a crumpled $50 note in one hand and a *Lottery Winner!* magazine in the other. It seemed like a lot of money for a magazine, and she seemed to take a long time at the counter. When she finally left I noticed she now carried her magazine and some lottery tickets in one hand (the apparent cause of the delay) and $5 change in the other. $45 for a magazine and a chance of winning a lifetime of luxury, wealth and, therefore, happiness. Under my breath, I wished her luck.

What does this have to do with GMOs? Unless you belong to one of the two extreme camps ('All GMOs are safe and should be released', or 'All GMOs are unsafe and ought never be released'), evaluation of GMO safety is a matter of risk assessment. Risk assessment is a matter of comparing chance. The chance of winning the lottery. The chance of getting hit by lightning. The chance of being harmed by a GMO. All involve manipulation of very large numbers, or very small numbers.

Like most people, I can handle about seven or eight digits (such as a phone number), or estimate about one in eight of a collection (cutting one-eighth of a pie is no problem), but beyond that uncertainty reigns. Then I must depend (sometimes to my regret) on external expertise—electrical, mechanical, or human—to provide direction. Big numbers baffle me. I don't often buy lottery tickets because to me, a one in a million chance of winning is too high to properly evaluate. A ticket agent with a sales promotion once approached me. The gimmick increased the odds of winning, from one in a million (for the 'big prize') to one in a hundred thousand. The ticket agent effused 'Buy now—you've increased your chances of winning by tenfold!'

'Wow!' I gasped, then calmly 'No thanks'. I notice he didn't try to hook me with 'You've *decreased* your chance of *losing* from 999 999 in a 1 000 000 to 99 999 in 100 000!' I can't comprehend a 1 in 100 000 chance, or even a 1 in 100 chance. Notice that, while the gimmick increases my chances of winning tenfold, it decreases my chance of losing by only 0.000 009. In the original draw, my chance of losing is 99.9999%; in the second, it is a mere 99.999%.

A variation of this gimmick is when lotteries offer a sale, giving two tickets for the price of one. 'Double your chance of winning' they claim. The problem, of course, is that everyone who buys one ticket gets two. The odds of winning remain the same (infinitesimal) because there are now twice as many tickets in the draw. Actually, if the promotion succeeds, more people buy more tickets, resulting in more tickets in the draw, so your chances of winning the Big One is reduced even further. If you really want to see a ticket 'sale', let's see the organizers increase the proportion of ticket revenue going into prizes. How often do the prize values rise above, say, 50% of ticket revenue? I'll buy tickets when it goes above 100%.

'What a spoil sport!' I hear. Sure, as long as you can afford to buy tickets for fun, and realize you aren't going to win big, go for it. 'Well, someone has to win. Why not me?' you might say. True enough, a few people do in fact win big on the lottery. My cousin was one. I don't buy lottery tickets any more because he obviously used up all the luck in our extended family.

I can grasp why, when I toss a coin, I can guess the result correctly about half the time. Or when I toss a single die, I can guess the correct number about one time in six. To me, one in a million or one in a hundred thousand is pretty much the same, even though I comprehend, intellectually and emotionally, that there is indeed a tenfold difference between them. I still see my chances of winning the lottery as so close to zero that it might as well *be* zero (especially if I don't buy tickets!). The continuing British–American debate over the meaning or value of 'billion' is similar. To me, the values are so high as to be beyond my comprehension. When I get to a point beyond my capacity to discern the numbers, I call them all 'zillions'.

Percentages are OK. I understand something divided into 100 parts, and 57% means 57 of those 100 parts. It's also fine with me that, when my favourite ginger marmalade jar says 'Made with 30% ginger'; I accept it is actually anywhere from about 27% to 31% ginger (they always claim toward the high end), depending on the batch. The point is it has substantially more ginger than the competitors' version. I don't expect them to be able to provide the exact figure for each batch. What difference does it make to me if it's actually 29.7333%

ginger? Will I not buy it if the last batch was 29.7334%? Can I taste the difference between 31% and 28% ginger? More importantly, am I willing to pay extra to help cover the cost of the more expensive industrial machinery required to measure that precisely? No.

I consider my own inability to comprehend large numbers to be advantageous. Many people don't understand that they don't understand the difference between a billion and a trillion (regardless of whether they're American or British). Perhaps this is why they keep buying lottery tickets.

Popular culture tells us that remote possibilities are in fact near certainties. A common theme has the down-on-his-luck hero walking into a casino and staking his last few coins in a 'one chance, last chance' attempt to gain enough winnings to overcome his opponents. In how many of these films does the hero *lose*? Paradoxically, overcoming the odds is *de rigeur* in movieland.

The probability of success doesn't even have to be minuscule. The overly emotional and frightened android C3PO, in the Star Wars movie 'The Empire Strikes Back', informs Captain Solo as their spaceship approaches an asteroid field, hotly pursued by the evil empire, that 'The possibility of successfully navigating an asteroid field is approximately 3720 to 1!' What does this figure mean? Several thousand and some isn't a huge number, but, for all real-world events, the chance against survival is (appropriately) astronomical. Yet they take the chance (wouldn't you, with the stormtroopers on your tail?) and do indeed survive unscathed.

DNA fingerprinting

A very interesting 'big numbers' debate, and relevant because of the DNA connection, is the evidence presented on DNA fingerprinting during the O. J. Simpson criminal murder trial in 1995. This one episode did more to teach genetics to the populace than any other single event in history. The arguments presented by the prosecution and the defence during this phase of the trial hinged on large numbers. Mr Simpson's DNA was compared with DNA from samples found at the crime site. The premise is that the sequence of DNA is unique to each person; no two people share exactly the same DNA base sequence (except identical twins).

In DNA fingerprinting (for which there are several different methods and procedures, all founded on a base sequence of portions of DNA of a given sample), certain regions of the genome are identified and compared with the same regions of DNA from other people, and from groups of people. Just as certain blood types are prevalent in people of certain human races, the DNA base sequences in these identified regions are more or less prevalent among certain races or groups of people. A specific short stretch of DNA may be very similar among all people (**highly conserved** is the technical term). Such a sequence would have limited probative value as evidence; if a suspect were found to have such a sequence, it would only indicate his or her companionship with most or many other people on Earth. A different region of the genome might have sequence variation, such that certain sequences are common among a particular race, yet rare in other races. This situation would be similar to our common ABO blood typing, where having a blood type of 'O' indicates, but does not prove, that you are white, as 'O' is the most common blood type for white people yet is also common in other races.

Statistical prevalence in DNA fingerprinting raises interesting hypothetical questions. If the crime scene sample DNA fingerprint for this one region was present in, say, one in one hundred men, and the primary suspect also had this sequence, would that be enough to convict? What if the sequence was then found to be relatively common among women? Should we set the male suspect free and search for a woman instead? What if the sequence was rare in the general population, but more common among people of the suspect's race?

DNA fingerprinting consists of analysing many sites on the genome in order to minimize the effects of statistical errors. But how do they come up with the figure that the suspect's DNA fingerprint would only occur in one person out of 10 billion (give or take a few billion), knowing there aren't (yet) 10 billion people on Earth? They look at the relative frequency of the sequence at each tested region of the suspect's DNA. If the base sequence at the first site is common to 1 in 10 people, and the sequence at the second is present in 1 in 10 000, then overall the incidence is likely to be (frequency at first site, 10, multiplied by the frequency at second site, 10 000) one in 100 000. Each additional site frequency multiplies, eventually generating astronomical figures. If the third site sequence is common to 1 in 1000 people, the figure becomes $10 \times 10\,000 \times 1000$, or 1 in 100 000 000 might be expected to share all three-region DNA base sequences. Arguments on these figures centre around the commonality of each individual region of the genome tested. For example, since the frequency of a particular DNA sequence at a given site often varies according to race, perhaps the calculation for the suspect should be based on his or her race, making the incidence not 1 in 10 000 but perhaps 1 in 1000, thus reducing the likelihood that this suspect is guilty. Other arguments can hinge on accepted frequency values, particularly for a given racial group. Perhaps not enough samples of DNA sequence data have been collected for a particular region of the genome to be confident that a sequence has a certain frequency. The defence is easy: if any sequence of the suspect's DNA does not correspond to the sequence in the same region of the DNA from the crime scene, the defendant is not guilty.

What is surprising is that the defence lawyers argue 'it's a one in a billion chance' versus the prosecution's 'one in ten billion chance' that the suspect's DNA was not the same as that found at the crime scene. Well, I suppose it's not that surprising. They have to argue something to try to get their client off. And it often works. It is ludicrous to be disputing these numbers. Even if it were one chance in a billion that it was someone else's DNA left at the crime scene, is that not enough to conclude the suspect's DNA and the crime scene sample DNA are the same? Of course, that does not by itself prove the suspect guilty. The sample might have been illegally planted (as alleged by the Simpson defence), for example, but it could *not* have been mixed with the real perpetrator's blood at the scene, because the blended DNA would give a pattern different from the suspect's and he (or she) would be freed. But many people remain convinced that a 'one in a billion' chance is a near certainty.

So it's not surprising that so many people are led to believe they comprehend big numbers. Now try cutting that pie into 100 thousand equal pieces.

An infinite number of monkeys . . .

There is great fun in debates about infinities such as 'If an infinite number of monkeys sat an infinite number of typewriters, eventually they would type out the Bible, or Shakespeare, etc.' What is the risk our belief system will be shaken or shattered by the knowledge that some primates pounded out the Bible? What are the chances? The answer, of course, is that there is zero chance; it is a certainty.

Look at it this way: consider one monkey (let's call him Mike) at one typewriter, simplified to have 26 keys, one for each letter of our alphabet. Also, let's for now ignore upper and lower case; we can add that condition later, if we wish, in an infinite time period. Mike types one key. If his selection is truly random, he has a 1 in 26 chance of getting the right letter. Let's wait until he hits the correct key, an 'I' (for the King James version of the Bible, starting 'In the beginning . . .'). Forget about all the previous events where he hit something else. Now, go onto the next letter; we're looking for an 'n' to complete the first word, 'In'. Again the chances are 1 in 26. After waiting a few more hits, we should discover he has 'In'. So, to get the first word would take approximately 26×26, or 676 two-stroke events. (Of course, we have to say approximately because this is a random series. He might have got lucky and hit 'I' on the first or second strike, then gone on to hit 'n' quickly also.)

A critical question is 'How long did it take to hit 676 two-stroke events?' Some of you might say, 'OK, let's assume Mike hits a key once per second. That makes 676 seconds, or about 11 minutes before we get the first word'. Perhaps, but in reality it doesn't matter, as we have no time limit. Whether it takes 11 minutes or 11 centuries is immaterial. The point is, eventually we will achieve the two-stroke combination 'In'. The next letter, 't' will come along eventually also, then the 'h'. There are 3 566 480 letters in the King James version of the Bible, so the number of events will be $26 \times 26 \times 26$ . . . for 3 566 480 times, until all the letters have been keyed in the correct order. That's a lot of events, but without a time limit, eventually it must occur.

What is infinity? Whether number or time, it means we are not constrained by usual earthly limits. We can play with the monkeys again, this time having an infinite number of them, each with a typewriter. In that situation, we don't need to consider the infinity of time. In fact, we can even set a time limit, say the time it takes for one monkey to hit one key. We will get the Bible typed out by looking for a sequence of monkeys, where the first in the sequence has used his single stroke to result in a 'I', the next hits a 'n' and so on. We would probably have to look at a huge number of such sequences, but there is no limit to the number of monkeys, remember?

Now, we can add back the other conditions, such as case and punctuation—go ahead, it makes no difference to the final result, all it does is increase the number of monkey sequences we have to inspect before finding the correct sequence of letters combined with the correct punctuation.

The relevance of this monkey business to our discussion of risk assessment of GMOs is this: Typical risk assessment is an analysis of chance, the likelihood of an event occurring. The monkeys illustrate that some chance events, as they approach infinity, cease being probabilities (or improbabilities) and instead become near certainties. An example is the chance of gene escape from a culti-vated GM rapeseed. As we'll see later, gene escape is beyond practical probability, it is a virtual certainty. The primates also illustrate another aspect of risk assess-ment. We've seen it doesn't matter to the result if one monkey pounds the keys for an infinite amount of time or if an infinite number of monkeys each strike the keys once. When conducting GM assessments, we could test a GMO on a small population or area over a long period of time (the 'long term'), or we could test the GMO on millions of people or acres over a few years. Although the approaches differ, both provide a substantial amount of data on health, safety, and environmental effects.

CHAPTER 8

'More wine, sir?': the role of science in regulation

- What are regulations intended to achieve?
- Are there regulations covering GMOs?
- What is effective regulatory scrutiny?
- What is 'substantial equivalence'?
- What is the 'precautionary principle'?
- What is the 'scientific method'?
- What are 'controls'?
- But shouldn't we consider the ethical questions?
- What about socio-economic considerations?
- How do countries differ in their regulatory approach?
- Doesn't anyone listen to the consumer?

Paving the road to hell: the purpose of regulations

What is the purpose of regulations? Most of us believe they protect the public by prohibiting inferior, unsafe, or otherwise harmful products. Most regulations achieve this. Some don't.

Sometimes politicians make regulations to show the public 'something is being done regarding a new threat to our society'. In 1989, Edwina Currie, the UK health minister, stunned the public by announcing that eggs and chickens carried *Salmonella* (actually, about one egg in 650 was infected with the nasty bacteria). Consumers stopped buying and farmers were understandably distressed. Currie resigned from the Cabinet in the ensuing hysteria. The bureaucracy hastily implemented several *Salmonella* control programmes, at substantial public expense. They changed the regulations governing battery hygiene and processing, resulting in millions of hens being slaughtered. Despite these costly measures, ten years later the incidence of *Salmonella* in UK eggs remains about one in 650–700, indicating a near-zero correlation between the problem and the bureaucratic response. Ordinarily, a problem arises first, and a solution follows.

Here, however, the political solution seemed unrelated to the scientific problem, indicating that Currie's political nightmare was no ordinary chicken and egg conundrum.

Based on this and other examples we have reason to suspect that at least some current regulations were designed and implemented simply to show the public 'something was being done regarding the threat to society' and that 'your government has the situation under control'.

Are GMOs regulated prior to commercialization?

Critics claim that GMOs are placed on the market quickly, with little or no regulatory scrutiny. According to the argument, any health safety or environmental assessments of GMOs are superficial and too hasty to be properly evaluated. Let's now consider the scientific basis of environmental and health safety risk and how GMOs are evaluated. We also follow the history of regulatory scrutiny of a real-life example, CDC Triffid, a GM linseed in international commerce. Since the assessments are scientific analyses of various forms of hazard, we start with the foundation: risk.

Two basic concerns with GM products

Earlier we noted two major sets of scientific concerns with GM products:

1 they might devastate our environment
2 they might poison us.

Consumers rightly demand reasonable assurances of both environmental and food/feed safety of new products. We depend on our governments to adequately, even vigorously, assess new products prior to commercialization. All jurisdictions claim their regulations are 'science-based'. But by what scientific means are new products judged?

Points of comparison

Regulators compare new products, not only GMOs but new pharmaceuticals, industrial chemicals, and food processing methods, with the most closely related conventional version possible. This gives a standard, a point of comparison to make measurements of similarity and dissimilarity. If the new product is similar to the standard for various important health and environmental characteristics, it is said to be **substantially equivalent** and poses risks similar to the conventional standard. If the standard version is considered 'safe', then the new version is also likely to be 'safe' and permitted on the market.

GMOs cannot be evaluated as absolutes; they need to be compared with some existing standard. When considering GM maize rendered insect-resistant by the insertion of a *B.t.* gene, regulators look at the parental variety of maize plus the conventional means of insect control in the crop. Legitimate questions of environmental and health safety are based on the differences between the conventional parent organism and the GMO. If, for example, the original or parent tomato is acceptable in the environment and in food, how did the modification change the tomato? What are the similarities, and what are the differences? Such an evaluation leads us to the concept of 'substantial equivalence'.

The concept of substantial equivalence is difficult for many people. It means, simply, when evaluating a novel product, you should compare it with similar but conventional counterpart products. Without a relative comparison, you have to evaluate based on absolute criteria, and we have none of those. For example, in evaluating Monsanto's Roundup™ resistant rapeseed, data are collected on the novel variety and on conventional rapeseed varieties currently in commercial production. In the comparison evaluation, the two varieties are said to be 'substantially equivalent' if all measured parameters—agronomic, environmental, health safety—seem equivalent. The chemical composition is similar, the yield is similar, disease resistance or susceptibility is similar, plant height, time to mature, oil content and quality, and so on are all similar, and the only difference is that one variety is resistant to a dose of the Roundup™ herbicide.

Other GM products are even easier to compare. A batch of maize oil can be analysed in any of many ways. A batch of GM maize oil can be analysed in the same ways. The two products should be indistinguishable from each other, substantially equivalent, regardless of the tests conducted. That is, there should be no way to ascertain that one batch came from GMOs and the other from conventional plants. If there is, they are not substantially equivalent. Cheese made from GM microbes, and sugar from GM sugar beet, are similarly 'substantially equivalent' to their respective conventional counterparts. If you can detect a difference, the product needs to be scrutinized further and perhaps discarded.

In addition, scrutiny is applied to the gene and gene product in the novel variety to ensure they present no health concern. According to the theory, if the conventional variety is safe for human consumption, then the novel one is also almost certainly safe.

Substantial equivalence is widely accepted internationally as a legitimate means to evaluate new products. It runs into opposition when people reject the underlying assumption that conventional products are safe. They argue, for instance, if the conventional variety is unsafe, then a substantially equivalent novel (GM) variety will also be unsafe.

Dr Pusztai invoked substantial equivalence in his GM potato project to reject his own subsequent interpretations. He noted that the nutritional composition of the GM potatoes was not 'substantially equivalent' to regular potatoes, and he questioned the validity of any subsequent results. With differences in major nutrients, he could not determine if the results were attributable to the GM or the originating differences in nutrient composition. In a properly designed experiment, we compare GM potatoes with potatoes identical in every respect other than the GM gene and its product.

Risk assessments

The precautionary principle

The principle of precaution, often waved as a banner of common sense, is not always what it seems. According to the principle, when you have a new product or technology, you assume you cannot predict exactly what will happen in every circumstance. Instead, you recognize there will be 'unexpected results'. You conduct a full scientific assessment of everything that might go wrong before allowing the product or process out into the world and marketplace. You do not give it the benefit of the doubt, where you might with a product of a traditional process. You remain prudent until satisfied the product or process is safe, or at least until satisfied you've identified the risks and can manage them.

At the same time, you make predictions of how the new product will behave, and you then check to see if it follows the predicted pattern. If it doesn't, you need to determine why it didn't and re-evaluate. If you insert a herbicide resistance gene into maize, for example, you predict the maize will acquire the new trait. You expose the GM plants, along with some conventional maize to serve as controls, to the relevant herbicide and observe the results. If the GM plants survive while the conventional ones die, the prediction is fulfilled.

The precautionary principle does not mean we assume the 'unexpected result' will be catastrophic, nor does it imply we wait until something goes wrong with the product or process before conducting tests and making decisions. We cannot arbitrarily demand as many scientific tests as we have or can think of. It is not scientifically valid to require a scientific analysis of an arbitrary parameter. Nor can we legitimately demand an answer to every conceivable problem that might be conjured up.

Instead, the precautionary principle is best applied in an aggressive, active fashion, where we consider the nature of the novelty in the product or process and base our investigations of logical assessments on those. We need a basis to investigate, a hypothesis to test. We start by establishing what we are going to scrutinize and why it is important to scrutinize it. We predict that a fungal disease resistance gene in a GM tomato will protect the tomato plants from the relevant fungal pathogen, so obviously we need to conduct tests to ensure that is the case and that it offers protection at a commercial level, one of interest to farmers. Prudence dictates we also test using other fungi to see if there is some effect on related organisms. But there is no need to test these other organisms if the transferred gene is designed not for fungal disease resistance but to delay ripening in the tomato. There is no scientific justification for conducting such tests.

I believe we've reached the stage of satisfying the precautionary principle with the GM process. The model of the GM process has been constructed with all of the results of thousands of experiments over twenty-five years. No fundamentally unusual, unpredicted, or unexpected results have emanated from the GM process.

I do not believe we yet have the same degree of confidence with all products of the technology. What's the difference between the model for the process and the models for the products? Let's explore.

The scientific method

Although often cited as 'the scientific method', as if there's only one, the number of acceptable scientific methods is probably unlimited. Many, many books discuss this, but in essence they all teach there is no one, true 'method' to follow for every scientifically valid procedure. Similarly, a scientifically valid procedure to test one hypothesis is not necessarily valid or even proper to test another. A light microscope is a wonderful instrument providing a multitude of scientifically valid and useful information. However, it doesn't tell us much about, for example, the fine structure of DNA. Using a scientific instrument or process does not necessarily make the interpretations of results valid. Any given scientific question can often be addressed in any of several acceptable ways. Conversely, there are many scientifically valid procedures inappropriate for or irrelevant in answering any given question.

However, all orthodox scientific methods have features in common. The most important is the controlled experiment.

The controls in a controlled experiment

Why do scientists make such a fuss over controls? What is a 'control'? Why do we need them? The scientific method dictates we have **controls** and **replicates** (or repeats). The justifications are several and compelling. A single experiment is not conclusive or convincing, because of the scientific phenomenon known in technical jargon as a 'fluke' result. We discount the possibility that a given result was a fluke only through repeats and controls. Another reason necessitating repeated experiments is the ubiquitous 'mistake'. We all make mistakes. We write the wrong word on a chart. We put the wrong data point in the box. We type the wrong information into the computer. Unaware of the mistake, we later look at the printout and see something remarkable—an unusual, unexpected, or unpredicted result. This event invariably causes great excitement in scientists, regardless of the gravity of the spurious interpretation, good or bad. The experienced scientist contains the excitement while checking to ensure no mistakes are apparent. The experiment is repeated with conditions duplicated as closely as possible to the original. If the same unexpected result arises, a colleague is asked to go over the results with an 'independent critical eye', to perhaps find alternative explanations for the result. The experiment may be repeated several times in order to verify the result. If, after a suitable number of tests and re-tests the unusual result remains, the scientific team may write a manuscript detailing the result. If the scientific team is in a private company, the manuscript is sent upstairs for review by the scientific management and/or the legal department for possible intellectual property protection proceedings.

A fundamental requirement in a valid experiment is to 'control' for each parameter or variable. In essence, this means you investigate only one factor at a time. The Showa Denko L-tryptophan tragedy involved more than one factor: they changed two things at once, the strain of bacteria and also the purification process. When people became ill, no one knew where to focus attention: was the problem with the bacteria, the purification, or perhaps some interaction between the two factors? If they had changed only one factor at a time, focusing on the single factor would have saved much time, money, and effort. And perhaps lives.

No small potatoes: the importance of experimental controls

Dr Pusztai at the Rowett Institute provides another example of the trouble we can get into when trying to cut corners. Shortly after appearing on TV to tell the world of his findings, he was drawn and quartered by his employers. In an effort to defend himself, Dr Pusztai posted his version of the experiments and data on the web, appended as an 'alternate' report to the official Rowett Institute web page (*http://www.rri.sari.ac.uk/press/*). Because of the public confusion and sometimes contradictory information emanating from Dr Pusztai and the Rowett Institute, the Royal Society conducted a thorough and comprehensive analysis of the incident, eventually publishing the report on their website (*http://www.royalsoc.ac.uk*). The Royal Society sent a set of 'all available' data and documents to six impartial reviewers with combined expertise in statistical analysis, physiology, nutrition, genetics, immunology, and clinical trials. The reviewers and the panel from the Royal Society concluded the research was faulty because:

- the experiments were poorly designed; the nutritional comparability of the GM and non-GM potatoes was uncertain
- different diets were enriched without adequate controls
- too few rats were tested and were given non-standard control diets

- data analysis was improper and there was a failure to account for inconsistencies in results between experiments.

Overall, the Royal Society cautions the work is '. . . flawed in many aspects of design, execution and analysis and that no conclusions should be drawn from it.' They conclude 'We found no convincing evidence of adverse effects from GM potatoes'. In effect, they said Dr Pusztai's experiments lacked the appropriate controls and replications to draw any conclusions. The stated objective of Dr Pusztai's experiments was to determine the effect of feeding GM potatoes to rats, but the experimental design did not allow that objective to be addressed because there were no suitable controls.

For example, the GM potatoes and their respective non-GM parent potatoes were analysed raw, boiled, and baked. This is an important point, because potatoes are normally eaten after cooking. Cooking destroys many common food toxins, and the background data provided by Dr Pusztai shows this for the GM lectin. Raw GM potatoes have between 12 and 25 micrograms of lectin per gram of potato, boiled potatoes less than 5 micrograms per gram, and baked potatoes less than 0.1 micrograms per gram. These values vary according to the specific line of potato and where the crop was grown. Ordinary potatoes, of course, have no GNA lectins (the kind added to the potatoes in the experiments), but they do normally produce their own potato lectins and other anti-nutritional factors. Dr Pusztai also provided some of the data on other nutrient composition. Unfortunately, only some of the measurements were recorded. Dr Pusztai's team neglected to compile some of the compositional data, particularly on the baked, non-GM parent potatoes. No meaningful comparisons can be made without these baked non-GM controls measured in the same way as the experimental group. Without this control, the results can only be described as half-baked.

The experimental treatments included regular potatoes, regular potatoes spiked with additional lectin, and lectin-producing GM potatoes. How hard would it have been to include a group of rats fed on a diet of potatoes genetically modified with non-functional DNA? Even with this additional treatment, though, the experiment would have to be repeated several times to generate meaningful valid data. Any indication that the problem was due to the GM would later have to be specifically challenged. If only one benign GM potato line was used, we wouldn't know if the problem was due to the GM process or, perhaps, the nature of that one GM line. Perhaps the introduced DNA had been inserted into the recipient potato DNA in such a way as to interfere with normal potato functions. Alternatively, perhaps that original potato line happened to be an off-type, or a spontaneous mutant. Another alternate explanation might be that the GM potato caused problems because of somaclonal variation (SCV) occurring during the transformation process, as is known to occur irregularly. This possibility was raised by Dr Pusztai himself, but he seemed to forget it when he drew his conclusions. In order to validly control for these factors, several different lines of GM potato would have to undergo feeding trials, but only if there was an indication the GM process itself was at fault, which there wasn't. At best, his controls seemed more appropriate for assessing the effects of lectin on rats, but even that was questioned and rejected.

Non-scientific considerations

Most risk assessments concentrate on health safety of the GMO—asking what are the potential hazards to human and animal health—and to environmental safety—asking the environmental impact and potential hazards to the environment. Both of these domains are well established and suitable for scientific analysis and assessment.

Other concerns are less well suited to scientific analyses. The ethical component, for one. Just because we can genetically modify something, ought we? Is it morally or ethically acceptable to insert a copy of a gene from one organism into another? Interesting as such questions are, they are not subject to scientific scrutiny. However, to debate ethical and other components requires factual, often scientific, background. Ethicists try to collect as much factual material as possible before engaging in a debate, as they have no desire to build an argument on factual errors or misunderstanding.

An excellent example is the report of the Nuffield Council on Bioethics. This group of distinguished scholars took the time to gather the scientific data relevant to ethical issues in biotechnology prior to debating the ethical issues. Their report, entitled *Genetically modified crops: the ethical and social issues* is a testament to common sense. Although it is written from a British perspective, the issues and arguments are relevant to everyone. They astutely expose the 'pseudo-science' behind many of what they call 'the alarmist media reports' and urge an informed public debate on the issues. Among other points, the Council report concludes, 'There are calls for bans on GM food and moratoria on GM plantings. We do not believe there is evidence of harm to justify such action.' Best of all, the report, all interesting reading, is freely available on the Internet (*http://www.nuffield.org/bioethics/publication/pub0010805.html*)

Socio-economic considerations

Some people demand GMOs be evaluated according to 'socio-economic considerations' before being allowed into the marketplace. Socio-economic considerations are under discussion at the Convention on Biological Diversity (CBD), the international group charged with developing a protocol for world-wide trade in GM products. There are legitimate socio-economic issues, but they are not in the realm of scientific discourse. Scientific evaluation of GMOs for socio-economic parameters was discussed but rejected by CBD delegates from the USA, Canada, and elsewhere, but is still on the table in many jurisdictions as regulators and negotiators grapple with the implications. One argument is that subsistence farmers in poor countries will suffer as GM technology appears to benefit mainly developed countries. For example, with genetic modification to and market domination by vegetable oils from the northern temperate zone (e.g. maize, rapeseed), traditional markets for oil products such as palm oil and coconut oil, grown mainly in poorer tropical countries, will diminish. Some delegates demand we take into account the socio-economic implications for the farming communities of these countries before allowing any GMO on to the international market. Simple economics (if there is such a thing) of supply and demand teaches that an increase in supply relative to demand of a commodity will result in a reduction in price. GM promises to increase the supply of vegetable oil, so the value of oil in general will drop. According to some, if it appears that GM oil will result in any market or income loss to the traditional producers of palm oil or coconut oil, either the GM oilseed must be disallowed or else the traditional producers must be compensated.

Beyond the economic implications, what about health issues? What if it turns out that the tropical product is less healthy than the GM product? Palm and coconut oils are high in unhealthy saturated fats. We demand health safety evaluations for GM products, with a view to excluding them from the market if they are less safe than traditional products. Is it not hypocritical to accept traditional products if we discover they are less healthy than GM products? We appear to include socio-economic consideration when regulating GMOs, but not when dealing with general health issues. In any case, it is not scientifically valid to consider socio-economic parameters in what is supposed to be a 'science-based' environmental risk assessment. The issues are too disparate and complex to evaluate together.

This is not to suggest these other considerations are not important components in the overall discussions of the risks and benefits of GMOs. Socio-economic aspects may well be important in the global debate, and ought to be discussed in a suitable forum. But they negate the credibility of any claim of 'science-based' procedures when they are inserted into the 'scientific' risk assessment.

Different definitions

Each jurisdiction has the sovereign right to regulate products in the manner best suited to satisfy the local political and natural environment. A problem arises when incompatible regulations intersect in international trade. Different countries have different concerns over food products and their domestic regulations reflect those differing priorities. With international trade in gross commodities, harmonization or at least compatibility in regulations is necessary to avoid substantial cost increases and confusion over safety.

It is possible to have compatible regulatory milieus while still respecting national priorities, as we have for so many commodities in international commerce. We could start with similar definitions for food products. GMOs are defined differently in different jurisdictions (see Chapter 1). Most countries use a single criterion: any product of rDNA technology. Others are less restrictive, focusing on the nature of the product. Considering that a food product poses the same degree of health hazard to people everywhere, it seems incongruous that in one country the product may be subject to no additional scrutiny, whereas in another country it is denied access to the market.

Going to market: Getting a GMO approved internationally

Regulators in different jurisdictions, and even in different departments in the same jurisdiction, can hold divergent attitudes. However, the real concerns remain the same. Legitimate food safety issues don't change from place to place, but attitudes do. Most regulations covering GMOs do require answers to appropriate and critical questions; the diversity becomes most evident in the extraneous requirements. One thing all regulators have in common: they all claim to apply 'scientifically valid' evaluation criteria to products of GM technology. The approach to applying the scientific assessment can vary substantially, though, and the attitude of regulators is a critical factor in determining the perspective. Although my experience is limited to a tiny sample from three jurisdictions, differences in regulatory attitude were evident.

To illustrate the pathway of what is an undeniably tedious process, we can conveniently use our GM linseed, CDC Triffid, and take up from where we left off in Chapter 4. At that point, you might recall, CDC Triffid had completed the approval process for variety registration and commercial release as a new crop variety. However, the launch was delayed because Triffid, having a 'novel trait', required additional regulatory scrutiny.

Canada

Canada is unique in that it regulates novel organisms on the basis of product novelty as opposed to process. During the early years of regulatory development, the Canadian bureaucracy accepted the argument that, while some GMOs might be hazardous, so might some conventional products. The hazard is related not to the method of production, but to the trait. It would be a mistake to single out the GMOs for special regulatory scrutiny while exempting the potentially hazardous other products with new traits. By the same argument, a benign GMO with traits similar to existing products would be exempt from the additional regulatory burden. Sounds good in theory, but practice is more difficult.

For products of conventional technology, we cannot fulfil the data requirements intended for GMOs. Scientists have no idea of the exact genetic changes in a 'conventional' mutation, so, in practice, different standards are applied for those mutated varieties. Scrutiny of a mutant variety is much simpler than for a GMO with a similar novel trait. Indeed, the Canadian regulations are more stringent for GMOs than for conventional products, but capture many still conventional products that are exempt elsewhere, such as Pioneer's Smart canola.

Canada: variety registration
After approval for variety registration is received, the Canadian Food Inspection Agency (CFIA), an arm of the federal agriculture department (AAFC), administers the paperwork. In addition to the results of the vote of the competent authority recommending committee, the breeder provides a sample of seed and a proposed name, along with a description. The bureaucrats ensure the variety name is appropriate and not already taken or likely to cause confusion. They inspect the seed sample to ensure it is clean and matches the description provided. If all is in order, they eventually issue the certificate of registration in the name of the agriculture minister. The process takes anywhere from six weeks to several months.

When the annual meetings conclude, newly approved candidate varieties are treated as if registered, with the formal certificate pending. The approved varieties are traded freely. Seed can be purchased, and marketing arrangements are made in anticipation of completion of the formality of certificate issuance. The University of Saskatchewan does not market its own varieties. Typically, new candidate varieties are put up for tender, with seed marketing companies bidding on each variety.

Triffid had several bidders, including one of the largest seed companies and some of the smallest. An 'arm's length' committee considered the bids and eventually awarded the marketing rights to Value Added Seeds, Inc. (VAS), a small local seed company operated by a group of cooperative farmers. In addition to buying the rights to market the variety, they also bought the actual seed. This transaction in 1994 marked one of the first commercial exchanges of GM seed. VAS arranged for their farmers to grow a seed increase of Triffid for the summer of 1994, blissfully unaware of the difficulties that lay ahead. When Triffid received its approval for registration from the official registration committee in February 1994, Canada still had not finalized its regulations dealing with GMOs, so Triffid had to await these new regulations prior to full commercial release.

Canada: environment
The Variety Registration Office (VRO), housed in what is now the CFIA, felt they could regulate crops developed using GM technology, despite being understaffed

to efficiently deal even with conventional variety registration. A commonly expressed opinion was that GM was a flash in the pan, a fad, and would be passé in a few years, so there might only be one or two such applications. This attitude started with the applications for confined release of GM plants in field trials in 1988, when there were 14 applications for field trials. However, the number grew quickly over the years. In 1998, there were 191 applications for 515 trials. It became apparent that this technology was not as ephemeral as some had predicted.

We characterized the inserted genes to satisfy the environmental review. One aspect was the likelihood of gene escape: outcrossing incidence, mechanisms of gene transfer in this species, flowering time, incidence of relatives capable of hybridizing, weediness of the plant or relatives, and so on. Most of the issues had already been addressed in the variety registration process.

The Agriculture and Agri-food Canada (AAFC) wrote a booklet on the natural biology of each of the major crop species undergoing GM development. Canola and flax (linseed) were the first, followed by maize, potato, soya bean, and wheat. These booklets, available from AAFC, describe the natural history of these species and serve as templates for comparison to use when evaluating the 'substantial equivalence' of GM varieties.

It took two years of negotiations, and a pile of public money, for AAFC to determine that the GM linseed was not significantly different from ordinary linseed. I was issued the letter allowing unrestricted environmental release and unlimited use as animal feed at the same time as my certificate of variety registration, in May 1996. It was a happy day. I could finally close the environmental file on Triffid. Figure 5 gives an indication of the amount of paperwork involved.

Industrial linseed for human food

Triffid was developed as an industrial crop, used to make linseed oil for paints, cricket bats, and so on, with the remaining meal (what's left of the seed after the oil has been squeezed out) fed to animals. However, linseed is now being promoted as a food crop, and some people do eat it, usually in very small amounts. I contacted Health Canada, the competent authority dealing with GM, and requested a food safety review for Triffid.

The regulatory people at Health Canada take a pragmatic approach in regulating food products. Health is too important to let politics interfere with a proper and science-based assessment of risks and hazards. An example of this is the scope of the product. Health officials wanted to know about dietary intake. If a food carries a potentially toxic compound (called an 'anti-nutritional substance'), they need to know how much is present, and how much people are likely to ingest.

- Is the food common, do the majority of people consume it regularly?
- How much is consumed on a daily basis?
- Is there a speciality consumption at particular times of year, such that a high concentration is consumed over a short period, then little for the remainder of the year?

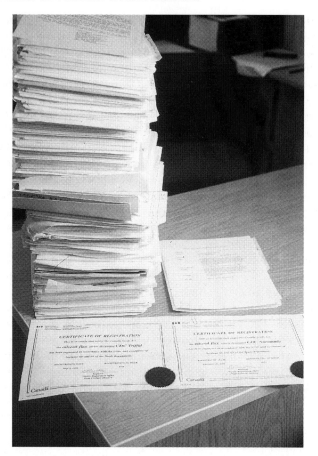

Figure 5   The documents necessary to support the registration of two linseed varieties. The pile on the left supported the application for CDC Triffid, shown with its registration certificate in front, which granted Canadian release only. The pile on the right supported CDC Normandy, with its certificate. The Normandy documents and certificate permit world-wide distribution, cultivation, and marketing.

- Is it a food popular with a particular ethnic group, demanding more intense scrutiny?
- Is it consumed more by children, who have special dietary considerations, or by pregnant women, also a special sub-group with legitimate need for special consideration?

These calculations are at the top of the priority list. Why spend the same amount of time and money assessing two products, one with minimal human consumption and no special dietary intake and one consumed by many people every day? Or comparing one product with a substantial amount of toxin and one with a minuscule amount of the same toxin? This dietary exposure approach to determining the degree of regulatory scrutiny is taken regardless of whether the product under scrutiny is GM or not. The agriculture assessment, on the other hand, seems more concerned with simple presence of a hazard, regardless of degree of risk. That is, if a stated hazard is presented in two GMOs, they receive the same degree of scrutiny regardless if one is a minor concern and the other a major concern.

It seemed like no time at all before the additional concerns were rectified and Health Canada sent a letter giving full human food clearance to Triffid linseed. As far as I know, this is the first linseed variety ever evaluated, let alone approved, as a human food. It seemed deliciously ironic that, although human consumption of linseed is primarily as 'health food' and organically grown varieties, the first linseed to be approved for human consumption was a GM variety.

With this approval, we had full regulatory clearance for the release of Triffid in Canada, encompassing variety registration, unrestricted environmental release, animal feed use, and human food use.

Linseed plants have pretty blue flowers so they have some commercial value as ornamentals (see Figure 6). With the unrestricted release approval, we started giving away sample seed in small envelopes to anyone interested who wanted to try growing Triffid in their gardens. I had a patch growing at home, and there are now hundreds of little garden patches of Triffid growing all over Canada. I also make it available to any teachers wishing to give students access to a real GMO.

Unfortunately, even with the full set of approvals, commodity farmers could not grow Triffid unless it was segregated from other linseed varieties. The majority of the Canadian linseed crop is exported, to Europe, to Japan, to the USA. None of these trading partners recognizes the GM evaluations by Canadian competent authorities (although there are now negotiations to improve harmonization with the US system); each jurisdiction conducts its own evaluation of each and every GMO. Because of the grain handling system, unsegregated GM linseed would end up blended with conventional linseed and exported. Triffid seed in grown in Canada was limited to domestic consumption, a very small market.

USA

The next step was to acquire approvals in the USA, our biggest trading partner and one from which our GM variety was attracting interest.

The Americans have the most experience with regulating GMOs and have the most clearly defined evaluation process coordinated across the different departments involved. All bureaucracies claim their regulations are 'science-based', but the American system comes closest to actualizing that ideal. The general attitude seems to be 'There may well be ethical, sociological, or political issues in regulating GMOs, but my office deals with the scientific data. Those other issues must be considered elsewhere.' The advantage to this attitude is that time can be spent on real scientific concerns.

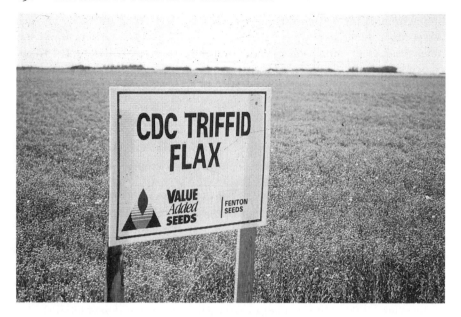

Figure 6   GM linseed flax growing unconfined in a farmer's field in Saskatchewan. The plants are just coming into flower. Fencing and protesters are conspicuous by their absence.

US Food and Drug Administration (FDA)

Variety registration in the USA is simple enough. There are no national trials or expert committees evaluating performance of candidate breeding lines. As with many products in America, the marketplace determines success or failure.

The US federal Department of Agriculture (USDA) regulates the importation of products of genetic engineering and, separately, the cultivation of genetically engineered crop cultivars to determine if they represent a risk of being plant or crop pest. The Federal Food and Drug Administration (FDA) regulates food products from GMOs in a voluntary fashion (which is 'voluntary' in much the same way that a murder suspect voluntarily assists police with their inquiries). The federal Environmental Protection Agency (EPA) regulates new pesticide uses in products of genetic engineering.

At this point, Value Added Seeds (VAS) had no interest in cultivating Triffid as a crop in the USA, but was interested in shipping Canadian-grown seed to crushing plants in the USA. This required an assessment and approval of the GM from the USDA. I called their office in Washington and asked what needed to be done. They told me to get FDA approval first, then call them back. I called the FDA and got that process going.

The FDA didn't want to see our actual data, they merely wanted to know that we conducted the experiments to compile the data, and that we interpreted the results as being benign. My interpretation of the FDA attitude could be summarized as:

You are going to get sued by somebody who eats your GMO and gets a headache or a hangnail. We will help you by ensuring you've conducted enough of your own assessments to be able to defend yourself from frivolous lawsuits. If you've forgotten to conduct an obvious test of risk, a victim's lawyer may use that lapse to show negligence and you stand a good chance of losing a petty suit in that situation.

I compiled the dossier for the FDA and submitted it. It was five pages long. After submitting dossiers consisting of hundred of pages to the AAFC, I was concerned that I had left out too much. I knew most of the documents submitted to the AAFC were either superfluous or meaningless, but five pages for something as important as human food safety in the USA seemed too little. I asked my contact if he thought it was too brief. He said, although it was short, considerably shorter than earlier submissions from others, it appeared to address all their concerns. A caseworker was assigned; she contacted me shortly after, introducing herself and acknowledging receipt of the dossier.

My caseworker studied the dossier and occasionally sent me questions, usually of clarification. None of these were novel or surprising, so I had no problem in providing the relevant answers. No question required my returning to the lab to conduct more or different tests. Eventually, my dossier was completed, and the FDA issued a letter, saying the 'voluntary consultation' was complete. Triffid was essentially approved for human consumption in the USA. Americans could eat Triffid, but were not allowed to grow it.

USA: USDA (marketing)
Within the USDA, the Animal and Plant Health Inspection Service (APHIS) regulates the introduction and cultivation of GM plant material in the USA. Once again I called USDA and asked what I needed to do to obtain regulatory approval to ship Triffid into the USA, not for cultivation but for marketing. They told me to send a letter asking approval for marketing Triffid in the USA, along with a copy of the letter I received from the FDA. I did. USDA sent me back a letter giving approval for marketing of Triffid in the USA.

This was the easiest regulatory approval I've ever obtained. The USDA explained that they have not seen any need to routinely scrutinize such GM products and it would be a waste of taxpayers' money to conduct unnecessary tests. If we were able to satisfy the health and safety concerns of their colleagues at the FDA, then that meant we had conducted enough of our own trials to provide assurance that we were aware of any problems that might arouse the interest of APHIS. I started thinking to myself that either regulators were becoming more sensible or I was getting better at negotiating approvals. In any case, I was now finished with my regulatory sojourn and might return to my lab. Triffid was approved for international trade, if only between Canada and the USA. It appeared to be the first GM product from a public institution cleared for international commerce.

My joy lasted about a week. John Allen, the manager of VAS, called and said they were getting considerable interest from US farmers wanting to grow Triffid.

I told John the recent USDA approval was limited to marketing, and that if he wanted to sell seed to US farmers, we'd have to seek another approval. Next day I called USDA again and advised them we were going to pursue cultivation approvals. They provided me with the information package I needed to complete and submit. Marketing is a very different business from cultivation. In marketing, the commodity is shipped in for processing. There are few real concerns about the product beyond the food and feed health safety aspects. Cultivation, on the other hand, necessitates environmental release. Many environmental questions arise that would be irrelevant to a food safety assessment. It would be inappropriate for USDA to rely on the FDA approval exclusively in granting approval for cultivation.

USA: USDA (cultivation)

The environmental risk assessment from USDA was another substantial document. However, it was clear and to the point. For the most part, the questions were limited to concerns of environmental safety. Since we had conducted the Canadian environmental assessment, we already had most of the questions answered and concerns addressed. The linseed growing area of the USA is adjacent to the Canadian border, and we had conducted trials with Triffid at several locations near those areas of the USA, so we had solid data easily applicable to the US environment. The legitimate environmental concerns had been addressed over the years of Triffid cultivation and so the data were available. It was a matter of putting the information into the format desired by USDA. Eventually, the file was complete and a notice published in the Federal Register. Two months later, in the absence of any public opposition comments, the application was approved.

There is no doubt that the US system was the easiest under which to obtain approvals for CDC Triffid. Of course, by the time Triffid went to US review, we had collected data to answer all the known legitimate health and environmental concerns. However, and especially with FDA, I was surprised when I was asked such questions as 'Do you have data on parameter X?' I would reply, 'Yes, I'll send it to you.' The reply was 'That's not necessary. As long as you have the appropriate data, we don't need to see it'. This means the reviewers didn't always review the data package relating to a particular issue. They did not actually 'approve' my data or my interpretation.

The USDA people are likewise pragmatic. They also have a well-developed regulatory machine that seems to run smoothly. Like the FDA, the questions asked of me were directly related to concerns and issues of science. I had no objection to any questions emanating from either the FDA or USDA.

Europe: the EU (stumbling) block

Most jurisdictions around the world, including the USA and Canada, developed their regulatory framework to deal with GMOs on a political level, largely independent of regulatory scrutiny in place for products of conventional breeding. In the European Union (EU), a GMO triggers regulation under Directive 90/220, which is primarily concerned with environmental assessment. The Directive is administered in the UK by the Department of the Environment, Transport and the Regions (DETR). European Commission (EC) Regulation 258/97 targets foodstuffs from GMOs, and is administered in the UK by the Ministry of Agriculture, Fisheries and Food (MAFF), at least until the responsibility is transferred to the new Food Standards Agency (FSA).

Proponents wishing to market GM products in the EU choose a member country to receive a dossier under the environmental regulations of 90/220/EEC. Although all countries adhere to the same legislation, there is regional variation in priorities and attitudes. In chatting with various people, I was given different advice on which member country should be the recipient of the GM linseed dossier. France and Belgium were suggested, in addition to the UK. The choice is important because the recipient country gets the first shot, and once the application is approved, that country is then responsible for negotiating it through the remainder of the European bureaucracy to achieve EU-wide approval. The applicant at that stage becomes simply a resource person, depending largely on the skills of the regulators of the recipient country to obtain the desired objective.

We ended up going to the UK for the simple reason that it appeared to have a reasonable regulatory protocol in place and we wouldn't have to translate any of the documents.

UK

The UK has a complex and comprehensive regulatory framework, which is completely different from that of, say, the USA. Regulators in the UK don't put much credence in US regulations or regulators. When I said my GM linseed had passed FDA and USDA scrutiny, various UK officials, including civil servants from the DETR and MAFF and academic advisory experts, stated emphatically that the American determinations didn't carry much weight in the UK. More than one even suggested I might omit the fact that we had US approvals from the UK application, implying that it might prejudice my case.

I noted a fair amount of enmity between MAFF in the UK and the US FDA, both agencies charged with similar responsibilities in food safety. The minutes of MAFF's advisory committee meeting on 24 September 1998 includes a reference to the FDA, but records it as the 'Food and Drink Agency' as if it were merely an industry support group.

A common attitude I encountered in the UK bureaucracy is that the FDA is in the pocket of the biotechnology industry, so it's not surprising FDA's approvals came so easily. One MAFF official told me 'We don't respect the FDA evaluations, as we're more rigorous and apply the precautionary principle. We don't want to be responsible for approving another thalidomide!' The irony of this attitude in

UK regulators is especially profound; some scientists at the FDA were suspicious of thalidomide from the beginning and refused to approve it. The drug was never marketed in the US because the FDA halted the approval.

The same people who denigrated the American regulatory system said the Canadian process was well respected and would carry considerable weight in the deliberations. I was surprised by the UK regulators' disdain for the US regulatory system.

UK: Environment

The DETR is responsible for administering the UK regulation of the EC Directive 90/220, a document hated by all GM proponents because of its unnecessarily complicated and often irrelevant requirements. When first preparing my application, I was filled with trepidation. My friends at AgrEvo and Monsanto who'd already filed under 90/220 told me it was huge and largely a waste of time, in that most of it had little bearing on the evaluation of real risk or hazard of the GM product. When I sent for the 90/220 document, I was informed it required my addressing only 36 points, suggesting it was a relatively straightforward matter. True, there were only 36 points, but adequately addressing them required hundreds of pages of data and supporting documents—far in excess of what was needed to satisfy US and Canadian officials.

The Advisory Committee on Releases to the Environment (ACRE) advises the DETR on the suitability of the data in the submission. Until recently, the committee was composed of a handful of the most capable scientists in the UK, with representation from industry and activist groups, but dominated by senior academics. This august group spends countless hours poring over the data for each submission, evaluating the results and suitability, and eventually passing judgement. If and when approved, the UK takes the dossier on behalf of the original applicant to Brussels for presentation to the Commission. Triffid is now caught in the *de facto* moratorium, along with a number of other applications, unlikely to be approved.

UK: MAFF

While dealing with the requirements for the environmental application under 90/220, I asked about food use. DETR make no determinations on human consumption, although they did require considerable information on nutritional composition and other aspects ordinarily related to food, as opposed to environmental, use. I was sent to talk with MAFF, who were responsible for evaluating GMOs as foodstuffs. Their responsibility is set to be moved to the new FSA, but Triffid's food safety dossier was compiled and sent to MAFF.

The UK maintains, under MAFF, an Advisory Committee on Novel Foods and Processes (ACNFP), which assesses novel foods in comparison with current foods, basing their judgement on the concept of substantial equivalence. ACNFP is an advisory committee composed of national experts, meeting regularly to deliberate on applications under the EC Novel Foods Regulation 258/97. When

ACNFP approves a particular application, the dossier forwarded to the Commission where it is distributed to other member states and evaluated further. MAFF (through ACNFP) is required to complete an initial safety assessment within 90 days. The ACNFP assessment is also sent to the Commission, where it is copied and sent to the other member states for their comments. Eventually, the product may be approved for human consumption throughout the European Union, but not before each member state gets a chance to object. Any objections from member states have to be made within 60 days, sending the consideration to the EC Standing Committee for Foodstuffs, who potentially consult the EC Scientific Committee for Food. If enough objections are raised, the matter may eventually be considered by the Council of Ministers. This time-frame suggests that applicants can expect no more than six months or so from submitting the initial dossier to MAFF to having complete EU marketing approval if no objections are raised. Few products are on this approved list, however.

The status quo

Triffid has been grown as a commercial seed crop since 1994, but only for seed increases and domestic use. Until we receive regulatory approvals for Triffid from European authorities, it will not enter the export stream. CDC Normandy, on the other hand, considered a 'conventional' variety, has been in international commerce for several years, even though, to my mind, it carries far more risk and has undergone far less scrutiny than Triffid. However, I see no concern in growing or eating either one.

Australia and New Zealand

Australia and New Zealand are somewhat behind North America and Europe in development of public policy. Australia is enjoying new markets in Europe for its rapeseed/canola, as it is the only country capable of guaranteeing non-GM production. Canada, the major producer of canola, no longer ships to Europe because half the Canadian canola crop is GM. However, GM canola is grown under trial in Australia *en route* to commercial release, so perhaps their fledgling EU market will be closed to them as well. Depending on the degree of contamination tolerated by Europe, it might be sooner, as GM pollen from the test lines will certainly have blown into commercial non-GM canola. At the same time, European regulators might recognize that the potential hazard associated with 'conventional' triazine-tolerant canola, which accounts for half the Australian crop, is at least as great as for GM herbicide-resistant rapeseed.

Food is regulated by a joint Australia–New Zealand committee on food safety. The primary concern there is with food and, unlike Europe in particular, it isn't so much food safety as food availability.

Public concerns are based mainly on labelling. The opposition groups are clamouring about all the GM foods already imported into Australia, and there are indeed many of them, mostly soya and maize products coming from the USA. Few, if any, of these products currently have GM labels, so political discussion centres around providing the labels so consumers can make their own decisions. Until recently, the debate, at both political and domestic level, has been subdued. The newspapers do not appear to have taken a particular position, but do report developments, both positive and negative. As in the media in other countries, it is not unusual to see a positive article applauding some GM research project at the local university destined to improve a locally grown commodity, across from another article arguing to ban all GM products. In general, the pragmatic Australians seem more concerned with what a ban might do to their food supply. The Brisbane *Courier Mail* headline of 10 March 1999 said it clearly: 'GM food ban will strip shelves'. Europeans, aghast at the number of products with GM ingredients on the shelves, are demanding at least labelling if not an outright ban. Australians and New Zealanders, faced with similar figures for GM foods, seem more concerned that a ban will eliminate many of their favourite food products from the shelves.

They also seem more confident in their regulatory structures than Europeans. In a Commonwealth Scientific and Industrial Research Organization (CSIRO) (Australia) survey released in April 1999, only 17% of Australians said they would be 'unwilling' to try GM foods, implying they were happy that the authorities would evaluate and not allow any clearly hazardous foodstuffs on to the market. Most Australians are willing to eat GM food if it provides an improved quality at the same price. The corollary to this is that people would buy GM products of the same quality as conventional ones if they were offered at a lower price.

It is somewhat surprising that the Australians have been so ready to accept GM food in the light of well-publicized concerns in Europe. The survey also noted, even emphasized the recognition by Australians that they are not as familiar with the technology as they would like to be, and would like more information on GM technology and its use in food production. Consumers in North America have an attitude generally similar to Australians, but benefit from several years of familiarity with GM products in the market with no major problems.

Smaller countries

What about imports of GMOs into small or isolated countries? Where do they get their soya, maize, or canola? Many countries lack the political and technical infrastructure to establish appropriate regulations, let alone conduct the molecular analyses needed for enforcement. Such countries are often satisfied to leave regulatory review to the exporting nation and accept the determinations of the originating country. The common attitude seems to be: 'If a certain kind of soya bean passes health safety review in the USA, and Americans eat it without problem, it is unlikely to harm our citizens, either.' Such countries defer regulatory functions back to the originating country. In this manner, many GMOs are in international trade already.

Although the governments (and citizens) of smaller countries might be satisfied with these provisions, what happens if the GM commodity is repackaged and re-exported to other nations with a regulatory infrastructure to deal with GMOs? With shipments from smaller countries, GMOs might slip through the system and into the marketplace unobserved and unregulated by the importing nation.

Consumer demand and acceptance

Most of the GM products are from big multinational companies such as Monsanto, Novartis, AgrEvo, and the like. None of these products to date addresses public demand; there is no 'pull' from the consumer to obtain these GM products. Instead, the novel features are of interest to the company because it will increase their sales of related products, such as their brand of pesticide. Or they are of interest to the farmer, who will enjoy increased pest control choices. Even the Flavr-Savr™ tomato, marketed as having longer shelf-life, and so of benefit to the consumer, was originally intended to benefit the processor, who could extend the harvest window time of the tomato crop.

An informal GM tomato taste test

I had the opportunity to visit Calgene (now owned by Monsanto) in Davis, California when Flavr-Savr™ was still in development. They kindly gave me a few of the special GM tomatoes to take home. When I arrived back in Saskatoon after smuggling the contraband through Customs, I went to my market and bought some regular tomatoes, then went to the lunchroom at work and set up an impromptu taste test. I cut the tomatoes into bite-size pieces and placed them in trays labelled simply as either 'Tomato cultivar no. 1' or 'Tomato cultivar no. 2', with a sheet asking people's opinions on several aspects of the different tomatoes, including appearance, taste, texture, and so on. Then I waited until the hordes descended for lunch. I wasn't concerned about any reluctance on the part of the unwitting subjects. Postgraduate students willingly eat anything offered for free.

Flavr-Savr™ won in only one category: appearance. It looked great. It was nice, big (even though it was cut into smallish pieces, you could tell it came from a large tomato), red, and mature. It didn't matter that it tasted like cardboard and so came a distant second in all other categories. Some people commented it was lucky to have come second. Tastes differ. American consumers like things big, and good looking. Even tomatoes. Consumers in the UK and, to a lesser extent, Canada, prefer tomatoes with more taste and texture; size and shape are of lesser import.

This was not a scientifically valid test. The sample size was too small (a few people) and not at all representative of the general population (students and faculty are hardly typical consumers). There was no control over what else the test subjects were eating at the time (eating a tomato with a chocolate peanut butter sandwich might skew the results). There were no replicates or repetitions of the trial because they ate everything in the first go. Nevertheless, it did provide some insight into the problems associated with Flavr-Savr™. And no one became ill or complained about eating GM DNA, even after I posted the results.

Another factor, though not evaluated by the *ad hoc* panel, was cost. I knew this would be a problem from the start. Just before Flavr-Savr™ hit the US market, I attended a conference in which a Calgene official gave a talk on the impending marketing release, saying it would be restricted to a couple of test markets first, including Calgene's home in Davis, California. He explained that the targeted market niche was in its 'fresh picked' taste, and that people would pay a premium to get that 'summertime flavour' in the winter. He said the cost would be about $2 per pound. Now, I live in Saskatoon, where nothing grows between September and May. Fresh tomatoes are at a premium throughout the winter, especially in January. We in Saskatchewan have our winter produce trucked in from California or Mexico and also have glasshouse production, primarily from British Columbia. Even in the height of winter, I paid only about $1 per pound for fresh tomatoes. This was going to have to be one terrific tomato for consumers to pay double when the competition, even the cardboardy winter imports, was a lot less expensive. Flavr-Savr™ wasn't a terrific tomato, and in fact, never made it to the Saskatoon market.

Flavr-Savr™ was the first whole-food GM product to enter the US marketplace. Despite the best efforts of some opposition activists to have it condemned, Flavr-Savr™ passed the regulatory reviews and was permitted to be placed on the supermarket shelves to be judged by ordinary consumers.

Consumers quickly discovered that whatever benefit they derived from Flavr-Savr™ wasn't worth the premium paid. No one was poisoned by Flavr-Savr™, and no environmental disasters befell the growing areas. Consumers were able to make a true choice to buy the product or not. They chose not to buy it. The marketplace was able to achieve what activists and regulations couldn't.

Risk assessment (revisited)

Every time you take a bite out of a tomato, you take a risk. Perhaps it has a spider in it. Perhaps it is GM for toxin production. Perhaps it has an excess of the natural tomato toxin, tomatine. What are the risks? Certainly we try to avoid risks where possible and to minimize those we can't. We depend on legislators to pass laws to these ends, but we must bear in mind that we cannot effectively legislate to preclude acts of lunatics or accidents of chance.

Overall, what are your chances of getting hit on the nose by an asteroid? Risk is a matter of everyday living. Genetic modification has been going on since the early 1970s. There are millions of acres of GM crops grown worldwide and the area is increasing rapidly. Tonnes of GM foods are consumed by humans each year. If we can detect a hazardous activity occurring with an adverse result frequency of one in six events (cigarette smoking—see p. 129), we'd be able to detect by now if GM was inherently hazardous.

Compared with similar products from conventional technologies, GMOs are highly regulated. Companies do not and cannot quickly generate a GMO and dump it on the market. Although each jurisdiction regulates GMOs somewhat differently, they all give intense scrutiny prior to allowing environmental and commercial release. Perhaps the opponents can argue the lack of *appropriate* regulatory evaluation, but the argument that there is 'little or no' regulatory scrutiny simply isn't true.

Particular GM products may carry unacceptable risks, but those are based on the nature of the product, not the process by which it was developed. That is, had the product been developed using conventional methods, it would present the same hazards. Let's focus on the risks associated with the product, not the process.

CHAPTER 9

Not on the table: the *really* scary stuff

- What should we be concerned about?
- Can GMO create new toxins or allergens?
- If a GMO is environmentally safe in one region, does that make it safe everywhere?
- What happened to the 'public' plant breeding effort?
- Do regulators always ask the right questions?
- Can't we just make the companies pay for all these tests and regulations?

Earlier, we exposed and discussed some common misconceptions of GM products and technology. Lest you now think there is nothing to be concerned about, let me now disabuse you of such thoughts. In this chapter I discuss some of the real and legitimate concerns. It is not an exhaustive listing, but there are legitimate issues that ought to be debated more fully.

When I talk with opponents of GM, I try to determine the underlying source of their concerns. Sometimes, it is a simple misunderstanding, like the fish gene in tomato, or the incorrect expectation that a GM plant really does look monstrous, part plant and part something else. Other times, it is a legitimate concern for safety, such as the inadvertent introduction of allergens into food. Most often, however, the underlying fundamental concern expressed by the activists is the domination of agriculture by 'big multinationals'.

When I discuss real concerns with regulators, I get different answers. Regulators are concerned with political interference in regulatory assessments. They are also more concerned with rising demands on their expertise and time while they face budget cuts. Oh, yes, they too are concerned with the domination of agriculture by the 'big multinationals'.

Academic scientists tend to be more concrete, focusing on explicit environmental issues, such as the management of *B.t.* or virus-resistant GM plants, or on specific health issues, such as the possible introduction of allergenic Brazil nut protein to soya bean.

There are indeed real concerns with GM, valid issues requiring serious debate and deliberation. Unfortunately, they tend to be obscured by the more attention-getting scare stories because they are more mundane and pedestrian scientific, management, or socio-political issues.

Novel allergenicity in GMOs

We've already seen legitimate concerns. Allergenic proteins in GM foods is one. Although Brazil nut storage proteins exist only in Brazil nuts, we have to screen GMOs vigilantly to ensure that novel genes do not make an allergenic protein. However, this does not always require complete feeding trials and allergenicity testing for every new GMO. Most allergens have common features and their allergenic properties and can be reliably predicted. Also, most genes being transferred are well documented as common genes and proteins occurring in food, so we already have a history of the gene and its protein in food uses. A non-allergenic protein in one food does not suddenly become allergenic in another food. Finally, a computer database of allergens and other substances of 'immunological interest' exists and is easily searched for comparative information on the transferred gene and its product. Although there's no guarantee, allergenic (or toxic) properties will surely be identified long before a GM product hits the market. Novel allergenicity remains a concern, but it's not something I lose sleep over because I have confidence any allergenic GMOs will be caught and eliminated long before they get near my kitchen.

Our knowledge of allergens and their characteristics not only provides a means of identifying and rejecting potential allergenic GMOs, it permits proactive targeting of natural allergens. We have the gene for the allergenic Brazil nut storage protein. We might turn that gene around and apply it to the Brazil nut tree to develop varieties lacking the allergenic protein. Perhaps we can do the same with allergens in peanuts, soya beans, wheat, or even fish and dairy products. Why not exploit our knowledge of molecular genetics to alleviate suffering? Because of my daughter's allergies, I know the anxiety of questioning every food item for the presence of nuts. The required vigilance is unrelenting. Kids at school share snacks ('Swap your chocolate bar for my broccoli and spinach tofu sandwich?'). Restaurant staff can be incredulous ('What's the big deal? It only contained little pieces of nuts. . . '). Even friends and relatives are not as diligent as they might be ('What? Marzipan is made with almonds?'). GM technology will not eliminate either the hazard or the anxiety, but could well reduce both substantially.

Keep in mind the presence of allergens (or toxins) is not limited to GM products—new conventional foods are also tested for elevated levels of naturally occurring undesirable substances. Prudence dictates we continue to monitor all new foods for the presence of undesirable components, regardless of their source.

Environmental release in different regions

GMOs undergo environmental assessments in countries where farmers intend to cultivate them. But every country, and every region of a country, has a different environment. An environmental assessment might conclude a GMO is environ-mentally benign and therefore allowed for cultivation in one place, but a similar assessment process in another region might come to a different conclusion for the same GMO. For instance, a canola (GM or conventional) may have no adverse environmental effect when grown in Canada, but wreak havoc when cul-tivated in the UK. Several different GM canola/rapeseed varieties have been approved and are grown over millions of acres in western Canada. Some GM canola lines are being considered for cultivation in the UK. We must account for different ecological features of different cultivation environments. Even more important, we must recognize that environmental release concerns are not lim-ited to GMOs.

The UK, with its unique natural as well as political environment, is probably not a suitable place to grow rapeseed, whether GM or conventional. The inten-sity of agriculture and the intimate relationship between wild and cultivated organisms in the UK presents a delicate environmental balance, perhaps more easily upset by the aggressive rapeseed *Brassica* species. Major rapeseed produc-ing countries include Australia, Argentina, and Canada, areas with huge open farmlands, often well segregated from natural wildlife areas and population cen-tres. The aggressive infiltration of escaping *Brassica* plants (GM or otherwise) into wild or natural environments is not a major problem in these areas. In the geographically compact UK, however, the environmental risks are greater. Renegade rapeseed need not travel very far to encroach and perhaps establish in previously native environments and wildlife populations.

In addition, *Brassica* pollen is allergenic. Many farmers and researchers develop hay fever working with oilseed rape. Growing the crops in close proxim-ity to population centres exacerbates urban suffering and widens any political rift between city and rural peoples. Is it really necessary to grow rapeseed in the UK? I recommend cultivation of even conventional, non-GM rapeseed in the UK be carefully re-evaluated. Many other countries produce canola/rapeseed, so market demand is easily satisfied from offshore production. However, the artificial sub-sidies, even if diminishing, make rapeseed an attractive option for UK farmers. It is interesting to speculate what would happen if the oilseed subsidies were removed, along with the stiff tariffs applied to rapeseed oil imports. In all likeli-hood, the UK farmer would return to growing more environmentally benign, less aggressive crops and the price of the oil in the market would not change dra-matically. UK consumers could reduce concern over GM rapeseed, as there would be little or no domestic cultivation of rapeseed, and market demand would be satisfied by imported oil (which, as we saw earlier, is DNA-free).

Another legitimate environmental concern comes from the new GM crops under development. New objectives include enhanced stress tolerance. When, say, a pesticide-resistant GM crop 'escapes' into the local wildlife, it usually dies out quickly. The GM attribute doesn't give it any particular advantage in the absence of the relevant pesticide. And since natural wildlife populations are not exposed to pesticides, the GM plant can't out-compete the wild residents.

However, give a crop plant the ability to withstand, say, a freezing cold snap—suddenly it acquires a valuable adaptive trait in areas where sudden cold snaps occur and cause damage to natural wild populations. If such a GM plant escapes the farmer's field and seeks refuge in the wild neighbourhood, it might establish itself if nature fortuitously clears some space by sending down a killer cold. With the local plants knocked out or off, the freeze-tolerant GM plant, which ordinarily wouldn't be able to compete with the wildlife, now has an advantage and exploits it. This is a real environmental issue we must consider and debate. Fortunately, we have a few years before seeing GM plants with such attributes. But they're coming.

Factory food: domination by big multinationals

Historically, public labs in agricultural research institutes and universities dominated plant and animal breeding. Government funding for such activities has declined dramatically in the past twenty years, and so private companies are becoming more prevalent. A major concern in the debate over GMOs is the apparent monopoly by private interests, particularly the 'big multinationals'. It is certainly true that the big companies have invested considerable resources into plant and animal breeding, and microbial manipulation. With the mergers and acquisitions in the private sector, there is legitimate concern about a few companies dominating the world food supply. Although the degree of domination by big companies in GM technology is often overstated, it remains an issue worth monitoring to ensure public institutions and smaller companies are not eliminated entirely.

It is ironic that the regulatory demands being placed on GMOs unwittingly assist the big companies in their domination, as few public institutions or small companies can afford to comply with the additional regulations. Because of the success by activists to establish the politically expedient (as opposed to the scientifically legitimate) regulatory regime in Europe, the GM playing field is left almost exclusively to those able to afford the fees: the big multinationals. Is this one of those 'unintended' or 'unexpected' effects we were warned about?

Sour grapes

Political intrigue

All bureaucracies have some excellent people who know what the real issues are but have to answer to political masters. Bureaucrats in all governments must toe the official line. Sometimes, government scientists 'go public' with information contrary to the political position of the government, resulting in considerable press activity. Unfortunately, that activity too often concentrates on the political ramifications of the 'leak' rather than on the merits, or demerits, of the scientist's concern. Government scientists, like their colleagues in the private sector, don't have the academic freedom enjoyed by university scientists to contradict their bosses. For one thing, it embarrasses the politicians. When the minister issues a position, the department ought not to release data showing the minister to be a fool. The minister is quite capable of that on his or her own. Second, and more important, maverick scientists going public usually have access to only a portion of the relevant data and, even if they have full access to all the relevant data, might well be wrong in their interpretation. In academic circles this is fine, as open discussion of scientific data and interpretation is a self-correcting phenomenon. Colleagues near and far will consider the data and apply their own interpretation. New information will be added from various sources and eventually the issue will be resolved. But in politically sensitive issues of science, like those surrounding BSE or bovine somatotrophin (BST), a contrary opinion from a government scientist serves only to confuse the public and engender non-confidence in the whole regulatory system.

Pollen escape studies

Trying to conduct a risk assessment based on gene escape via pollen is a waste of time and resources. In my petitions to place Triffid on the market, I needed to provide a complete data set, requiring a substantial expenditure of public funds to acquire. The data set addressed concerns of gene escape, the interpretation of which required another expenditure of public funds on submission to the regulatory authorities. All wasted.

The UK government spends a considerable amount of money conducting research into the likelihood of a GM plant pollinating nearby plants to measure the risk of genetic escape. The hazard is the gene escape under a certain set of parameters. The exact species of GM plant is critical to the research. Rapeseed, especially *Brassica rapa*, is by nature promiscuous and will, left to its own devices, spread pollen all over the countryside. By contrast, wheat is almost completely self-pollinating. The risk of escape of a gene from a GM wheat is lower than the risk of escape of a GM rapeseed.

One component of these studies is the calculation of possible pollen recipients. This involves finding the populations of the same species growing nearby that might serve as recipients. This calculation has to account for managed, as well as unmanaged, plants of that species and related ones. Are any potential recipients weeds that might become more 'weedy'? Are there any rare or endangered species that might become even more endangered? The scientists must also consider pollen vectors. Is this pollen spread by wind? If so, what are the weather patterns in that geographical area at the time of pollen shed? Perhaps insects transfer pollen from this species. We need to know what, if any, insects serve as pollen vectors, and what their populations are in the area at pollen-shed time, where the insects are likely to go, distance, location, and so on. Differences in pollen biology between species account for the differences in risk of gene escape. While the pollen grains within each plant species look the same, pollen from different species displays remarkable variation. Pollen grains identify plant species as accurately as fingerprints do us; they're reliable enough to be used extensively in forensic research. There can be substantial differences in shape and size, influencing wind and other vector dispersal type and range. Pollen grains can be heavy or light, also influencing dispersal mechanisms. Some species have long-lived pollen, others have a very short period of viability, a matter of minutes. Some species complete pollination even before the flower opens, ensuring self-pollination. Other species have self-incompatibility mechanisms to preclude self-pollination, ensuring cross-pollination. If we are going to measure risk of gene escape through pollen at all, these differences in pollen biology account for the need to analyse each species separately.

When these questions are all answered for each GMO in each intended geographical area, we have piles of scientific data collected by some of the best scientific minds at the best universities and institutes in the country, for which taxpayers have contributed equally huge amounts of money. But at least the public can rest assured that scientifically valid risk assessments can now be determined for the risk of escape, via pollen, of genes from these GMOs.

But that's only part of the equation. Don't we have to know what will happen in the event of pollen escape? Will it result in an environmental disaster of biblical proportions? Or will it be a benign, mundane event? Surely the magnitude of the consequences influences the assessment. Back to the scientists, back to the public trough. Science will calculate what will happen to the environment in the event pollen does escape and fertilize some unsuspecting plant across the road. Again, we have to consider the parameters. If the trait is a pesticide resistance, we have to determine how each potential mate might act having acquired the pesticide resistance. All of these questions are complicated by the fact that, in many cases, we have to make guesses—educated guesses, indeed, but guesses nevertheless about how the gene might affect fecundity in the new recipient plant. Maybe the population of the weedy relative will explode and we will be overrun with them. On the other, equally disastrous hand, perhaps the presence of the novel gene in the plant will cause the population to diminish to extinction. More money. More time. More public scientists employed.

In most jurisdictions, including the EU/UK, risk assessments of GM plants place immense and (in my view) superfluous emphasis on questions of gene escape. Pollen flow, the type described above, is only one mechanism of genetic escape. Some plants exercise gene escape by vegetative means. That is, a piece of the plant might snap off, blow away, or be dragged by a passing animal, and take root in a new location, starting a new population. The preponderance of such vegetative mechanisms of genetic escape needs to be determined for each species.

Potatoes are a common and well-known example of a plant with a predilection for vegetative reproduction. Strawberries can reproduce by runners. Leaf pieces from begonias can easily be propagated on soil. Other means of gene flow are known in the plant world, and each needs to be considered for each GM plant being reviewed. What about birds and animals munching on the GM plants? They don't always fully digest the seeds before dropping them, complete with a dose of natural fertilizer to give the germinating seed a competitive head start, some considerable distance from where the 'confined' crop was growing. As you can imagine, calculating the incidence of all of these potential escape routes involves a huge amount of money to provide the background information on these issues.

None of it is money well spent. Regardless of how much genetic escape will occur from pollen flow or other mechanisms, it's still immaterial and a waste of everyone's time and effort, not to mention our public money.

Why is it a waste? Don't we need to know about the likelihood of gene escape? No, we don't. Gene escape is a fact of nature. Period. Save the money. Cancel the projects. Let those top brains do something useful instead to trying to find hypothetical phantoms. The genes have already escaped.

Regulatory mistakes

Gene escape via spillage

For those few genes that don't already exist in the natural environment, gene escape will occur within one year, and it won't happen predominantly through pollen. It will happen through a source that no major regulatory body has identified as a source for genetic escape—seed. No regulator has ever asked me about the likelihood of GM seed spillage from, for example, agricultural equipment. We spend immense amounts of money trying to figure how long it will take for pollen to cross the road, but nothing to study mechanism virtually guaranteeing gene escape on day 1. When farmers plant seeds, they spill some, every time. They spill seeds when loading their seeding equipment. The seeds get stuck in the machinery works, only to dislodge the next day or week, with the equipment on a different field, perhaps a considerable distance away. Spillage also occurs at harvest. Some of the harvested seed gets stuck in the machinery, only to dislodge on the way home, along the road. It is a clear regulatory mistake to place so much emphasis on pollen-based gene flow and nothing on the most obvious route for gene escape.

I pointed this inconsistency out to an official of MAFF, who promptly replied they would have to establish a mandatory monitoring system for seeds, under which a farmer would have to account for each and every seed at planting and at harvest. The image of anyone trying to enforce such a ludicrous regulation was hilarious, but I didn't laugh as I noticed my counterpart wasn't.

Using GM regulations to access and regulate conventional products

We discussed earlier that 'prove the GMO not hazardous' is not a scientifically valid demand, because it requires a proof for a negative, and science cannot prove negative assertions. Instead, we must compare the risks of the product in question to those of a known and accepted product. This is the basis of substantial equivalence, or now, in regulatory parlance, simply **equivalence**. To establish safety of a GMO, scientists and regulators ordinarily compare the GM version with the parental version. CDC Triffid GM linseed is compared with its parental conventional linseed variety, Norlin.

An official in MAFF is one, but I've encountered some in other countries, who object to the use of 'substantial equivalence' because they see the conventional products as potentially unsafe. However, the regulators have no statutory or regulatory authority to recall currently available products in the absence of tangible evidence of their potentially hazardous nature. These bureaucrats see regulatory oversight of GM products as a conduit to scrutinize all suspect products, GM certainly, but also the products currently on shelves of which they have some unsubstantiated suspicion. But because it assumes the conventional product is safe, using substantial equivalence as a base for safety evaluation precludes pursuit of their agenda.

Why do they think current products might be unsafe? In MAFF, it's probably because of the BSE crisis which arose out of beef products that were assumed to be safe, but weren't. Others express similar sentiments and extend them to a wider range of commodities. Many of our common foods were developed long before technical advances in testing and evaluation. It's commonly said that potatoes, if proposed today, would not pass regulatory scrutiny for health safety. But it's too late now, the tubers are firmly entrenched in our society. Many commonly consumed products contain various quantities of chemicals toxic when presented in large amounts. When first used as foods, the toxins went unnoticed. It is only with the refinement and increased sensitivity of many of our assays we can detect the toxins in our common, assumed safe, foods. Should we use modern technology to reconsider and re-evaluate the health safety aspects of current and traditional foods as we do with GM products? Or should we continue in blissful ignorance to enjoy potatoes, tomatoes, coffee, chocolate, fruit with stones, beans, and other potentially hazardous foods we now know to contain such toxins? If we do want to apply modern analytical methods to health safety evaluation of conventional foods, is it appropriate to try to 'piggyback' the regulatory authority for the review on to regulations specifically designed for GM products? Or ought we develop regulations to cover all potentially hazardous food products?

Basic faults in the regulatory approval process

I mentioned earlier that an unexpected or unintended consequence of the regulatory process is to ensure public institutions and small companies don't get to partake in the new technology. Only the big multinationals have the resources to play the political regulations game and they eventually get their money back.

Close scrutiny before large-scale environmental or market release is a good idea, but close scrutiny of what to scrutinize is more important. The problems with requiring detailed studies of aspects for which there is little scientific basis for concern (such as gene transfer from plant to bacteria in the gut, for which there is no scientific basis) are several, It

- distracts from what might be real issues of concern, such as allergenicity,
- gives the public a false sense of complacency, that regulators are really scrutinizing these products closely,
- sets a benchmark that others need to follow, regardless of the nature of the product in question. It is ludicrous to evaluate a small, generally non-consumed crop like linseed to the same degree we scrutinize a large crop designed for human consumption, like maize or soya, finally
- it allows mischief by big players to try to keep competition down, especially from small players. One Canadian regulator, on receiving a huge dossier of largely irrelevant data from a big company, decided every applicant should provide the same quantity of information in their application packages. Most small companies and public institutions simply couldn't afford to generate all the meaningless information, and so were unable to comply with the demand. Through simple flummoxing of a gullible regulator, a big company was able to eliminate potential competition.

Who pays for development and regulatory compliance costs?

You do. Tax monies go to create the regulatory bureaucracy, they support basic (and sometimes the actual applied) research; they also support potential opposition from activist groups through grants. Companies invest in particular projects. All of the monies spent on research and development, testing, regulatory compliance, marketing, advertising, production and distribution, legal costs, financing, profit, etc. are taken into consideration in the determination of the price you and I pay for the product when it hits the market. The companies are quick to point out that very few of their products are ever commercialized. Glyphosate, the active ingredient in Roundup™ herbicide from Monsanto, is a simple and inexpensive chemical to manufacture, yet was quite expensive when it first came out. Now that the patent has expired and other manufacturers are making generic versions, the price is quite reasonable, more reflective of the cost of manufacture. Companies justify the initial high price of new products by pointing to all the costs of the thousands of products that they have investigated but never brought to market. A new chemical needs to be discovered, purified, evaluated, developed, and undergo years of expensive testing, not only for efficacy but also for toxicity and other health and safety criteria. The costs of these tests and the salaries of the staff have to be paid whether or not the new chemical ever reaches the market. Thousands of chemicals are evaluated, some making it right to the edge of the marketplace before being dropped. The successful ones, like glyphosate or AgrEvo's glufosinate, have to pay the bills accrued by all the other products that never generate any income. When we buy a product, we consumers pay a share of the costs for every failed product.

Final comments

The real issues facing the GM debate are several and varied. In this chapter have we explored some of them, including the scientifically legitimate safety concerns in GM foods and the need to consider the ecology of different cultivation environments for certain GMOs. We also considered some of the problems of establishing a credible regulatory bureaucracy, from chronic underfunding and political interference to 'hoop-jumping' and basic faults in the regulatory process. Unnecessary regulation and regulatory mistakes are endemic but serve no one. They debase proper regulatory oversight and cost all of us. We've seen that taxpayers and consumers end up footing the bill, one way or another, for every aspect of GMO development and regulation. We pay for meaningless research programmes as well as the unnecessary regulatory processes. We pay for GM product development, including the cost of regulatory compliance. Many expenditures are legitimate and, as consumers, we must expect to pay when we demand assurances.

Some of the more extreme activists will note that the easiest way out of all this cost and bureaucratic blundering is to simply ban all GM material. True, regulatory costs will be minimized and consumers won't bear the brunt of all the different charges. Unfortunately, this solution presumes each nation is entirely self-sufficient and capable of dropping out of the world of international commerce. But even apart from the international trade legal obligations, the solution is unworkable. When you leave the table, you lose your seat. Within a few years, citizens of a 'GM-free' nation would observe the benefits accruing to neighbours enjoying properly regulated GM materials and demand them domestically. By then there would be an even bigger price to pay to regain a place at the table.

CHAPTER 10

'Waiter, what do you recommend?': who's serving my best interests?

- Does anyone care about the public?
- What's the connection between BSE and GM?
- Are all academics in the pocket of private industry?
- What do farmers think of GM?

Finding good reviewers

Where do we obtain trusted information?

A recurring theme in the GM food debate is that ordinary citizens have no clear source of credible information. How can the public contribute to an informed debate without reliable information? How can consumers exercise informed choice in the market if there's neither information nor choice? Consumers appear to lack a champion with the specialized knowledge representing the public interest. Government agencies are supposed to represent the public, but are often stifled by widespread distrust of government policy. The companies developing GMOs are obviously biased, as are the pressure group opposition activists. Public academics are all but invisible, and the media seems to present contradictory stories on the risks and benefits of GMOs. The major participants in the debate so far have failed to establish credibility with the public. No wonder there is such confusion and uncertainty; we don't know whom to believe. In this chapter we look at the problems faced by the public in the search for credible information on which to assess the real risks and benefits of GMOs.

'Multinationals give me a pain'

The big multinational companies, the major proponents of GM products, tell us GM is simply an extension of traditional breeding methods. Most of us then think: But you need to sell these products to make money for your investors, and it certainly doesn't seem like a simple extension of old methods. Weren't you also telling us that GM is wonderfully powerful new technology that will revolutionize food production? It doesn't seem consistent that a such a power-ful new technique set to revolutionize an entire industry, especially one as big and important as food, is simply an extension of old methods.

The pro-GM food industry, based in North America, is flabbergasted at the reluctance of European consumers to embrace GM foods. 'After all', they say with an all too common note of exasperated arrogance, 'if Americans don't have a problem with it, why should Europeans?' They blame the well-organized Green movement and anti-business lobby for conducting a campaign of misinforma-tion against GM on a gullible EU public. They make much of the Zeneca tomato paste, placed on sale in the UK in 1996, and insist if only the public were exposed to other GM products, they would accept them into the marketplace as readily as they did the GM tomato paste.

The single most important predictor of a purchase decision is cost. According to surveys, most people don't even look at the label. Given a choice, most go for the least expensive item. Several years ago I attended a farm meeting where one of the speakers was talking to the audience, a public gathering in a small town in Canada, about the prospect of GM milk coming to the market. The speaker was addressing the concerns of the public, or at least his perceived concerns, when he suddenly took an impromptu survey, asking the audience how they would respond to see-ing GM milk in their supermarket side by side with regular milk. He was astounded when majority said their decision to buy depended almost entirely on the price. The ensuing discussion revealed that most consumers, at least in this small community, trusted the bureaucracy to keep unsafe products off the shelf. After that, if the quality of the product was maintained and the price was less they had no hesitation in buying the GM milk. Especially if the price was less. Of course this was not a scientifically sound survey for a number of reasons, but it did pro-vide a glimpse of what at least a sample of ordinary consumers were thinking.

Monsanto is another big company. They are probably the best-known (if not best-loved) 'life sciences' company (as they like to refer to themselves) in the world. They certainly have the highest profile. Monsanto has some of the best scientific minds money can buy. They've hired some of my own students, and I know several other excellent scientists in their employ. They are certainly not short on brainpower. And, as we've seen earlier, they have a unique method of dealing with intrusive competitors. They buy them. Through corporate acquisi-tions, bright individuals have been sucked inexorably into the fold through direct or indirect procurement.

Monsanto also has some excellent products and projects. Aside from Roundup™, arguably the most popular and effective herbicide in the history of chemical farming, they also have some imaginative ideas on increasing the nutri-tional composition of potatoes, wheat, and other crops. They will certainly continue to be a dominant player in the GM foods industry if non-scientific fumbles don't cripple them.

Why, if Monsanto has corralled such excellent scientists, and developed such creative products, do they keep making such stupid mistakes? Their UK news media blitz of 1998, intended to calm the widespread public fears over largely Monsanto GM products, was a disaster. Taking full-page advertisements listing opponents' contact numbers in major national papers was certainly an innovative and dramatic idea. But even I could have advised Monsanto that, although such a ploy might work well in the US, the more subtle and sophisticated readers in the UK would not be impressed. It might look like slick public relations in the US, but in the UK it appeared more like crass commercial manipulation.

Monsanto also ran into trouble in the UK for improperly conducting a field trial with GM rapeseed. Apparently, the field plot didn't have the required six-metre 'buffer zone' around it and, in fact, there was as little as two metres in some spots along the perimeter where GM plants were grown. The point of a buffer zone is to ensure there's no 'escape' of GM material from the precise location of the approved test. The financial penalty was large by normal standards, but piddling to Monsanto, who pleaded guilty to the infraction in an effort to get it over with as soon as possible. Of course, some people use this as an indication of Monsanto's (and, by extension, the entire industry's) cavalier attitude toward regulatory compliance. Monsanto were guilty of, if not gross environmental negligence, then sheer stupidity and technical sloppiness. They were not the only ones to violate environmental release conditions, whether through defiance, incompetence, or accident, but they knew their trials were going to come under close scrutiny by hostile activists and regulators. They could easily have ensured a six-metre buffer zone through routine site monitoring. But they didn't.

This incident was the last straw for some of the more responsible players in the industry trying to establish public credibility. Apart from being competitors, some executives from other large companies suggest that Monsanto would make a valuable contribution to the industry as a whole if they would just go into hibernation for a few years.

In addition to annoying their competitors, Monsanto also has a knack for getting into trouble with their customers. Their innovative 'technology' use agreement (TUA) obliges farmers to give up farmers' traditional rights to re-grow saved seed from one season to the next. Monsanto does not provide their seed to any farmer not signing the contract. Although Monsanto did a credible job of explaining the TUA, some farmers signed on to get the new seed but chose to save some seed for next year anyway. Monsanto then initiated a truly innovative approach to business by suing their customers. The courts will decide the legal aspects, but, win or lose, this novel practice is unlikely to promote their public image.

Recently, in the light of the various public relations disasters, Monsanto officials decided they would no longer try to influence public opinion. Instead, they say it is up to governments and regulators to convince wary consumers that the products passing regulatory review are safe. In the past few years, Monsanto has spent a lot of money to be the international leader in genetic technology. It seems that, while they may have achieved that goal, they are abdicating the major responsibility of leaders—to provide responsible leadership.

Despite the often slick public relations campaigns, many people feel uneasy about trusting big companies. Perhaps Monsanto would fare better if they made a point of doing the 'little things' better. Building trust and providing leadership grows from the ground up and takes time. Shortcuts don't often work.

'Activists and pressure groups give me indigestion'

Some opposition activist groups are sincere and well-meaning but lack the scientific knowledge or communication skills to convey their legitimate concerns. Others operate behind a thinly veiled agenda to rid the world of the capitalist scourge. Many activists are excellent media manipulators, experts at attracting microphones and cameras with dramatic and sometimes imaginative stunts. Unfortunately, on closer inspection, the substance to their argument is all too often lacking. Occasionally it is pure disingenuousness. Some activists continue to flog the story of GMO L-tryptophan poisoning innocent people, or the Brazil nut in soya bean causing new allergic reactions, even after being shown the facts (see Chapter 6).

Even when appearing sincere, some opponents find making corrections and apologies difficult. One newsletter from the Natural Law Party included an article entitled 'Blindness, mad cow disease and canola oil', by John Thomas, warning of the dangers of rapeseed oil—not GM, but conventional rapeseed oil.

Rape (canola) causes emphysema respiratory distress, anemia, constipation, irritability and blindness in animals and humans. Rape oil was widely used in animal feeds in England and Europe between 1986 and 1991 when it was thrown out. You may remember reading about the cows, pigs and sheep that went blind, lost their minds, attacking people and had to be shot.' 'The 'experts' blamed the behavior on a viral disease called scrapie. However, when rape oil was removed from the animal feed, 'scrapie' disappeared.

The subsequent issue carried this understated 'correction', provided by the editor '. . . there is no evidence linking canola to scrapie or mad cow disease.' Needless to say, we were all relieved by this update, but we're still wondering when the other afflictions will strike, as the newsletter implicitly stands by the remaining claims.

A coalition of environmental activist groups in Canada launched a media campaign asserting government-sponsored 'secret tests' of GMOs several years ago. When a local journalist asked me for a response, I asked him 'How many of these tests (documented in the press release) did you as a journalist know about?' He replied 'All of them. We don't publish the notices of GM trials anymore, unless there's something new or unusual'. With the media subsequently dropping the coverage, the discredited coalition campaign ended.

Some activists simply like to go along for the ride. For these 'rent-an-activist individuals', joining the protest is more like a social occasion or an opportunity to get on the news. How can you trust someone who seems not to be dedicated to the cause? Despite these problems of dishonesty, activist groups in the UK enjoy a high degree of public credibility. Surveys sometimes ask 'Where do you obtain your scientific information?' Astonishingly high proportions of people claim to get their most credible scientific information from groups with few or no recognized scientific advisers.

I'm reluctant to afford trust to a group with an inconsistent track record. Sometimes they're right in bringing to public attention, for example, an issue on a pollution problem due to waste dumped by ships at sea. But when the next issue comes up, they miss the boat altogether. How do we know, when a groups cries 'wolf', whether or not it's just another mistaken fish gene in tomato issue?

'Regulatory agencies make me sick'

Government agencies suffer the most, perhaps because of the depth of the bureaucratic morass. The companies are doing what's best for their shareholders; we know their motivation despite Monsanto's claims that they they're only trying to feed the burgeoning world population. The activists serve as the 'loyal' opposition, we expect them to oppose and raise potential problems that others might not see. But government agencies are supposed to represent the public interest. We pay them to protect us.

Why does FDA in the USA have Monsanto people on the advisory board? Even if there is no undue influence or favouritism, the image presented is not one to instil confidence concerning objectivity. Why do cabinet ministers of departments regulating GMOs hold shares in GM proponent companies? Even if there is no political interference and the investments are all 'arm's length', it raises suspicions. We face a dilemma. We want those people most knowledgeable of the science and the agriculture industry offering advice and working on our behalf. But few of the most capable people are completely independent of industrial connections. If we insist that none of our senior advisers have any industrial ties, we won't have many capable advisers. One practical solution is to require a candidate's full public disclosure of industrial ties (including those with the 'activist' industry!) prior to appointment to any 'public interest' body. This will simplify monitoring for conflict of interest while allowing the most qualified minds to serve the public interest.

Public opinion surveys in the UK consistently put government regulators near the bottom of the credibility tables. The 'reassurance' attitude provides an exemplary indication of the ivory tower arrogance that destroyed whatever credibility the public had in MAFF's ability to regulate emerging technologies in agriculture. It's such a shame that such attitudes prevalent within certain departments tar all civil servants with the same brush. Too many capable civil servants are rendered impotent by having to 'manage the damage' instead of doing what they ought to be doing in the real public interest. It will be a very long time before

MAFF recovers public credibility in the aftermath of the BSE crisis. And it will happen only when they learn the lesson of truth and openness and transparency instead of misguided paternalistic protection schemes.

The connection between BSE and GM foods

Both BSE ('mad cow disease') and GMOs seem to result from or in the intensification of agriculture. Industry drives the fastest, most efficient possible route to generate food, for example, feeding cattle with whatever is readily available or cheap.

In the BSE fiasco, public sector scientists were scapegoated by the populace and blamed for the entire problem. It was the superb work of scientists in the UK that provided the information on the BSE mystery. They didn't cause it, yet were roundly blamed for it. In any earlier era, even just a few years ago, there would probably be no indication of the connection between BSE and CJD (Creutzfeld-Jacob Disease): it would simply be another of those mystery diseases that people have died from all through history. AIDS would be in the same boat: it took modern molecular genetic analyses to track it down, but scientists aren't blamed for spreading AIDS.

But the award for the most successful public relations manipulation coup must go to the activists who managed to link GM with BSE in the public mind. BSE was not caused by genetic manipulation. BSE might be relieved by appropriate molecular genetic technology, but there was absolutely no indication that GM was in any way involved in causing or continuing BSE. Nevertheless, the responsible government bureaucrats and scientists in the UK do not command the respect and credibility they have earned and often deserve.

'Academics give me heartburn'

Who else might we trust? Academics? The common image of professors is that of doddering old men hiding in ivory towers, having been out of touch with the real world for decades.

Academic scientists used to command public respect, but now they have lost credibility. They were once seen, and respected, as independent experts. That independence is now questioned, as more and more academics must turn to industry to provide research funds to replace those lost through government cuts. Governments have stripped basic research budgets dramatically over the past fifteen to twenty years, encouraging or requiring public academics to seek private sponsorship. As a result, very few of our best public scientists conduct their experiments exclusively on public funds.

Certainly, some scientists are unduly influenced by their sponsors. Most, though, design the collaboration to benefit both public and private interests simultaneously. Over the years, I have collaborated on specific research projects with many of the big names in industry—DuPont, Monsanto, Rhône-Poulenc, and others. In each project, my motivation was to help provide the public with a useful new product or service. If that condition cannot be met, the project cannot run. At least not with my contribution. Most public academic scientists share this attitude. My loyalty remains with the people who pay my salary—the taxpayers. Nevertheless, these collaborative projects expose me, and the vast majority of my public sector colleagues, to charges of conflict of interest. I am not opposed to the charges—prudence dictates we investigate the extent of the connection and possible divided loyalty. But I am opposed to simply rejecting anyone having any industrial ties. Such a move is counterproductive, as we'd exclude many of our best and most qualified champions.

Another problem with academic scientists is that, although knowledgeable, they are notoriously poor communicators. They use too much detail, they are too precise, and use too much technical jargon for public consumption. Scientists, especially public sector or academic scientists, are often naive about political issues (ivory tower syndrome), whereas private sector scientists are usually censored by their bosses.

Why are academic scientists such poor communicators?

Scientists' lack of communication skills is no simple coincidence or freak occurrence. By and large, scientists are poor communicators with a general audience. Any students of science who might have natural (or especially highly developed) communication skills have these skills actively beaten out of them during their training period. 'Never say anything unless you support it using data derived from well-designed and well-executed experiments. Otherwise it is mere speculation'. (To be accused of speculation is a particularly nasty insult in the scientific community.) 'Write only in the third person, passive voice to avoid any personal attachment, which would adversely impact the impersonal objectivity of the work.' Scientists are taught to be precise and accurate, and the distinction between the two. 'You must support any and all assertions with sound experimental evidence and provide sufficient technical detail to enable the reader to repeat your experiments and obtain essentially the same results.'

Fortunately, scientific articles are much easier to read and understand, even for scientists, than they were twenty-five or thirty years ago. The 'Plain English' movement has made some inroads even in the scientific literature. We still have a long way to go to eradicate unnecessary technical jargon and obfuscation, and to allow scientists to proffer an unsupported hypothetical opinion without denigrating them to the 'speculators' rubbish bin.

Activists, having no such constraints, have the system down pat. Certain activists can pose questions, even irrelevant ones, but do not feel any obligation to partake in the debate by having to answer questions themselves. Asking such simple and apparently sincere but unsubstantiated questions as 'Is there any concrete proof the GMO is safe' will send the scientists and bureaucrats to work for quite a while coming up with some attempt at a reasonable answer. The answer, however suitable, doesn't end the debate. By this time, the opponents to the technology will have created another question from their fertile collective imagination. The satisfactory response to the previous question is ignored as if past history. These activists do not care for the answer and do not care to debate. They do a disservice to the responsible sceptics who sincerely want to know the risks and benefits of the technology and point out potential problems and solutions perhaps overlooked by scientists and regulators.

In any case, academic scientists keep too low a public profile and are often overlooked when people are searching for credible advice.

'Media? Not enough nutrition, too many empty calories'

Can we trust the media to provide guidance and leadership? There are indeed some well-informed and popular journalists covering the GMO beat. Unfortunately, the well informed are not very popular, and the popular are not very well informed. It is not unusual to open the newspaper and find a gloom and doom story about the imminent environmental or market release of some GMO across from a glowing article about research into using genetic technology to overcome some health or environmental obstacle. This is no regional aberration; I've seen such articles in news media in North America, Europe, and Australia. The media often seems to support the research, but not the application. Am I the only one to detect a contradiction here? How can we trust an institution that says a technology is wonderful and beneficial in one column and negates it in the next? It seems there's a lack of informative consistency in the popular media.

On occasion, the media also seems to have difficulty in finding the real story. When Monsanto was discovered with the inadequate borders around their GM rapeseed field test, the incident was widely reported in the press, but the press missed the major issue. The oversight was, what was a rapeseed plot doing with a prescribed 6-metre buffer zone? Earlier I mentioned it was important to know which particular species was used, as oilseed rape could be any of two or three different species. Well, regardless of which species, 6-metres is far too little to provide any assurance whatsoever of genetic isolation. Seed growers, professional farmers who have been concerned with isolation distances for ages, will use 200 to 400 metres as a buffer to minimize (not eliminate) cross-pollination in rapeseed. If reproductive isolation was a prescribed requirement for this test, who suggested 6 metres? Who approved 6 metres? Why? This seems a sham, to merely let people know, 'Yes, we are ensuring Monsanto is conducting their test under reproductive isolation requirements'. A journalist might be excused for not knowing exact appropriate isolation distances for a crop, surely it is apparent that 6 metres is too little in any event.

Even well-respected sources are not immune to occasional sensationalism. In summer 1999, BBC TV covered the story of John Losey, from Cornell University in New York state, who reported findings that pollen from GM maize was potentially lethal when fed to Monarch butterfly larvae. The BBC reporter described the findings as 'unexpected', dealing an astounding blow to proponents of GM and vindicating opponents to the technology who assert GM will present unpredicted and negative biological consequences. The report seemed to present the first verifiable evidence of such unexpected and negative consequences. The GM maize carried the inserted *B.t.* gene, conferring resistance to insect pests. The *B.t.* was supposed to kill pests, not 'friendly' and attractive insects like the Monarch, or ladybirds, or lacewings. The interview with Dr Losey was informative. The *B.t.* gene produces a crystal protein toxic to lepidopteran insects. Many crop insect pests are *Lepidoptera*, including the corn borer, the main target in this GM maize project. When the corn borer (or other lepidopteran insect) eats the crystal protein, an unpleasant reaction in the insect gut kills the bug. Where, you might ask, was the sensationalism? Well, *B.t.*, a natural insecticide, is toxic to lepidopteran insects. Monarch butterflies are lepidopteran insects. Why was it 'unexpected' that a lepidopteran insect toxin was found to be toxic to lepidopteran insects? Instead of vindicating the opposition argument about unexpected results, the actual data supported the orthodox prediction: *B.t.* toxin is toxic to lepidopteran insects. Even 'friendly' ones. The point here is to illustrate how even respected media can present misleading stories.

So it appears we have little choice in where to place our trust. We might choose to trust the companies, who have some of the facts but don't share them. The activists, while sincere, have a tendency to muddle the facts. The government has many of the facts but often looks at the wrong ones. Academics have some of the facts but don't share them in a manner the public can understand.

So where's the leadership?

Where's the leadership? So far in this chapter I've discredited pretty well every source of information. Public and private, proponent and opponent, even the supposedly objective and disinterested media are suspect sources. Fortunately, it's not that bleak. Credible and objective information does exist. My point is that everyone is potentially suspect, everyone has biases. We needn't disregard everyone with a bias, we simply account for them.

We already do this. When considering a new consumer product, we critically evaluate the spiel from a salesperson to separate the wheat from the chaff. We mentally reject the puffery and use the real information to determine our interest. A Novartis scientist is obviously biased in favour of, and will pitch, Novartis GM products. I recommend you apply the same procedure as with a consumer product sales rep. Discard the promotional material and keep the meaningful information.

What about the other end of the spectrum, the opposition? Activists present a different perspective, raising issues proponents might overlook or actively suppress. Take the same approach as with a sales rep. Recognize the bias, uncover and reject any hidden agenda, and critically evaluate the kernels of truth found hidden below. There are legitimate health and environmental concerns with GMOs and other products. The activists often miss the mark because they're aiming at the wrong target. The proper target might be present but obscured by the antics and rhetoric. We can miss the real concerns if we reject outright everything the activist groups say, and we can miss them if we unquestioningly accept everything they say.

This brings us to the supposedly neutral—the government, academics, and media working in the public interest. They too carry their own baggage. How do we minimize the biases and acquire meaningful information? A number of public sector groups have both the expertise and integrity to represent the public interest.

The Advisory Committee on Releases to the Environment (ACRE), for one in the UK, at least until it was (genetically?) modified by the government. Because ACRE receives and evaluates data dossiers on all GMOs intended for commercial release in the UK, they collectively know more about GMOs than anyone or group anywhere. Even the American FDA, USDA, and EPA do not see as much scientific data on as wide a range of GMOs as ACRE.

The Royal Society is another highly regarded and capable group issuing balanced analyses and press releases on the GM debate. The Fellows span a wide range of political and social interests. The one feature they share is a dedication to scientific excellence. This is exemplified in their thorough, objective, and careful analyses of Dr Pusztai's GM potato feeding trial data.

The House of Lords Select Committee report (January 1999) is one of the most comprehensive and balanced analyses I've seen on the subject. It was roundly criticized on release because it was 'too positive towards the industry'. The Lords, in a massive document, exhort us to conduct a rational debate on the risks and benefits of GM technology. Among many other points, they note there are indeed real risks, but that appropriate regulation and management might enable benefits to accrue while minimizing hazards. They also note that current and accepted agricultural practices also carry risks, some of which might be alleviated by GM technology. I see no polemic and have no argument with any of the points raised in the report. This does not mean I agree with every recommendation, I don't. But all are valid starting points for rational discussion.

The British Medical Association (BMA) recommended a moratorium on GM foods to the cheers of various activist groups, as this respected body became one of the first scientifically credible bodies to endorse such a notion. However, the report also said:

The BMA accepts that there are potential benefits of GMOs and foods, but believes that it is most important that a comprehensive cost benefit and health impact assessment, comparing genetic modification with other agricultural techniques, is implemented.

Here, we have a major medical body recommending a scientific comparison between GM and 'other agricultural techniques', presumably conventional technologies. The BMA might be surprised to find many of those studies are already completed. And the activists might cease their cheers when the results of the comparisons are publicized. Also salient is the confusing rationale for their position. The BMA deservedly commands respect as a medico-scientific group. But their justification for calling a moratorium is not on scientific or medical grounds, but on social and political grounds. They admit as much, saying in a press release

The BMA agrees there is no evidence to suggest that GM food technologies are inherently harmful but says there is also insufficient evidence to reassure policy makers and the public that they are completely safe.

Certainly, every one (and group) is entitled to advocate any position, but when one uses a reputation gained in a particular area of expertise to support a cause in a different sphere, it misleads and confuses. In this case, ordinary citizens, if they don't read the entire report (and who does?), may be excused for thinking the British Medical Association has a medical reason for calling a moratorium. For the BMA to rely on its medical reputation to advance a political cause is as inappropriate and extraordinary as a political group advancing a scientific cause. The confusion, in the long run, jeopardizes the BMA's reputation, contributing to the decline in credibility of all public institutions.

Scientists active in the public interest convene at regular meetings of their various associations to discuss GMOs. The International Symposium for the Biosafety of GMOs is a major series attracting delegates from around the world. Senior academic and government scientists, industry scientists, and environmentalists deliberate on the science of biosafety and how to deal with the potential problems posed by GM, especially in the environmental sphere.

Down on the farm, farmers usually endow leadership on other farmers. Regardless of flashy ads, field days, subsidies, free meals, and extension specialists from governments and universities, the best way to get a message to farmers is to convince a local leading farmer. Farmers in any given region keep an eye on their farm leaders and usually follow their example.

Steve Wentworth is a prominent maize and soya bean farmer in Illinois. He and his family have farmed the same area for generations, becoming extremely successful in the process. They are what sociologists call 'early adopters', quick to try the latest toys and gadgets. Every community has at least one middle-aged adolescent who buys the newest most expensive stereo equipment or computer available. Steve and his family are the farming community version. They use satellite and global positioning system (GPS) technology to map out the farm. With a satellite receiver and computer in the cab of the tractor, Steve is able to identify soil conditions on the farm as he drives across the fields in order to apply pesticides only where needed. It might look like a toy to some, but Steve and other pioneers say it saves a lot of unnecessary pesticide usage. Steve also was one of the first to try GM crops, including some of Monsanto's GM varieties. He claims to be a small businessman, that he will try a new product and continue with it only if he sees a business advantage in doing so. It has to pay for itself. As long as regulators have approved the new toy, he's willing to give it a go and continue with those that work. GM crops make money for Steve Wentworth. He and his followers will continue to support approved GM crops as long as they continue to make farming worthwhile.

Addressing the leadership void

Clearly, there's no 'one-stop shopping' for good information. No one source is completely unbiased, and no one source is expert across the wide range encompassed by GM technology. But, overlooking the limitations, almost all offer something of value. Despite the tendency to be too specialized in their individual expertise to be of comprehensive use, public sector scientists can be excellent sources of accurate and largely unbiased information. Scientific committees and societies are valuable sources, as the inadequacies and biases of individuals are buttressed and balanced by assigning the challenge to broad-based committees. The Royal Society in the UK and the National Academy of Sciences in the US are good places to start. Another valuable source of objective information is the American Council on Science and Health (ACSH). The website of this consumer-orientated non-profit organization (http:www.acsh.org/) is a virtual goldmine of balanced information on everything from food safety to environmental health. They have been known to lose industry funding by releasing information critical of the sponsor's products. This kind of integrity and dedication to the public interest is indicative of the endangered species it is, and deserves the support of consumers everywhere.

Companies and activists both provide useful information, but they often make you work for it by hiding it in the detritus. Take advantage of the 'knowledgeable' media. The journal, *New Scientist* is an excellent source aimed at the general but scientifically inclined reader. If you're feeling more adventurous, pick up *Nature* or *Science* and their associated imprints. The take-home message is that good information is available and flowing, but there's no one spring from which to drink. Sample several.

CHAPTER 11

More small fry and red herrings

- GM technology is brand new and untested, isn't it?
- Won't antibiotic resistance genes get into germs?
- What about all the unintended or unexpected results with GMOs?
- Don't GM insecticide-making plants kill 'friendly' insects, too?
- What is this awful-sounding 'Terminator technology'?
- Do multinational companies control all GMOs and GM technology?
- What about genetic pollution?
- Can we predict the long-term consequences of GM technology?

We've had a closer look at some of the major controversial issues in preceding chapters. Here we step back into the scientific debate and look at some other aspects serving to cloud and otherwise obfuscate the legitimate concerns.

Gaining experience

When GMOs were first coming along, GM microbes, such as experimental modified bacteria, *Pseudomonas* species, were released in California. Activists were screaming because they believed (incorrectly, as it turned out) that these microbes, individually invisible, could escape and devastate the natural environment. After substantial negotiation and regulatory review, the proponent agreed to conduct the release under very tight environmental conditions. For example, the technicians actually releasing the bacteria had to wear space suits for protection. When the environmental release took place, the media released the pictures of the technician looking like an astronaut in the awkward and uncomfortable environmental containment outfit.

The experiment went well, data were collected, and the bacteria didn't devastate the world. The environmental containment suit worked well, in that the technicians remained healthy, but the workers probably would have remained equally healthy if they used their regular work clothes. The space suit was scientifically valid in that it protected the workers, but perhaps regular clothes would have also. Wearing the space suit was bad science, because there was no evidence it was needed in the first place. The only reason it was worn was that it was part of a negotiated deal. The activists won. The picture of a scientist spreading bacteria while wearing a space suit scared the wits out of people, who figured, 'If this scientist is wearing it, it must be for a reason. A scary reason. Why can't they be honest with us and tell the truth of the dangers? There's a logical inconsistency to say it's not hazardous, yet put on a moon suit while handling it. Smacks of a cover-up.' This one incident did more to support the anti-technology activist cause than any other argument for years.

Despite the negative publicity of the early 1970s, GM experiments continued. Recombinant DNA technology has been around for over 25 years, with thousands of environmental releases of genetically engineered microbes, plants, and animals. Millions of acres of GM crops are grown annually. No major problems have been documented with any GMO. Some did not perform as well as hoped. Some gained notoriety for failure of the company to observe details of the trial approval conditions. Others, like Showa Denko's GM L-tryptophan bacteria, were falsely accused of causing harm. In the meantime, thousands of other GMOs went along doing exactly as they were intended without the glare of the public spotlight. Most of the trials were designed to test the effects of the GMO in the environment. A few are in widespread environmental release, growing over millions of acres and over several years. None has been recalled.

Small fry: antibiotic resistance marker genes

The recent scare in Europe involves antibiotic resistance marker genes. Some responsible and knowledgeable groups call for a complete ban on the use of antibiotic resistance markers; others recommend phasing them out. What's the story behind this? Antibiotic resistance markers have been used from the very beginning of GMOs and are almost ubiquitous because they facilitate identification of microbes carrying transferred DNA. Scientists used the microbes to ferry sequences of DNA around until we were ready to combine the sequences for insertion into the host. We also use certain kinds, like the *npt*-II gene conferring resistance to kanamycin, to identify transformed plant cells early, as described in Chapter 3. However, once we successfully identify the transformed cells and plants, the antibiotic resistance marker gene becomes useless and superfluous— it is just carried along in the plant's DNA. The concern is that antibiotic resistance genes might transfer from the residue of the GMO during digestion in the human gastrointestinal tract to microbes living in the gut, thus providing the bugs with immunity from therapeutic agents. From the naturally domiciled gut microbes it's easy to speculate on their transfer to other microbes, including pathogenic ones that might happen to be around. After all, we've seen microbes in the lab take up DNA fragments from their surroundings, and we know the ordinary process of digestion cuts DNA into small fragments. What if one of those fragments happened to be an intact antibiotic resistance marker? And what if the hungry bacterium happened to be a pathogen? Would the gene confer antibiotic resistance to the bacterium? Progeny of the bacterium would also become resistant. The antibiotic would cease to be useful.

Markers of some sort are still needed to monitor construction and movement of DNA fragments. The antibiotic resistance marker genes were chosen because they worked well and were readily available. They were readily available because they are common in nature. Because they are common in nature, most of the relevant antibiotics have little therapeutic value in the first place. Furthermore, the current concerns were conjured out of hypothetical scenarios, there being no evidence of gene transfer from foods to gut microbes or from decaying plants to surrounding microbes. Nevertheless, it is difficult to disprove, to the consternation of many. The easy way out of the conundrum is to invoke caution.

The Advisory Committee on Releases to the Environment (ACRE) in the UK approved a number of applications for release of GMOs containing the markers, but admonished the developers for using them in the light of the concerns over transfer to microbes, either in the gut of consumers or in the wild during natural decomposition. Some regulators suggest an outright ban on antibiotic resistance markers, considering the potential damage they could cause and that they are unnecessary in the GMO. Why are the developers continuing to use these markers when alternatives are available? Why are regulators in North America apparently unconcerned about them? Regulators in Canada and the USA have not overlooked the concerns and arguments against using antibiotic resistance markers, but they respond differently. Essentially, the North Americans say there's no point worrying about hypothetical situations and spending limited resources chasing phantoms.

The majority of GMOs currently under regulatory review were generated ten or more years ago—such is the time lag between the DNA insertion and the commercial release. The markers in use ten years ago were antibiotic resistance markers. To ban antibiotic resistance markers in GMOs now would result in a lag of several years before the crop variety could be re-evaluated by the regulatory committees, not just a few months as some seem to believe. Developers must return to the labs, reconstruct the foreign DNA segment using alternatives to antibiotic resistance markers, re-transform the parental organisms, re-evaluate newly derived progeny lines for performance, for efficacy of the novel gene, and to ensure no undesirable features, and advance the best lines to commercialization stage. Then, who's to raise the concern ten years hence that the alternative markers present an even greater risk to environment or health than the antibiotic markers?

The *npt*-II gene

The most commonly used antibiotic resistance marker, *npt*-II, has been used in experimental and commercial GMOs since the early 1980s. The gene, originally isolated from a bacterial colony, is often coupled to a 'gene of interest' in a DNA segment destined to insertion into a target crop plant. The *npt*-II gene is used exclusively to identify and select those (few) plant cells successfully transformed. Those cells are regenerated into whole plants, the progeny of which will be evaluated for the activity of the gene of interest. The *npt*-II gene, having fulfilled its duty, is then carried along as excess baggage in the prospective new commercial cultivar.

The *npt*-II gene is in several commercial GMOs, including the first GM whole food, the Flavr-Savr™ tomato. By the early 1990s, the *npt*-II gene and its product were the subject of several scientific accounts concerning environmental and health safety. None of these accounts, published in the peer-reviewed scientific literature, exposed any expected or unexpected problems with the use of *npt*-II in food or the environment. Earlier, Calgene submitted a substantial data package to the Food and Drug Administration (FDA) concerning the fate of ingested *npt*-II DNA and protein. The concerns expressed about antibiotic resistance marker genes are simply not supported by scientific evidence in spite of substantial efforts to seek such data.

How real is the risk?

Just how real is the threat imposed by antibiotic resistance markers? What is the chance of gene transfer in the gut or the dump? A number of steps are involved in order for this scenario to unfold in the real world.

- The GMO has to be consumed or discarded.
- The intact gene would have to be released.
- The surrounding and opportunistic bacteria would have to take up the gene.
- The bacteria would have to express the gene to confer resistance.
- The antibiotic would have to be present to provide an advantage to the recipient bacteria.
- The initial recipient bacterium would have to transfer the gene to a pathogen.
- The recipient pathogen would have to be previously deficient in this gene.
- The antibiotic would have to be present to provide selective advantage to the newly emboldened pathogen.
- The pathogen would have to infect a person.
- The therapeutic treatment would have to include only the relevant antibiotic.
- The antibiotic resistant pathogen would have to spread.

The incidence of each of these steps is subject to debate, as no one has good data supporting any particular and reliable figures for any of the steps. However, there is general agreement that each of these steps, beyond the first, is an extremely rare event. One absolutely critical event, that of intact gene transfer from food to bacteria, has not been reported, although it has been hypothesized and artificially created in an experimental synthetic stomach. Combining the probabilities of these events occurring in the sequence and time-frame required resulting in a therapeutic compromise results in such remoteness that it is ludicrous to take preventive measures.

On the other hand, there *is* reasonably good data to support the figure for spontaneous mutation resulting in antibiotic resistance in bacteria. The probability is somewhere between one in a million and one in a thousand million. Spontaneous mutation giving rise to antibiotic-resistant bacteria is, using almost anyone's figures, several orders of magnitude more likely than transfer from GMOs. It seems incongruous that we are concerned only about the GMO transfer mechanism when, if antibiotic resistance is going to occur, it is far more likely from other mechanisms.

This is evident in the natural populations of microbes displaying antibiotic resistance, acquired long before GMOs could have provided the genes. One authority estimates humans consume over one million kanamycin-resistant bacteria each day, as a natural, if unintended, component of ordinary food. Zillions of kanamycin-resistant bacteria live inside you right now, whether or not you consumed any GMOs. If pathogenic bacteria are to acquire a kanamycin resistance gene, they are more likely to obtain it from one of these naturally occurring kanamycin-resistant bacteria, either in our gut or in the environment.

A sample of naturally occurring bacteria in a random soil sample collected in GMO-free New Zealand revealed hundreds of different bacteria. Almost a third were resistant to ampicillin and two-thirds were resistant to penicillin. These microbes did not acquire the antibiotic resistance gene from GMOs. If pathogens were to acquire antibiotic resistance genes, would they not be more likely to have already acquired them from current antibiotic-resistant microbes rather than from eukaryotic food digestion? After all, the DNA in food consists of far more genes than the microbial DNA. And why haven't we seen more eukaryotic gene sequences in microbes if they are so readily acquired from partially digested food?

If regulators really were concerned about development of antibiotic resistance developing in bacteria, they would not be looking at GMOs; they would be looking at far more mundane situations. In addition to the natural populations of antibiotic-resistant bacteria, physicians prescribing unnecessary antibiotics and patients not completing their course of drug therapy are far more effective at creating and offering selective advantage to resistant microbes. We are concentrating on a tiny fraction of the risk, while largely ignoring the most probable sources of problems.

Regulating GMOs to avoid compromising therapeutic use of antibiotics is like building a huge dome around the Earth to protect against giant meteors. Both involve a crippling cost to taxpayers, in one the cost of construction, in the other, regulation and regulatory enforcement. The chances of the untoward event happening are extremely remote in both cases. Finally, it's unlikely to achieve the goals in either case. A giant meteor bearing down on us is unlikely to be slowed, let alone stopped, by any shield we can construct. And antibiotic-resistant microbes are going to occur regardless of regulatory restrictions on GMOs, because they arise spontaneously and are already here among us. Like many of the stated concerns with GMOs, they have to be considered not in isolation but in perspective and relative to the status quo. In this case, we have to consider the likelihood of the events leading to compromising therapeutic uses of antibiotics from all potential means, not just GMOs. When we conduct the proper assessment, including analyses of all the various processes by which pathogens may become resistant to our therapeutic antibiotics, we readily see the futility of trying to restrict that acquisition by restricting only GMOs. The worry over GMOs contributing to antibiotic resistance in the pathogens is another red herring.

Famous last words: what about 'unexpected or unintended results'?

Initially, many people demanded a full moratorium on GM environmental releases. They argued that because GMOs had never been released before, we need to know if something unexpected or unintended would happen. This was a fair point, as no one had evidence of either expected or unexpected results in the early days, so most scientists went very slowly and cautiously in the early years of field trials (about 1986–9).

According to this argument, since the product and process are novel, we cannot predict all of the results with any degree of certainty. Scientific models of experimental systems are constructed not of plastic and glue but of results of past experiments. Each model is modified by the results of each subsequent experiment. If verifiable results are new or unexpected, that portion of the model dedicated to that aspect is modified to accommodate them. If the results are similar to those of previous tests, the relevant portion of the model is stabilized with the addition of this supporting data. After a sufficient number of experiments and results, the model is stable and strong, not only able to accommodate new results but also to predict results of subsequent experiments. Models have turned out to be remarkably accurate and reliable in their predictive capability, but not infallible. In the case of GM technology, the starting model was unstable and unsupported, based largely on information extrapolated or borrowed from related disciplines of microbiology, breeding, and genetics. This preliminary model was insufficient to apply in making confident predictions of results with GMOs. In some respects, all of the initial results of experiments with GMOs were, if not entirely unexpected, then low in confidence.

Unexpected results fuel the engine driving scientific knowledge acquisition. Scientists noting an unexpected result are usually thrilled, because they get to bask in the glory of describing the phenomenon and modifying the relevant model to account for and accommodate the novel result. The professional accolades accumulate after peer review of the analysis and verification by other scientists. Paradoxically, most research experiments are expected to generate 'unexpected' results.

Any particular 'unexpected result' only occurs once. After that, the phenomenon will have been documented, such that any new results will be repetitions or variations of previously documented unexpected results. They cease to be 'unexpected'. GMOs intended for marketing have passed through the 'research' phase and entered into the 'applied' phase. Because of the intense scrutiny under which all new plant varieties and animal breeds are subjected, it is unlikely an 'unexpected result' will first be noticed during commercial production. Those products displaying 'unexpected' or untoward results are usually eliminated or modified to remove the undesirable characteristics years before getting to commercialization. The precautionary principle will have been satisfied.

Scientists sometimes have to modify the theories to account for events they did not predict. We have now completed thousands of GMOs release trials, the vast majority having no commercial intent or application, because scientists developed them to study and look for 'unexpected' events. The type of unexpected event to arise includes those things that would be caught in the normal scrutiny of candidate cultivars anyway. The most common undesirable feature to arise in GM plants is the new gene not being expressed strongly enough. An inserted disease resistance gene provides only partial protection against the pathogen. This 'unintended' failure is usually caused by one of two things. One, the gene simply isn't strong enough to provide the degree of protection necessary. In this situation, the breeders have to decide whether the protection afforded, even if incomplete, is sufficient to justify commercial release. If not, it's back to the drawing board. The second reason is that the inserted gene is poorly expressed because of its particular location in the genome. In this case, the breeder eliminates this plant and chooses another with the same gene inserted elsewhere.

The most common 'unexpected' manifestation is the instability or inactivation of the inserted gene. That is, the inserted gene starts out functioning properly, then later ceases activity. If this inactivation or instability occurs early, the GM plant will lack the desired trait and will not be identified as a candidate in the first place; if it happens early enough, we may not even notice it as GM. If the inactivation occurs later, the GM plant line will be noticed to be 'variable' or 'heterogeneous' and eliminated from the development track. In either case, the unstable line will not make the market. We don't need additional regulatory scrutiny to eliminate any unstable crop varieties. Gene instability typically means the introduced gene becomes inactive, thus the plant reverts back to the parental appearance. Genetic instability does not mean the entire genome becomes unstable (such events are rare, usually noticed quite early, and are eagerly studied by geneticists as 'mutators').

For most novel genes, consider what happens if the gene is unstable. This means one plant out of, say, 100 000 loses the novel trait in any given generation. (Instability only works on individuals; you do not see instability working on an entire population at once, to result in an entire field losing the trait.) If the trait is a herbicide resistance, for example, what happens if that the farmer sprays the field with the herbicide, killing the weeds and 1/100 000 of the crop plants? This number of dead crop plants goes unnoticed. Similarly if the trait is *B.t.*, insects are able to consume one plant in 100 000 in a field. This goes unnoticed while contributing (insignificantly, but nevertheless) to the 'refuge'.

Genetic stability is an international requirement for new crop varieties, whether GM or 'conventional'. Therefore, genetic instability is not a health or safety issue for foods, GM or otherwise derived. In any case, the normal plant breeding process will eliminate genetic instability long before any line goes into commercial production.

Consider, also, that genetic instability, at least over many generations, is a natural phenomenon required for evolution. Nature devises mechanisms to encourage genetic instability, including spontaneous mutations and 'jumping genes'. All living things are subject to natural genetic instability, so if it were inherently hazardous, we'd know about it by now.

Another not entirely unexpected effect has the GM plant express the new trait adequately, but with a loss of agronomic performance. In this situation, we go back and look at many different transformation events, plants that each has the same new gene inserted in different locations in the genome. If all the plant lines have reduced agronomics (say poor seed yield), it's likely that the gene and its expression interfere with a critical aspect of the plant's basic physiology. If only a few lines have the reduced agronomics, it's likely due to the location of insert, not the gene itself. In this situation, as earlier, we select the best performing line for further scrutiny and assessment.

The data collected from the initial trials in the mid-1980s were essentially as expected, consequently the trials increased in size and in number, but remained very stringently regulated. Again, nothing dramatically unexpected was observed in any of the trials. Over the years, the trials became larger and more diverse. Thousands of different GMOs have been released to the environment. In 1999, GM crops covered a hundred million acres in North America alone, and the area is expanding rapidly. There are no documented dramatic or adverse 'unexpected effects' from any of these GMOs. Some activists continue to demand a full moratorium.

The Monarch butterfly

Earlier (p. 178), we mentioned the BBC report on the Monarch butterfly incident, in which it described the potentially lethal effects of *B.t.* pollen on Monarch butterfly larvae as 'unexpected', although the *B.t.* toxin is known to be lethal to lepidopteran insects such as Monarch butterflies. It might have been unexpected to the BBC, but not to scientists. They might have meant 'unintended', as no one intends a pesticide to affect any other than the 'intended' target pests. But as we've seen, Nature doesn't feel obliged to follow human definitions of pest. Or anything else, for that matter.

This recent case, along with other reports that *B.t.*-producing GM plants were adversely affecting ladybirds, lacewings, and other non-target species, illustrates the complexity of the potential environmental hazards associated not with GM, but with *B.t.* First, not all GM plants kill insects, so it's not a question of GM process, but of product. And the specific product in this case is *B.t.* toxin. Second, the Monarch experiments were fed milkweed leaves dusted with pollen from *B.t.*-producing GM maize. Another batch was fed the leaves dusted with ordinary maize pollen. But were they fed ordinary maize pollen spiked with *B.t.* toxin? No. The conclusion drawn by many, other than the authors, is that GM is to blame for the increased mortality of the larvae. Unless ordinary *B.t.* toxin (available at any organic farming supply centre) sprinkled on ordinary maize pollen is *not* lethal to Monarch larvae, the GM aspect is incidental, it serves only as the delivery system. Unfortunately, as with Dr Pusztai's GM potato experiments, we don't have the proper experimental controls. The only valid conclusion is that *B.t.* may be responsible, GM isn't. And we know from many previous studies that, yes, ordinary *B.t.* toxin from organic supply outlets is lethal to non-target insects. Unintended, yes, for both GM and organic versions of *B.t.*; unexpected, no, again for both GM and organic.

The butterfly work also suffers from other problems. The initial report by John Losey, Linda Rayor, and Maureen Carter in *Nature*, less than a page long, also identifies some of them. It was a preliminary report, based on a single, unrepeated experiment. Ordinarily, without either the GM aspect or the Monarch aspect, such a letter would not have been written, if written it wouldn't be published, and if published it wouldn't be cited. Especially not in the popular media. As a preliminary experiment, it was fine—it serves to provide some basis for conducting proper experiments involving complete controls, replications, verifications, and other hallmarks of good science. Related issues need to be addressed and explored. There was a noted difference in feeding behaviour. Like Dr Puzstai's rats finding potatoes unpalatable in general, the larvae here didn't enjoy eating pollen, GM or otherwise. Essentially, and again like the rats, they had to be force-fed, they were not given a choice of foods. We also have a problem in translating force-feeding experiments in the lab to the reality of the open fields. Milkweed is not common amid cornfields, so it's unlikely Monarchs would lay eggs there. Maize pollen is relatively heavy and doesn't travel very far, so milkweed in nearby fields wouldn't get exposed to much maize pollen anyway, GM or otherwise. In real life, maize sheds pollen over a short period of several days. Those days do not typically coincide with Monarch larvae feeding periods. If the Monarch larvae hatch and feed a few days either way of the pollen shed, they're unaffected. In the lab, of course, they're not given a choice.

To draw a conclusion based on this one experiment that GM crops will accelerate the decline in Monarch butterflies is, simply, wrong. The authors know and state this. It seems disingenuous for activists to support increased use of 'organic'

B.t. while demanding a stop to *B.t.* in GM crops when they both pose the same hazard to non-target insects (like the Monarch, lacewings, and ladybirds). Even more interesting is what will happen in the future. Most of the current GM-*B.t.* crops produce the toxin in pollen as well as other parts of the plant. New GM crop lines are coming along with no *B.t.* toxin in the pollen, so negating any adverse effects from pollen feeding.

The acceleration of insect pests resistant to *B.t.* toxin through the increased use of GM plants is a legitimate issue of considerable import. Ecologists, population geneticists, statisticians, and many other experts are trying to figure out not if, but when it might arise and how to manage the problem to minimize the threat. GM plants with the *B.t.* gene are also a rich source of confusion and misinterpreted science, especially by the media.

Genetic deprivation

The following anecdote relates to the public misconceptions of science, and also to the sometimes poor communication skills of scientists dealing with non-scientists.

When genetic engineering was first an issue in the popular press, a general reporter for the local newspaper interviewed me. She was sent to do a story on local scientists conducting research in genetic engineering, I was merely one of her interviewees. After she explained her objective and that she had no scientific background whatever, I assured her she could ask for clarification whenever I said something confusing or of particular interest. Well into the interview I was talking about our method of generating transgenic linseed. One of the genes we had available at the time had been isolated from a mouse. In standard but casual scientific parlance, I mentioned that we had taken a gene from a mouse and were attempting to put it into the linseed plant. After droning on a few minutes, I noticed her eyes had glazed over in a manner different from most people pretending to understand. I stopped to inquire, she said simply, quietly, '. . . poor mouse . . .'. Puzzled, I said 'What? What poor mouse?' She replied, a little more assertive this time 'The mouse you took the gene from. You deprived it of a gene. How is it getting by without its gene?'

I was taken aback, but it taught me a lesson. Don't assume people know what you're talking about. I hastened to assure her we only made a copy of the gene, that no mouse was deprived of its genetic heritage, and 'taken from' is only an expression scientists use in casual discussions. In retrospect, it certainly did seem to imply an illicit theft of genetic property.

Terminator technology

What scares farmers more than any other aspect of GM is probably the patented seed destruction system dubbed Terminator. The US federal Department of Agriculture (USDA) teamed up with Delta and Pine Land Co. in the USA to develop a seed suicide method. The Terminator system introduces genes that, when triggered in the GM plant, precludes the seed from sprouting. When a patent was issued on the system, the farming world went ballistic. Many farmers believe it is their God-given right to save seed from one harvest to plant next season, thus accessing a perpetual supply of seed. This 'right' of farmers is entrenched in various national and international laws. With Terminator, the farmers will have to buy fresh seed each year. I support the option of farmers to save seed if they so wish. I also encourage them to buy fresh seed each year, not so much to support the seed companies, but because of the other benefits of using fresh seed. In most cases, the additional cost of fresh seed is more than recovered later, through increased yields, better quality seed, and cleaner crops and fields. If it wasn't, farmers simply wouldn't buy fresh seed at all.

If Terminator technology is such a hot and feared item with farmers, why do I have it in the 'red herring' chapter? Because it *is* a red herring. Terminator was such a scary concept that the United Nations and Food and Agricultural Organization set up an international *ad hoc* committee of independent experts to analyse the patent and the technology to assess its potential impact. After conducting their investigations, the international committee concluded that farmers have nothing to fear from Terminator. Although a patent was issued, no one has ever put the theory into practice. There are several complex genetic modifications to make the system work in a plant, and so far it isn't practicable. No doubt, technology with a similar effect will become functional one day. In the meantime, we can discuss it rationally and not panic.

Terminator (along with Terminator 2 and subsequent incarnations) precludes farmers from growing saved seed. So does ordinary hybrid seed. Hybrid seed, developed in maize earlier this century, is preferred by most farmers, even though they have to buy fresh seed each season. Why do they prefer it? Because it gives them a superior product resulting in an income premium that more than compensates for the additional annual seed cost. When Terminator technology hits the farm, it will have to be packaged in a way to entice farmers to pay for it. No farmer will pay only for the Terminator system seed. Instead, they will continue to grow what they grow now. No, a Terminator technology, with a more generic if less memorable name—genetic use restriction technology (GURT)—will have to promise farmers an advantage to make it worth their while to buy the seed each year. Hybrid seed does not concern most farmers; GURTs will not concern them either.

Some aspects of Terminator-like GURT technology can be environmentally attractive. GURTs will be developed in two forms—one a variety or V-GURT, the other a trait or T-GURT. The GURT gives a measure of control over the activation of the restriction. The V-GURT will allow farmers to pay a fee and continue to use the variety, but a T-GURT might be an option, in which a farmer pays only if the option is exercised. Say, for example, that a T-GURT variety carries a GM fungal disease resistance gene. The relevant disease occurs irregularly in the locality. If a farmer grows the crop and there's no sign of the disease that season, he pays nothing extra for the T-GURT. If the disease blows in, he gladly pays the fee to activate the gene while the crop is standing in the field. On payment of the fee, the farmer is given a substance to spray on the crop. The substance activates the gene in the crop and the crop becomes immune to the disease. This way, the farmer has the choice to use or not use the technology. It's almost like being able to buy retroactive fire insurance after your house burns down.

Domination by multinationals (again)

The press is filled with stories, usually negative, about Zeneca and its tomato paste, about AgrEvo and its GM rapeseed, about Monsanto and its GM maize, soya, and canola. It is understandable if one thinks all GM products are from the big companies. A common concern is that the entire industry seems to be the big multinational companies. Are no public institutions or small companies involved?

Products from public institutions and small companies

In addition to the University of Saskatchewan's CDC Triffid linseed flax, there are other GM products in the market or *en route* from public institutions and smaller companies. These include GM papayas, bananas, and cut flowers.

GM papaya
Dr Dennis Gonsalves is a plant pathologist at the University of Hawaii. His work interests include viral diseases, especially papaya ring spot virus (PRSV). Not all of Hawaii is dedicated to tourism. A substantial component of the economy is agricultural, including fruit production. Papaya has been grown on the islands for some time, but diseases such as PRSV limit production. In fact, PRSV is like the AIDS of the papaya world. There is no cure, and the only treatments merely slow the progression. Like AIDS, the best advice is prevention of spread and avoidance of high-risk activities. Once the disease has entered an area, however, it is only a matter of time before it infects and destroys all the papaya trees, taking with it the livelihood of many indigenous farmers and farm workers. Oahu was once a major papaya growing area until PRSV wiped out the plantations. Papaya production moved to more remote regions in the islands, but, as expected, the virus eventually

found the hidden plantations and invaded with a vengeance, claiming 38% of the crop in just four years between 1993 and 1997.

Gonsalves and his colleagues at University of Hawaii, Cornell University, and USDA, with help from the Upjohn company, had been monitoring the spread of the plague and had the foresight to start working on a GM strategy to battle the disease in the early 1990s.

Fortunately, virus resistance is an objective within the capacity of genetic modification. Viruses are extremely simple organisms consisting of a few genes (encoded on a single short stretch of nucleic acid, either RNA or DNA depending on type of virus) wrapped in a protein coat. When the virus invades a susceptible host, the host cell machinery expresses the viral genes, resulting in the diseased state. Earlier basic science work had shown a copy of one of the virus' own genes, the recipe for the protein coat, when inserted into a host cell, could confer immunity on the host organism without causing the disease itself. Gonsalves and his colleagues acquired a protein coat gene from a virus and worked to transformed papaya with the viral gene.

The team hoped they might be able to develop a new, hopefully immune, variety without going through the usual time-consuming breeding and selection work necessary when using a non-commercial or obsolete variety as a host. They used a commercial papaya variety called Sunset as their recipient. The first GM papaya plants were placed in the fields and the researchers waited for the virus to appear. Fortunately, or unfortunately depending on your perspective, the virus showed up in that same year (1992), infecting the conventional papaya trees in the region the first test GM papayas were planted out. The GM trees, although young and tender, displayed a high degree of resistance to the disease.

The resistance was monitored and found effective and stable over the several years of testing, and is continuing. The papaya fruit from the GM trees is apparently indistinguishable from the fruit of the conventional parent. The local farmers were understandably overjoyed, as they were well aware the virus would leave them bankrupt and unemployed as it did farmers in other virus-infected regions. All that was left before commercial distribution of the GM variety to local farmers was to convince regulatory authorities the GM papayas were safe.

Regulatory compliance always takes longer than expected, even for relatively straightforward cases such as this. The PRSV-resistant GM papaya variety, named Rainbow, was eventually cleared by USDA-APHIS in 1996, followed by FDA and EPA in 1997.

Another hurdle was the intellectual property. In developing the papaya, Gonsalves and friends applied information contained in several patents. Each of the patent holders had to be recognized and rights negotiated before the GM fruit could be commercialized. A special agreement was negotiated with each of the patent holders to allow the use of the patented technology in Rainbow, but restricted to the Hawaiian growers. An association of papaya growers (PAC) organized the negotiations and distribution of 200 pounds of seed by September 1998, enough to seed almost 900 acres. Farmers had to attend a briefing to explain the GM variety and their rights and restrictions prior to receiving Rainbow seed, at no premium charge.

The disease-resistant papaya is the first commercial GM whole food generated by a public institution in the USA. Most people outside Hawaii are unaware of it, as it is a minor crop to all but the people of Hawaii, and media coverage seems to prefer private sector GM activities.

Concerns over the food safety of Rainbow papayas have been largely addressed satisfactorily, but viral disease resistance is still a crucial environmental issue. There are outstanding concerns over distribution of viral genes into the environment and the possibility of speeding the evolution of PRSV to overcome the resistance. For these reasons, academics debate the wisdom of releasing virus-resistant GMOs into the environment, but there is no such debate among the farmers of Hawaii. In their real world, the GM papayas provided them with an economic lifeline. As far as these indigenous farmers are concerned, debates on the hypothetical scenarios conducted in academic ivory towers halfway around the world may as well be on another planet.

Carnations

Florigene is a small company in Australia. Although it started life as an adjunct to one of the big companies, it was jettisoned several years ago during one of the frequent 'reorganizations' and set about establishing an independent existence.

The niche Florigene carved focused on cut flowers, concentrating on roses, carnations, and chrysanthemums, the most important flowers in the market. Florigene's 'holy grail' objective was a blue rose, and the company continues to pursue it as diligently as a crusader. Along the way, however, as often happens, other opportunities arose. The small but experienced group of scientists had to learn the genetic and molecular basis of blue pigmentation as well as the basics of genetic modification with the plants.

A sideline of the research was a blue carnation. Not their holy grail, but enough of a curiosity in the marketplace to attract attention and sales. Florigene set up a branch in Europe to pursue the European market. Most of the regulatory legislation in Europe concerns environmental issues, particularly in cultivation of the GMO, and in food safety of novel GM foods. Because the blue carnation was developed and marketed as an ornamental, it did not require food safety clearance. Since it was to be grown elsewhere and marketed in Europe as a cut flower, it passed environmental review, becoming the first GM plant approved for commercialization throughout the European Union. This achievement was a substantial coup for a small but well-focused company having to compete with the big companies in seeking regulatory approvals.

Now, in addition to varied flower colour, Florigene is interested in providing another positive attribute to buyers of cut flowers: longer vase life (the equivalent of shelf life for perishable fruits and vegetables and, fortunately, regulated by the same genes).

Unfortunately, although Florigene was successful in acquiring the European approvals for one of their GM products, the company is thinking of abandoning the European market. The regulatory compliance is too expensive and onerous, and much of it is irrelevant to their flowers. For example, why should cut flowers have to undergo a full environmental impact assessment if they're not going to be cultivated in the EU and, in a sense, are already dead? Although they did eventually obtain European approval, it came after France objected because there was no guarantee the dead flowers would not get into the perfume market, potentially endangering an unwary public.

More recent applications for marketing GM flowers are being delayed as EU officials demand more unnecessary information, including irrelevant DNA sequence information. Instead of continuing to fight European regulators, according to an official, Florigene is planning to concentrate its business in Japan and North America, where the regulatory regime is based on science and is more sensibly applied.

Rice

Many other GM products developed at public labs and from small companies are currently undergoing regulatory review prior to commercialization. These products are coming from government labs, especially the USDA in the USA, as well as from university and non-profit research foundations. The Rockefeller Foundation and other international philanthropic organizations support an impressive research effort in rice biotechnology to assist the predominantly poorer rice-producing countries generate not only more food but more nutritious food. Sponsored primarily by public funds, Swiss scientist Dr Ingo Potrykus leads a team developing 'Golden rice'. This GM rice is modified to help provide two crucial nutrients, vitamin A and iron, to combat leading causes of death and blindness in the developing world. The GM rice is provided to public plant breeders to incorporate into local breeding programmes. Details of collaborations between such agencies and labs in the Third World don't often reach the public's attention, unfortunately. For some inexplicable reason, they aren't very newsworthy.

Bananas as vaccine delivery vehicles

Medical and food objectives can coalesce. A number of debilitating diseases can be pre-empted by vaccination, but in many parts of the world, the vaccines cannot be delivered efficiently because of a lack of proper equipment and storage facilities (and local distrust of unhygienic hypodermics). Charlie Arntzen and his colleagues at the Boyce-Thompson Institute, associated with Cornell University in upstate New York, are developing a vaccine delivery system based on GM banana instead of hypodermic syringes. Everyone likes bananas, even children, and they can be easily delivered to remote areas and eaten raw (cooking usually destroys vaccines). With proper regulation, GM fruits could deliver effective vaccines and other therapeutic agents to fight the myriad of diseases prevalent in developing countries.

Public and private GM products

Within a few years, there will be a good mix of public and privately derived GM products on the market. Those consumers wishing to avoid products from the big companies will be able to do so yet still enjoy the fruits of GM technology. Especially banana and papaya.

Large international companies are certainly dominant in the biotechnology industry. Domination of any industry by any singular component is a legitimate concern in itself. But, the smaller companies and public institutions are indeed in the game, bringing forth creative and useful GM products. Many public institutions have GM products in various stages of evaluation. But public institutions tend to maintain a lower profile. They certainly don't have the advertising budget or PR personnel of the big multinationals, and tend not to be targeted by activist groups as aggressively as the big companies. In addition, many products associated with a big company originated in a public lab, but few public institutions, especially universities, have the means to take a product of a research programme to commercialization. Zeneca's GM tomato paste, for example, started life in the lab of Dr Don Grierson at the University of Nottingham, UK. Zeneca bought the marketing rights to the tomato and now pays a royalty to the university based on sales of the paste. There are other examples where public institutions work 'behind the scenes' to help in the development of commercial GMOs. AgrEvo developed its first GM canola lines when their employee, Dr Michael Oelck, was working as a guest scientist in the public lab of Dr Wilf Keller, at the National Research Council of Canada in Saskatoon. The concern over multinational domination of the technology is an issue, but often overstated.

What is genetic pollution?

Genetic pollution is a nonce-word, an expression coined to elicit a negative emotional response to GM. It implies a gene located somewhere it should not be, as a gene from one species in the genome of an unrelated species, placed there by scientists. It is often used to support the position that GM is unnatural, because (according to the argument) nature does not allow gene intermingling across species. However, this position is easily refuted. Wheat, as just one example, is the result of an evolutionary combination of genes from different species, and no humans were around when it occurred. And it is a phenomenon not just on an evolutionary time-scale. Natural gene recombination between species, even unrelated species, occurs every day without human intervention. Is it also 'genetic pollution'? The human genome carries several fragments deposited by marauding viruses. *Agrobacterium* transfers bacterial DNA into cells of higher plants. Transposable elements, the so-called 'jumping genes' are pieces of DNA that naturally move about genomes. Human intervention, via GM directs which genes get moved where, but gene transfer itself is a natural process. Also, as we know from the concept of gene homology, many genes are common to many, unrelated, species. I know of no scientific society that recognizes the concept of 'genetic pollution'.

Now what?

So far, there are no documented untoward results from the release of any GM product. But what about 'long-term' effects? There are rising demands for a moratorium on field trials until we have a better understanding of the longer-term effects of releasing GMOs. Both the proponents and the opponents were well aware that the best way to collect meaningful scientific information on the long-term effects of an environmental release was to have this over the long term. Obviously, if there is a moratorium on releases, there cannot be a long-term study, and without a long-term study (with appropriate results and conclusions) there could be no releases. Opponents meet their strategic goal (of banning GM crops outright) simply by success in the apparently reasonable call for a moratorium until long-term studies are concluded.

Other modern developments are marketed and accepted without moratoria. GMOs have been around about as long as microwave ovens. Consumers did not demand, or even want, microwave ovens. There were, and are, concerns about microwave ovens, and they certainly have had unintended consequences. When first introduced, manufacturers expected (hoped?) they would replace regular ovens. They haven't, but they've become essential adjuncts in many kitchens.

Even new foods are introduced with little public opposition (as long as they're not GM!). News of several new foods appeared in my newspaper the other day. One caught my attention: macaroni and cheese on a stick. I remain fascinated. Who would think of such a bizarre food? Who would eat it, other than curious children stuck at that age where everything goes into their mouths? I wonder who regulated and approved the new food. After all, we're used to eating mac-and-cheese, but not combined with a stick. If we can justify regulating a GM tomato with a bean gene because it's a new combination posing perhaps unforeseen risks, why not regulate the stick food on the same basis? And why, oh why, can't protesters target this unnatural, unnecessary and unappetizing nauseant instead of properly regulated and approved GM tomatoes?

Consumer acceptance of new products and new technology can be rapid, even when the technology is highly scientific and erudite. This includes DNA technology. Earlier we discussed how, just a few years ago, DNA fingerprinting evidence was suspect in courtrooms, with defence lawyers convincing judges and juries of the uncertainty of DNA technology. Now it is widely accepted and convincing, requiring defence lawyers to create more elaborate and imaginative arguments. For example, my morning newspaper carried two such stories recently. In one, a man was charged with sexually molesting and murdering a young girl, on the basis of DNA fingerprinting linking him with semen found in her vagina. The defence? Apparently, the defendant masturbated one morning, then went for a run in the local park, where he found the victim's dead body under a bush. Overcome with curiosity, he stuck his still semen-laden finger into her vagina, then continued his run. He did not deny the DNA, or semen, was his. Even if the DNA evidence indicated only two people on Earth having the same fingerprint, he might have been better off to argue mistaken identity. He's now behind bars.

In the second case, a physician was charged with drugging and sexually molesting his patients. Asserting his innocence, he cheerfully cooperated with police when asked for a blood sample, even going so far as to assist the technician in finding an appropriate vein to extract the sample. He appeared vindicated when the DNA fingerprint differed from that of the semen at the crime scene. But police became suspicious when the physician's DNA fingerprint exactly matched that of another local resident, not an identical twin brother. Another sample, this time hair from the physician's head, matched with the criminal evidence and differed from the genetic 'twin' across town. How could DNA from one person differ between hair and blood samples? After the Court heard expert testimony of how simple it was for a medically trained person to insert a thin plastic 'vein', loaded with someone else's blood, down an arm, the physician admitted doing this. He's now behind bars.

These two cases illustrate how quickly a new technology can move from suspicion to wide acceptance. Instead of arguing the legitimacy of DNA technology (a defence which served O. J. Simpson so well), we have defendants now having to contrive bizarre (if not ludicrous) situations to explain or avoid DNA matching that of the criminal evidence.

Waiting for Godot?

How long do we wait? How do we evaluate the long-term consequences of GMOs? An untoward effect in the 'long term' is hypothetically due to one of two events: either a gradual accumulation of minuscule and unobserved short-term effects, for example toxins, or the realization of a very low frequency, but single catastrophic event, unlikely to occur in a short time-frame.

We can condense the analysis of the hypothetical 'long-term' events into observation of a large population over a short term instead of a long term on a small population. This is rather like buying a large number of lottery tickets at once, instead of one at a time for years. You actually improve your odds of winning by going for the large packet.

What happens is that we evaluate the entire GM acreage. If we are concerned of a small amount of some toxin in each seed, the bulk commodity will carry enough accumulated toxin to detect. No adverse toxins have been reported from the millions of acres of GM crops. Similarly, we can also use the accumulated GM acreage to test the single event hypothesis. Each plant is an individual, grown from a separate seed. If the GM nature of the line does harbour a single catastrophic 'time bomb' hazard, each plant in the plot will have a more or less equal chance of activation (explosion) at any time. If the chance of the bomb exploding is one in a zillion, each individual plant has a one in a zillion chance of going off. If we grow a plot of one plant each year, we need to observe for over a zillion years until we start gaining confidence the bomb doesn't exist (presuming, of course, the existence of the bomb doesn't make itself evident). The total number of GM plants grown on all the millions of acres is astronomical, far greater than would be grown in small plots over several years. None has yet blown up.

These scenarios are models and, like most models, are subject to technical debate. Thankfully, the 'long-term' concern over GMOs will remain an academic exercise. Older GMOs have been in existence for over 25 years. Younger GMOs, for example the GM maize and soya in the USA, cover millions of acres each year. There are no reports of environmental destruction or health hazards from these older or widespread GMOs. It seems unlikely, then, that the mere genetic modification will be problematic in the 'long term'.

This doesn't mean I believe all GMOs are harmless. I have concerns over certain GMOs and their possible adverse effects on the environment over the long term, see Chapter 9, for example. There are certainly traits requiring cautious evaluation in an environmental release.

Fortunately, crop cultivars have a fairly short-term commercial life. Most new cultivars reach a peak of popularity about five years after release, then slowly recede as they are replaced by newer, better cultivars. Ten years might be the average life of a crop—GM or otherwise. This gives us a benchmark with which to evaluate long-term effects of a given new GM product.

CHAPTER 12

'Waiter, I can't understand the menu': labelling problems

- Isn't GM labelling an easy and effective means to placate wary consumers?
- Why are companies refusing to label their GM products?
- Will GM labels really provide consumers an 'informed choice'?
- What are some current misleading food labels ?
- How will street vendors cope?
- Can't we use 'May contain GMOs'?

In one of the few unified features of the worldwide GM food controversy, consumers support mandatory labelling for products of GM technology. The justification for GM food labelling varies. Some people want labels in order to avoid certain GM products. For example, vegetarians might want to know if the GM food contains an animal gene or protein. Some people want labels to enable them to avoid GM foods entirely. Another large contingent supports labelling for political expediency. They don't feel strongly about labelling themselves, but see it as an inexpensive concession to those holding strong feelings. 'What's the problem?' they say. 'Let's put a label on the foods and spend our time on more important issues.' Regardless of the personal justification, the common worldwide theme is to allow an 'informed choice'. Many people assert 'Consumers must have the choice to avoid GM foods they don't want . . . ' followed by '. . . so we must have mandatory labelling for GM foods!' as if labelling were the only route to achieving consumer choice. It is not. I fully agree with the first part of the assertion, providing consumers an informed choice, but the second part does not logically follow and, in actuality, will diminish the very informed choice they demand.

In most cases, a mandatory 'GM' label will be, from a public policy perspective, counterproductive, impracticable, or both. Considering the almost universal support for GM labelling, this may sound as if I'm arguing against motherhood, but I'm not. I'm trying to preserve it. Product labelling is one of the best achievements of the consumer movement. I am in full support of appropriate product labels, but indiscriminate labelling of GM products is inappropriate and will debase legitimate food labelling policy.

I strongly support 'informed choice' and, in Chapter 13, propose a mechanism to accomplish that objective while maintaining credibility in overall labelling policy. First, though, let's consider the purpose of labels, why they don't always serve the intended purpose, the impracticalities of indiscriminate labelling, and other difficulties. Along the way I raise questions concerning implementation of labelling policy and practical considerations. 'Let's label all GM products' sounds simple enough, but questions largely unanswered by the proponents of labelling illustrate the obstacles in implementing and enforcing comprehensive mandatory GM labelling.

'What's that small print on the menu?' GM labelling regulations

The international body charged with discussion of food issues is the Codex Alimentarius Commission, established to administer the joint Food and Agricultural Organization/World Health Organization Food Standards Program. The Codex has a committee reviewing the GM labelling debate. They review the issues and advise the 165 member country governments on regulatory policy.

The Codex world breaks into two camps on GM labelling. One camp wants to require mandatory and comprehensive labelling of all products of biotechnology. This camp includes most of Europe and India. The other camp says only those products carrying new health or safety concerns, of different nutritional composition, or intended for new uses ought to be labelled. That is, if a product is substantially equivalent, or, in the official parlance, 'equivalent', to the conventional version, there is no need for a GM label. In this group are Canada, the USA, Australia, New Zealand, and some South American countries.

Like most international multilateral negotiations, the Codex process is quite long and involved, so don't expect to see consensus reached soon. In the meantime, we can look at some individual markets.

Both Canada and the USA have several GM food products in the market; few are specifically labelled as GM. The practice in North America is to require a label where there is a new and identifiable health concern or a substantial alteration in the nutritional composition compared with the 'conventional' food. It is important to note that the regulations apply to any food, not just those from GM technology. That is, a food with new allergenic properties carries the label, regardless of how it was produced. Consumers in North America do not have a simple mechanism to avoid routine GM products.

Europe also has regulations on labelling GM foods. The European Commission Regulation 258/97 on novel foods requires labelling for all products of GM technology. The labelling-specific regulation, EC Regulation

1139/98, carries the detailed rules based on the review for GM maize and soya, but will be applied to all subsequently approved GM food materials. The UK led the way with implementing legislation in 1999, requiring labelling of all GM food products, whether judged safe or not. As Food Minister Jeff Rooker said, the '. . . legislation will apply to everyone who sells food—from all the main supermarkets to restaurants and caterers, and even Mr Happy's hot dog stand.' Notable exemptions from the labelling requirement include small packages such as individual pats of butter or small packets of condiments, as well as food products where GM DNA or protein cannot be detected.

Several groups are lobbying to re-establish mandatory labels for undetectable products. They've yet to enlighten us on how officials will enforce such a regulation, because in most democracies an accused is innocent until proved guilty, and legal proof ordinarily requires some evidence. How will the prosecution detect an undetectable GMO? Without detection, there is no evidence. Since the accused need only respond to the prosecution's evidence, without evidence there can be no case. With the revelation of legal technicalities dating back to the Magna Carta apparently interfering with effective prosecution, a number of amendments are already under discussion, as are technical and enforcement rules.

Australia and New Zealand are in the process of establishing labelling regulations, even though they are only just starting to grow their own GMOs. Their major concern is with imported GM material. US soya is imported into Australia and abundantly used in processed foods, as it is almost everywhere. The public concerns include the absence of labels on such foods and apparent absence of local regulatory scrutiny.

Why are companies refusing to label GM products?

'Why are they making such a fuss, unless the companies just want to restrict our choice? Do they think the products just won't sell if people know what they are?'

Certainly some consumers will avoid products with a GM label, so that is part of the companies' concern. In general, though, the companies are not refusing to label, they are complying with regulations or even voluntarily labelling their GM products. Why do so many regulatory authorities agree with the companies that labelling GM products is unnecessary? In North America, regulators and companies agree that mandatory labels should be reserved for those products carrying a documented health risk or substantial change in nutritional composition. If the GM products are 'substantially equivalent' to conventional counterparts, the companies argue, the GM label would be misleading. Labels intended to warn ('cigarettes will kill you!') or to provide nutritional information ('low in sodium'), usually assist in health or dietary restrictions. If the GM nature of the product has no bearing on either of these, regulators see it as misleading by consumers who interpret labels, often unconsciously, as warnings.

The purpose of labels

Consumer products are labelled for two reasons: to inform us of nutritional information ('119 calories per serving'; 'a good source of vitamin A)' and to warn ('caution: may cause drowsiness'). Other labels are used for advertising and marketing.

Is the intention of labelling of GM foods to warn consumers that the product is a GMO and possibly carries some health hazard? Regulations in North America do demand GM product labelling where they present an increased health risk over the equivalent conventional product. All GM products must undergo a rigorous health safety evaluation before entering the marketplace. If a GM food carries a health risk not carried by conventional but otherwise equivalent foods, the GMO must be labelled. It would seem a warning label on an approved GM product would be contradictory, in conflict with the determination of the health safety evaluation. Moreover, to put a safety warning on a product judged safe by health authorities would undermine their credibility.

Alternatively, perhaps the GM label is intended to inform, not necessarily about direct health risks, but generally, such as information on calorie count per serving or nutritional composition. Again, current regulations in North America require labels on GM products with a substantial change to nutritional composition compared to the 'conventional' version.

People want to make an informed choice about buying GMOs. An informed choice means, for example, a consumer chooses 'low sodium' foods on the advice of a physician as part of a therapeutic diet regime. The consumer's positive and informed choice enables a healthier diet consistent with the prescribed plan. A label indicating 'low sodium' enables such a choice. A label saying 'contains nuts' is useful information to a person allergic to peanuts. The informed choice allows the consumer to avoid the food in order to avoid an allergenic reaction.

The proposed 'general' GM label ('this product contains ingredients from GMOs' or similar wording) does not appear to contribute nutritional information. It informs only that the product contains GM ingredients. That is undoubtedly information, but how does the information contribute to an informed choice? How does a consumer weigh and evaluate the information in formulating a decision to buy or not buy? Some people want simply to avoid products of GM technology (we'll see how best to avoid GM foods in Chapter 13). Once again, we need to determine if we are concerned with the method or the product of the method. If we are concerned with the method, and demand a label based on the GM method, we end up painting all products of the method with the same brush. Then we are faced with the question; do all products of GM methods present an equal risk? If not, then having the same label on every product fails to distinguish the potentially hazardous GM products from the more benign. How can consumers make a legitimate informed decision if both hazardous and non-hazardous products carry exactly the same label?

Few consumer products are labelled according to their method of production. Champagne, for one. Top designer fashions are advertised as individually tailored. Finest quality confections are hand-made. It seems ironic that the method of production seems to be a label feature only for our most desirable and highest quality commodities, and for GMOs.

Labels can and do provide meaningful information and help consumers in making informed buying decisions. However, labels can also be perverted from being consumer tools into marketing tactics.

Labels can be accurate, but misleading

A label may fail to satisfy our need or desire to know about a product. Our supermarket is full of products and, although many do carry good informative labels, some product labels are deficient or even misleading. Such labels do not contribute to making an 'informed' choice. Different jurisdictions have differing regulations controlling the composition as well as the language of labels. For example, does your supermarket carry 'low fat' or 'reduced fat' vegetable margarine? 'Light' might mean reduced in calories to at least a (locally) prescribed degree, or light in colour, or perhaps reduced net weight of the package, compared with an earlier version. Perhaps your supermarket has 'reduced fat' products instead of 'low fat'. This 'low fat' margarine '. . . made with 100% canola oil' attracted my attention when I first saw it in my supermarket. Reduced fat oil sounds wonderful; like almost everyone else, my family and I want to reduce caloric intake without giving up content (in this case, the oil). I was immediately sceptical, however, as I know that fat and oil are the same thing: if, at 'room temperature', the product was liquid (e.g. sunflower oil), it was called oil; if solid (e.g. lard), it was called fat. I picked up the container and looked at a curious product indeed: something that billed itself essentially as reduced fat 'fat'. The only apparent difference compared with the 'regular' oil was the fancy label and the price (about 20% higher cost for the 'light' product). How could they reduce the fat without reducing the volume?

The answer, it turns out, is water. Water has no calories, so 30 calories is saved for every gram of fat replaced by water. Water is blended into the margarine. Obviously, 500 millilitres of liquid containing a higher than usual proportion of water to oil is going to have fewer calories than 500 millilitres of pure oil. Hence 'reduced fat'. No wonder it doesn't work very well when people try to use it for frying—the water boils off leaving too little oil to do the frying.

Is the label 'reduced fat' misleading? It is factually correct; there is less fat per unit volume. But most shoppers end up compensating for the reduced oil content by using more (and thereby having to buy more) of the product to get the same amount of oil as they used previously. Not only that, but they're often paying about 20% more for the privilege of getting less oil. I'm not aware of any place where water costs more than cooking oil, other than in these 'reduced fat' butter, margarine, and similar products.

Another example is a 'calorie-reduced' peanut butter labelled 'light' in my supermarket. Closer examination reveals the product does indeed have fewer calories. A standard serving (14 grams) of the 'light' carries only 79 calories, while the regular has a whopping 86 calories. Let's put this difference in context. Take Susie and Johnny, two growing twins who enjoy, among other things, a peanut butter sandwich for lunch every day. Hitting adolescence, Susie, in response to social pressure, becomes weight conscious so demands the 'light' peanut butter. Johnnie, similarly responding to social pressure, demands the full-bodied regular version. Assuming all other factors are equal, and based on the caloric difference between the two types of peanut butter, how long will it take for Johnnie to gain one pound over Susie? A week? A month? Three months?

Let's figure it out. We assumed that one pound is attributable to the caloric difference between the light and regular peanut butter, and the difference is 7 calories per serving. Well, one pound is 3500 excess calories, so 3500 calories divided by 7 calories per sandwich equals 500 sandwiches. It will take over a year and a half before Susie can gloat over the single pound advantage.

Or, put another way, Susie can eat more peanut butter sandwiches without gaining additional weight. Of course, she also increases her chances of getting cancer from eating more peanut butter. But then, that's not on the label.

Is it worth it? Is the 'light' product truly beneficial and is the label truly informative?

No free lunch

There are plenty of misleading labels. 'Reduced' or 'lower' implies a relative comparison and therefore easy to fudge, but what about the absolutes 'No' or 'Free'? Surely they are unambiguous terms immune to equivocation? Unfortunately, no. 'No cholesterol!' shouted the label on the package of processed potatoes in Australia. When my wife first saw this, as an ordinary consumer, her first thought was, 'Great—either they've developed a new type of potato that doesn't have cholesterol, or they've altered the processing to eliminate the requirement for adding cholesterol. I'm willing to buy such an obviously improved product.' She interpreted the label to indicate that something had changed, that previously this type of potato carried cholesterol and now it doesn't.

In fact, potatoes do not contain cholesterol and the type of processing does not introduce cholesterol. Potatoes, like all plants, do not have the

genes necessary to synthesize cholesterol. No vegetable product contains cholesterol unless it was added from animal sources during the processing (which
was not the case with this product). This company, instead of 'responding to
public demand for healthier foods', was misleading consumers into buying
their product by making them think it was now different from, and better than,
their or their competitors previous products. Potatoes certainly do contain
lectins, alkaloids, protease inhibitors, and other anti-nutritional substances,
but these are not recorded on any label I've ever seen in the market.

Another attention grabber on the shelves is 'free'. No one is mistaken in
thinking that this means the product is free of charge, even when the pitch
says, for example, 'free pizza'. We know, perhaps through bitter disappoint-
ment, that this offer means you get product free of charge only if you buy one
or more at regular price. This might represent good value, but in reality offers,
at best, two items at half price but only when you purchase two or more (try
asking for one pizza at half price). For some reason that might make sense in
the often bizarre world of advertising, the items on offer are often the type of
commodity for which there is rarely a need or desire to acquire two or more at
a time. In any case, they are not free of charge.

Free typically means 'without'. 'Cholesterol-free' means the product contains no cholesterol. This may be misleading and an abuse of proper
labelling, although factually correct. Some jurisdictions now prohibit claims
of 'cholesterol-free' on vegetable or other products where cholesterol is not
ordinarily present. The UK is not one of those jurisdictions. The label on
St Ivel 'Vitalite Light' margarine, emphasizes that the product was made from
'cholesterol-free' sunflowers. It also indicates, in much smaller print, that the
primary ingredient is water, that only 27% is sunflower oil, that it contains
pork, soya lecithin (almost certainly from GM soya), and a range of other
ingredients.

The label on Perrier™ water bottles in Canada proudly proclaims 'sodium-
free', right under the listing of sodium content as being 0.02%. Since when is
0.02 equal to zero? In practice, it might be very low, it might even be the lowest amount of sodium available in any consumable (it isn't), but in any case, it
isn't zero! Yet some people read the label proclaiming 'sodium-free' and buy
the product on that basis.

'No means no'

I heard this phrase often, growing up as a sometimes mischievous lad. More
recently, the expression has evolved to 'What part of no don't you understand?'
Although I still understand no to mean the absolute no, today's modern and
more astute children know that to today's modern and more permissive parent,
no means 'Well, maybe just a little'. Apparently this is the case with labels as well.

The converse is the 'contains 100%' claim. Several Australian brands of fruit
jams proudly proclaim 'made with 100% fruit' in large letters on the front
panel. In small letters on the back, I learned that Australian fruit contains fruit

juice, pectin, colourants, and other goodies. Although it is true that fruit does contain these ingredients, the impression was that I was buying only strawberries, not strawberries plus these other things from other, different fruits. This is another reason labels can be misleading and sometimes, as here, self-contradictory.

Although the USA has the most comprehensive labelling and advertising regulations, companies there are not exempt from questionable tactics. The inside back page of the popular monthly magazine *Consumer Reports* features misleading labels and ads sent in by readers. The sheer audacity and creative ingenuity of some is both amusing and frightening.

Other forms of advertising can be accurate, but misleading. Last week I received a flyer from a US firm offering me a postgraduate degree from a 'prestigious, non-accredited' university. Although flattered, I decided to decline, figuring that if my current qualifications from merely accredited institutions were insufficient, I probably couldn't meet their evidently higher standards of prestige.

Labels can be factually informative, but ambiguous and useless.

I reached for a bottle of vegetable oil in the shop. The front panel said, simply 'vegetable oil'. I turned the bottle to read the ingredient label. In small print, it said, simply 'contents: vegetable oil'. No argument from me. I had no doubt it contained vegetable oil; I wanted to know what *kind* of vegetable or vegetables provided the oil. Consumers have different needs in their pursuit of knowledge. Was it peanut oil? Those allergic to nuts need to know. Perhaps you want to know the kind of oil because you're limiting intake of saturates, and canola oil, for example, has half the saturated fat content of olive or soya oil. With this product, you just don't know, although the label is factually informative.

The problem with this oil is not the label, and legislation will not solve it. First, it is not peanut oil—regulations do exist to ensure such potentially allergenic products are properly labelled. Of course, this useful titbit of information is not found on the label, so it's not much help to consumers trying to exercise 'informed choice'. Second, the label merely states 'vegetable oil' because it can't be more specific, at least not without increasing the cost substantially. The processor is providing a generic product to the lower strata of the market. The oil is almost certainly a blend of whatever was cheapest by the tonne in Rotterdam the week it was processed. You might buy this bottle, enjoy the product, and decide to get it again next time you need vegetable oil. But you're disappointed because, for some inexplicable reason, the second time around it doesn't taste quite as good. Now you know why. It's a different batch, a different blend.

I fully support this product, even with an inadequate label. If you prefer safflower oil and can afford it, great. If you find you enjoy a blend of sunflower and rapeseed oil, buy a bottle of each and blend them yourself, to your own exacting specifications. But not all of us can afford the luxury of paying premium prices for premium products, and the generic 'vegetable oil' is a valuable, inexpensive product. Besides, if this product was not on the shelf (the cost of labelling each batch might raise the price sufficiently to make it non-competitive) the perfectly good oil would probably be discarded, and I hate seeing good food wasted.

Another example includes processed food products. The label on my package of chocolate mousse raises several questions. What is 'spray dried vegetable oil base', or 'modified starch'? These terms may mean something to the food industry, but not to the consumer. Relevant to our concern is the modified starch. Does this mean it's genetically modified? It might, but it probably refers to another industrial food process applied to ordinary starch. We don't know. The label, although compliant with the law, is ambiguous. Further, if the starch isn't GM, how can we be sure the modification, whatever it was, is safe?

Labels can be factually informative and unambiguous, but still useless

Labels provide much factually correct information, but the interpretation is sometimes beyond most of us. Some are simple enough: 'smoking causes lung cancer' is unambiguous and most people understand the warning correctly. Yet they still buy the product. Other items on the label are more difficult to interpret, and we continue to buy the product nevertheless.

Many people insisting on GM labels under the banner of ensuring informed choice don't seem to know much about either labels or choice. How many people actually read the labels before choosing a product? Of those, how many are informed enough to interpret the contents of the label accurately? And of those, how many buy the product anyway, in spite of a 'questionable' ingredient?

Let me take a test. Like most families, we keep a few prepared food packages in the freezer for those evenings when we're too tired, hurried, or indecisive to prepare a proper meal. Grabbing one of the packages at random, I inspect the label. Of the several ingredients listed, one towards the bottom is 'sodium benzoate'. I've seen that on labels often enough, but what is it, exactly?

- Is it a preservative or a flavour enhancer?
- Is it mined or manufactured?
- Is it natural or synthetic?
- Does it cause cancer in lab rats?
- Are there any other health hazards?
- How toxic is it if I eat a large amount at one sitting?
- How toxic is it if I eat small quantities over a long period?

The point is, I can't make an informed decision about buying this product based on the label information unless I can answer those questions. If I don't know what 'sodium benzoate' is, I can't make an 'informed decision'.

A more relevant point is, I already bought the product. Moreover, even if I read the label and knew sodium benzoate was an antimicrobial preservative used in a wide range of products from pickles to toothpaste, I would in all likelihood still buy the product.

One of the manufacturers of sodium benzoate, Hummel Croton Inc., of New Jersey, provides useful information from the Material Safety Data Sheet (MSDS) and publishes it on their Internet site (*http:// www.hummelcroton.com/*). According to the MSDS on sodium benzoate:

Ingestion may cause gastroenteritis (inflammation of the lining membrane of the stomach and intestines) with abdominal pain, nausea, vomiting and diarrhea. Systemic effects may follow and may include ringing of the ears, dizziness, elevated blood pressure, blurred vision and tremors.

The MSDS form also warns:

To the best of our knowledge, the chemical, physical, and toxicological properties have not been thoroughly investigated.

and

This product is hazardous under the criteria of the Federal OSHA Hazard Communication Standard 29 CFR 1910.1200.

The good news is there is no evidence linking sodium benzoate with cancer. However, the LD_{50} (see Chapter 5) for oral consumption in rats is 4 grams per kilogram of body weight. This means, if you fed 1 gram of sodium benzoate to each of 100 rats weighing 500 grams apiece, about 50 rats would die from the consumption. One gram of any foodstuff is not very much, even for a rat. Yet sodium benzoate is considered one of the safest preservatives. According to another manufacturer, B. F. Goodrich, a relatively new use for sodium benzoate is as a corrosion inhibitor in automotive engine coolant systems. And by the way, the official European warning for sodium benzoate is simply 'harmful if swallowed'.

A closely related chemical, potassium benzoate, is also used as a food additive and has MSDS data similar to sodium benzoate. The chronic exposure data has not been determined for either product. What are the long-term effects? No one knows—long-term studies haven't been conducted.

If the health risks are similar, and the properties of the preservatives are similar, why are some manufacturers switching from sodium to potassium benzoate in their food formulations? Is it less expensive? No, the two chemicals are similar in cost. If anything, potassium benzoate costs a bit more. Do they know something about safety we don't? No, it's not that sinister. Processors switch from sodium benzoate to potassium benzoate not for reasons of cost or safety, but because they can then label the products 'reduced sodium!'

Well, now we can make a true informed decision on whether or not to buy that toothpaste with the 'reduced sodium' label.

Some people argue that placing a GM label on GM products will allow 'informed choice' for consumers. Implicit in the argument is that, given the 'informed choice', consumers will shun GM products. But labels, even those seen as 'warning' labels, do not always put buyers off the product. Few smokers quit because of the dire and explicit labels on cigarette packages. And most of us still buy consumer products labelled to indicate such ingredients as sodium benzoate, even though we don't know what sodium benzoate is.

Not all food products are labelled

We know some, but not all, of the ingredients in popular food items. Are any of the 'secret ingredients' harmful? We have no way of knowing. What about ingredients we do know about? Most carbonated soft drinks, such as Coca-Cola, contain phosphoric acid. In high concentrations, phosphoric acid can dissolve steel. In less concentrated form, it burns our skin and irritates our innards. The toxicity of phosphoric acid is about the same as for sodium or potassium benzoate, an LD_{50} of roughly 4 grams per kilogram when consumed orally by rats.

This can be scary stuff. An 'informed decision' might be to avoid any foods with phosphoric acid, sodium or potassium benzoate, or other chemical or artificial-sounding name based on information gleaned from the label. An informed choice would also require we avoid food items with 'secret ingredients', such as Kentucky Fried Chicken and Coca-Cola, because, in the absence of complete disclosure of ingredients, an informed choice is impossible. Some people have made this choice. They eschew 'fast foods' and processed foods, eating only fresh, non-processed foods. But they are still making non-informed choices. For example, fresh produce is not required to have a label indicating the residue level of various pesticides. Nor do meat labels indicate residual hormone content. Without this information, we delude ourselves in thinking we're making an 'informed' decision. Without complete disclosure, we cannot make an informed decision. So what do we do? One popular alternative is to consume organic products, as they lack all these additives, preservatives, and pesticide residues (or at least they're supposed to). But they might carry 'organically approved' contaminants, like *B.t.* powder or nasty copper compounds, and they don't lack natural contaminants. There's no label on organic products warning us about the amount and type of fungal spores, bacterial toxins, and other 'organic' items. What about labels for cadmium content in organic durum wheat, or the amount of mercury in fish? Organic producers do not provide this information. We can't make an informed decision because we don't have full information on the complete composition of organic products. If we demand complete labelling to enable an informed decision on GM foods, why are we not making exactly the same demands, for exactly the same reasons, on organic foods?

Advertising of consumer products is a cut-throat business. Claims are often stretched to obtain an edge over the competition. We consumers are used to this, hence don't place much credence in such advertising claims as 'Vastly improved using our exclusive secret patented formula X50!' This type of claim is especially prevalent in health and beauty products. Does anyone really wonder what X50 is? What does it mean that it's patented? Many people presume, wrongly, that if it is patented it must be really good and work really well. We'll deal with patents in a later chapter. For now it's sufficient to note that,

- if it's patented, it isn't a secret
- it was probably patented forty or fifty years ago, making it now public domain, no longer exclusive to that company
- 'secret formula X50' is almost invariably this manufacturer's name for a common industry standard compound plus perhaps an unusual but inert ingredient to make it different.

Many consumer products in the market appear to be unique, but aren't substantively different from their competitors' products.

Not all components are on the label

For the most part, foods in our marketplace are cleaner and purer than ever before. However, no food is truly 100% pure. Even pharmaceutical products, employing the highest and most costly standards of production cleanliness and purity, are allowed certain levels of impurities. Contaminants are present in all foods. A batch of food is rejected when the contaminants reach the threshold level. But an approved batch of food doesn't provide purity information or the composition of the impurities on the label. Even something as pure and uncomplicated as flour is measurably less than 100% flour. As we noted earlier (Chapter 5), 21% of 567 cereal-based foods tested in the UK, including flour, contained mites. Perhaps these animals should be listed on the label. After all, strict vegetarians, among others, might be interested, particularly as these contaminant animals contribute far more animal DNA and protein to the food than GM will.

Another perspective on purity concerns the EU mandatory GM labels. Suppose we have a batch of conventional rapeseed oil approved at 99% pure. Presumably, it would avoid triggering the mandatory GM label. Can the remaining 1% be GM rapeseed oil without requiring a label? If yes, doesn't that defeat the purpose of the indiscriminate GM labelling? If no, doesn't that defeat the purpose of the 1% impurity allowance? What if we don't know exactly what the impurity is? Does the approved batch get a GM label on the chance that it might be GM material? I can foresee an opportunity for mischief here. An unscrupulous processor might be tempted to carefully blend oil from GM varieties to below the threshold level in a 'conventional', non-GM batch and sell it as 'non-GM' oil.

Impact of mandatory labelling costs

Segregated whole foods, such as Flavr-Savr™ tomatoes or varietal wine grapes, are easiest to regulate and label, if necessary or desirable. However, the lower end of the market, typically the mixtures of various qualities and sources blended into the 'no name' product, will be the most costly to label and regulate because of their uncertain provenance, and will therefore have the greatest price adjustment. The Prince of Wales and I have at least one thing in common. We both can afford to pay extra to buy non-GM food if we so wish. Many people do not have that luxury and must buy at the bottom of the market. Unfortunately, these are the consumers with least purchasing choice in any case and simply buy whatever's cheapest, whether out of ambivalence to the potential dangers or out of penurious necessity. Raising the price on these products through unnecessarily and largely ignored labelling will not help them.

According to the proponents, the major argument in favour of mandatory and comprehensive labelling of GM products is that it will enable informed choice. However, indiscriminate GM labelling will not enable informed choice for most consumers. The examples and scenarios noted above show how labels don't always enable informed choice and don't work to the benefit of consumers, even when they do provide accurate information. In addition, focus group studies show most consumers obtain product information from media, advertising, word of mouth, and recipes well ahead of labels. I prefer the model requiring labels only on new hazardous or allergenic products or those substantially changed in nutritional respect, regardless of method of production.

The impracticalities of indiscriminate GM labelling

I will probably lose the argument, at least in Europe. Well, I'm enough of a democrat to accede to the will of the masses and say, 'OK, if we must have mandatory and indiscriminate GM labelling, how can it be most effectively implemented?'

Let's consider how blanket GM labels might be applied. Using real examples, we draw up scenarios and ask questions concerning labelling practicalities. In a stepwise fashion we encounter increasing complexities, demanding increasingly complex answers. We learn that it is facile to simply say 'Let's label all GM products'. Opponents to indiscriminate GM labelling don't have the answers to all these questions, so it is up to the proponents to provide answers and practical mechanisms to address the concerns. Let's start with an easy one.

Under what situations will GM products be required to be labelled? Consider an example of a whole food product such as the Flavr-Savr™ tomato. We all agree the GM tomato would trigger any blanket labelling requirement covering GMOs. Does each individual tomato get its own little sticker? Or would it be satisfactory to have a sign on the bin in the supermarket? One practical problem with the bin label is that tomatoes in different bins will, inevitably if inadvertently, become mixed. We'd have to either set a 'tolerance' limit or increase bin security.

Let's complicate the situation slightly. Consider tomato paste. We have an example of GM tomato paste in the UK, a product of Zeneca, made with tomatoes grown in the USA. The company has voluntarily labelled the product. It went on sale in the UK in 1996, preceding the mandatory labelling regulation. This product, clearly labelled as being made with GM tomatoes, was a market success for several years.

Let's complicate matters a bit more. Many tomato paste manufacturers use whatever tomatoes are available when they are ready to make a batch. The Zeneca tomatoes were segregated and used exclusively for the UK-labelled brands, but in many brands the cultivar origin of the tomatoes is mixed or unknown. Should these tins from blended tomatoes of unknown variety origin be labelled? With what? 'may contain . . .'? This wording introduces its own problems, as we'll discuss later.

The next step in our complication series is to combine cultivars. The lower end producers and 'no name' brands may acquire small loads of many different cultivars and have to blend them to make enough for a commercial batch. What labels should the resulting tins have? Finally, the really low end may be local 'farmer's market' type product, where unsold but over-ripening whole fresh tomatoes are combined in a batch to salvage a saleable sauce, puree, or paste. The cultivar origin might be not only unknown but unknowable because of the varied sources and the advanced state of ripening.

Next step. What about when the tins contain 'product of more than one country'? On its own, this is not too hard to deal with. We already see many such products in the market with this notice. What do we do about a GM ingredient produced in one source country? Presumably that would invoke the label requirement. A problem arises if the product is not considered a GM in that source country, but is a GM in the consuming country. Does it make a difference if the situation is the other way round, that the product was considered and produced as a GM in the source country, but not in the consuming country? What if it is processed (and labelled or not, as appropriate) in the source country but consumed in the other country with conflicting definitions of GM? Then the situation can become even more complex by asking about the country of origin, a second country of processing, and a third country of consumption.

The oil from an oilseed crop presents a different issue. Suppose GM maize or canola is properly grown and regulated in one country, the oil extracted and shipped as oil to a second country for consumption. There is no conflict in the determination that the plants themselves were indeed GM. But the oil does not contain GM DNA or novel protein. Does the bottle of oil have to be labelled? Similar questions can be asked concerning starch or flour from GM potatoes, wheat, maize, soya, and other GM starch crops.

Motivation behind calls for labelling becomes important here. A person may object to eating GM foods on health or safety grounds because they believe, for whatever reason, the foreign DNA is potentially harmful. They should have no objection to consuming the oil or flour from GM plants because the foreign DNA and protein was left behind, unconsumed (at least not consumed directly by that consumer). For people holding this view, labelling of the derived food product should not be necessary.

On the other hand, people who wish to avoid GM foods for ethical or religious reasons might still see the product as undesirable, even in the absence of the foreign DNA or protein. These people object to the original method. To them, any product derived from an objectionable method, is also tainted.

Continuing the 'derived from' scenario, consider the plant breeding process. There is no demand or even interest in labelling food products based on the method of breeding when the method is a 'traditional' one. Plant breeders often start the process with a registered cultivar as a parent in a subsequent cultivar. A breeder may start with a GM parent, but use conventional crossing to develop, in twelve or so years' time, a new cultivar. This new cultivar has a new name and identity and was clearly produced by a traditional breeding method. Again, we run into the problem of jurisdictional definitions, in that some places do not see the new cultivar as GM but other do. We also have a labelling problem. Is the new cultivar guilty by genetic association? Presumably by the time of its release we will have become aware of any health or safety issues with the GM parent. Such events, if substantial, would have precluded commercial release of the progeny cultivar. What, if any, criteria do we apply to labelling food products from such derived cultivars? Some people might say if we have a history of this type of GM in the parent cultivar without problem, perhaps we should exempt the progeny from the labelling requirement. Others might argue that the basis for labelling should be the presence of 'foreign' DNA. (I would ask such people about the oil and flour situation.) If the criterion were simply the presence of 'foreign DNA', food products from the conventional cultivar would have to be labelled. Or would they? What constitutes 'foreign DNA'? Similarly, in human society we grapple with immigration and legal or illegal incursions into a country or society. When does a human foreigner become assimilated into and a welcome member of the local society? How many generations need pass before they are 'one of us'? How many generations need pass before a 'foreign' gene is no longer foreign?

Another complication arises when the 'foreign DNA' isn't foreign. Once again, we can consider the Flavr-Savr™ tomato. Clearly, the Flavr-Savr™ was produced using rDNA methods, so if the sole criterion for labelling is method based, it triggers the label requirement. Let's say we use rDNA methods to develop a similar GM tomato but insert only another tomato gene. The GM criterion is met, we used rDNA to develop the cultivar, and so the product must be labelled. We then continue our tomato breeding programme, but revert to traditional breeding methods and use the GM cultivar as a parent. What is the labelling requirement for the resulting progeny cultivar produced using traditional methods? If we apply the 'method' criterion, the progeny cultivar does not trigger the requirement because it was generated using conventional methods, not rDNA. Nor does it carry any 'foreign' DNA from a non-tomato species, so any criterion based on DNA from a different species would similarly not trigger the requirement. I'm not aware of any practicable criterion to apply to this tomato variety to require labelling. The proponents arguing the tomato ought to be labelled will have to provide a better set of criteria.

Let's look at yet another complication. Suppose a clearly GM cultivar is used as a parent in a conventional breeding programme. The breeder may develop a new progeny cultivar but 'breeds out', and thus eliminates, the foreign DNA of the parent. CDC Triffid GM linseed carries positive attributes other than those introduced by the inserted DNA. For one, it is quite early-maturing, a positive and desirable trait in the Canadian short growing season. A breeder might like to use the GM linseed as a parent in a conventional breeding programme not for the GM features but to provide early maturity to conventional cultivars. In this situation, the breeder would select progeny with early maturity and exclude progeny carrying the foreign DNA. The new cultivar, produced using conventional methods, would contain only linseed genes with no trace of the foreign genes. Although it must admit to a GM parent in its genetic lineage, the GM features of the parent were eliminated. Do the new cultivar and its food products require labels? The proponents of blanket labelling provide no criterion by which this cultivar could be distinguished from 'conventional' cultivars. Furthermore, no enforcement or verification test would indicate the linseed to be GM. Regulations are meaningless without verification and enforcement measures.

Another complication involves labels for meat from animals fed GM grain. The animal itself isn't GM, but it will have proteins and DNA made from GM building blocks, provided by digestion of the GM grain DNA and GM protein. Complicating the issue further, we may not know for sure the genetic source of the feed for the animal. Even free-range animals might be exposed to GM plants, the GM plants or pollen having escaped from the confines of the cultivated fields where it or an ancestor was sown under 'controlled' conditions.

Another avenue to confound the 'derived from' scenario includes clothing made from GM fibre crops such as cotton or flax. Linen is particularly suspect, as it is made from whole living cells, containing a tiny amount of DNA and protein. Does that expensive linen shirt really need a warning label?

What else gets labelled?

Tomatoes are fairly easy. We all know what they are and what they look like in the shop. Earlier we asked if the label is to be placed on each individual tomato or if a sign on the bin is sufficient. It is technically feasible to place a sticker on each individual fruit—many apples, bananas, and other fruits already have labels on each individual, usually a brand sticker.

Let's complicate life again. Some products (e.g. GM maize) are more difficult to label. Maize comes in many forms, from individual seeds to entire shiploads. Both examples would present a problem in effective label mechanics. How do you place a label on a single grain of maize? How do you place a meaningful label on the cavernous hold of a ship?

Mr Happy's hot dog stand

The government said labelling provisions apply to all, including Mr Happy's hot dog stand. Here we have all the practical problems mentioned earlier, plus new ones. For one, how is Mr Happy supposed to inform all prospective customers about every ingredient in every item? The UK regulation allows signs, but they must indicate verbal capacity also. Most vendors don't have time to go through the spiel about menu options and costs, and most customers don't have time to listen. How long are you willing to stand in the queue while Mr Happy delivers the requisite speech to each customer ahead of you?

Again, the proponents of blanket labelling have to provide answers to practical problems. For example, if labelling and segregation are required, how is Mr Happy supposed to keep the GM tomato sauce from slopping into the non-GM tomato sauce, and vice versa? The current regulation allows zero cross-contamination. Most labelling discussions seem to demand absolute segregation. If a single drop of GM sauce is observed slipping over, what then? Is the whole batch to be discarded? If not, how much slop will be tolerated before the sauce is considered contaminated? If contaminated sauce is to be discarded, where can it safely be disposed? Into a hazardous waste container? Who monitors the contamination level? The regulations say local food safety authorities, but it seems impracticable for anyone other then the vendor to regularly monitor the contamination from one sauce to another. It is also unlikely vendors will strictly enforce the regulation if it means throwing out their profit margins. Also, regardless of who gets to monitor the tomato sauce, contamination must be measured somehow. There is no currently accepted and reliable measuring system to detect and quantify GM components. Considering the elaborate and expensive tests required, a mammoth monitoring and enforcement bureaucracy would have to be established to sample and test every batch of tomato sauce for every conceivable GM product. Mr Happy will probably have to change either his name or his business.

Let's assume a batch of conventional tomato sauce is tested and a small amount of GM sauce is detected in it. Mr Happy faces steep fines (£5000!) or incarceration. If we are truly concerned for the health and safety aspects to consumers, we would also have to notify customers exposed to the un-labelled sauce. How far back do we go—to the time the last test showed non-contaminated sauce? In practice, this will require more and more frequent testing, as the ability to track down past customers drops dramatically with time.

These complications were based on the tomato sauce example. GM mustards are on the way, bringing with them the same concerns and more. Not only will we have to consider contamination of conventional tomato sauce with GM tomato sauce, we'll have to guard against contamination of conventional mustard with GM mustard, plus GM tomato getting into GM mustard and vice versa. After all, there may be people who have no problem with GM tomato sauce but avoid GM mustard.

The impracticality of this ludicrous situation is that street vendors exist by offering an inexpensive and convenient snack. Their prices, and therefore their costs, must be kept to a minimum. By forcing vendors to segregate their tomato sauce (and, eventually, their other condiments, buns, and even meat as more and more food products include GM ingredients), they will not comply, they will instead provide only one. Now, no doubt at this stage some of you will be clapping hands and saying 'great', on the assumption that if only one tomato sauce is to be stocked on the vendor's wagon, it will be the non-GM version. After all, with so many people expressing concern over GMOs, street vendors won't risk alienating a substantial segment of customers.

In all likelihood, if only one tomato sauce is stocked on Mr Happy's wagon, it will be the GM version. Only one factor is more important to a street vendor than attracting as much custom as possible—cost. Despite possibly alienating some prospective customers, street vendors live on survival mode, and will stock the least expensive product available. Under the EU regulation, in order for a tomato sauce to avoid the GM label, it must have documentation to show it contains no GM products. Because of the requirement to identify cultivars and derived products as being GM or not, we lose the bottom, unidentifiable source of the least expensive tomato sauce. Instead of being the 'generic', non-GM tomato sauce, the bargain basement sauce gets labelled as GM (whether it has GM cultivar contribution or not—who's going to check?) and available at the lowest cost. The GM product becomes the 'default' status. So what if they have to post a notice on top of the umbrella? Most people will ignore it within a few weeks anyway, and then it can blow off in the breeze.

GM becoming the default status will become apparent far beyond low-end food retailers. What happens if a small- or medium-sized food processor honestly and sincerely doesn't know the pedigree of a load of tomatoes? The tomatoes may be a mix of many different cultivars gleaned from local communities or overripe imports from retailers. Local entrepreneurs might use various batches of tomatoes from local markets to make up 'home-made' tomato sauce. Individuals might buy properly labelled GM tomatoes, but then use the seeds to start a tomato patch in the home garden, with the resulting product passed around the community and selling in local markets. Obviously, passing of GM foods without a label will require severe penalties, so no one would want to take a chance if they didn't have complete documentation. Because such documentation is expensive, most small operators likely won't bother with it. Without documentary assurance of 'non-GMO' status, all of these products will, by default, be labelled as GM, making the label useless. We still won't know for sure if the product contains GMOs or not.

One beneficial consequence of this GM label confusion may be the market opportunity in speciality, non-GM snacks. After all, we can't expect seriously rich people to stop at Mr Happy's hot dog stand. Seizing the chance to make big money and cater to a higher class of clientele, some enterprising young environmentalist might set up a speciality, non-GM snack shop, in direct competition with Mr Happy. Of course, the prices will be higher, but we've seen other consumer goods offered very successfully at the high end of the market for speciality service and perceived quality. Under this scenario, free enterprise will have prevailed and all will profit!

What about this simple solution?

Donald Bruce is director of the Church of Scotland's Science, Religion and Technology Project, which looks at ethical issues in technology. Dr Bruce has a simple solution: label all foods with any GM-linked ingredients. The government has missed the point of mandatory labelling and essentially abandoned people with their legitimate anxiety, he says.

Unfortunately, as we've seen, it isn't always simple to identify all sources of all ingredients. It appears Dr Bruce is assuming we already know all of the cultivars going into all of our foods. What happens if you just don't know all of the cultivars represented in the batch of tomatoes you're about to make into paste? Do we dump these 'no name' foods into a sanitary landfill? Do we ban all such foods? We'd end up banning many of those 'bargain' brands on the shelves, or else forcing the price up sharply and substantially. Before taking such drastic action, let's ask Dr Bruce to consider the consequences on the less affluent sectors of society.

The other 'unintended' effect of Dr Bruce's suggestion is that we'd lose the benefit of labels by inundation. Warning labels are useful only as long as they're relatively rare. We've heard that 60% of the foods on our shelves already have GM ingredients from GM soya alone. What proportion of foods will contain GM ingredients when they start to include by-products of GM tomato, maize, potato, sugar beet, canola, and linseed? If and when GM crops are grown in the UK the proportion will be even higher. When the majority of products carry the same label, the labels cease to provide any benefit for consumers. Implementation of mass label regulation will dilute the value of warning labels on all products. But what worries me particularly is the effect on those products for which they really do serve a health and nutrition warning purpose, and on the poorest segments of society.

What wording to use?

Another pragmatic problem with the 'label all ingredients' camp is what information to put on the label. Is it simply 'contains GM ingredients'? Or we could provide more detail, such as 'this tomato contains a tomato gene, inserted backwards'. Or perhaps we need to include the specific method of transformation, as some people recognize *Agrobacterium* as a 'natural' method and therefore acceptable, but not other mechanisms of gene transfer.

Most people seem to have no problems with the simple 'contains GMOs'. This might be useful for those who object to all GMOs on ethical or moral grounds, but not those for whom the issue is one of health.

I know Orthodox Jews who eat only kosher foods. The onus is on them to determine the nature of their foods. Orthodox Jews do not demand all food products be labelled as 'kosher' or 'non-kosher'. If people object to GM food on an ethical or religious basis, that's their privilege, but, like orthodox Jews, the onus ought to be on them to determine the source and propriety of their foods. Labelling foods to satisfy religious preferences would set a dangerous precedent. It would probably lead to a profusion of similar demands from many different groups with concerns or prohibitions of various types of food product.

Society has more sympathy for labelling requirements based on health issues. For these cases, more information than simply 'contains GMOs' is needed. For example, beans containing a gene for Brazil nut protein would need accurate labels to inform those people allergic to Brazil nuts. The simpler sign 'contains GMOs' could mean almost anything—an inserted gene from another bean, for example, which would not be of concern to people allergic to Brazil nuts.

Vegetarians or members of certain religious groups might not be concerned with a GM food unless the introduced gene comes from a prohibited animal. Tomatoes with a tomato gene inserted, in reverse orientation or not, may not be an issue to vegetarians. But a tomato with a pig gene might cause considerable anxiety and interest, not only to vegetarians but also to Jews, Muslims, and others. A simple 'contains GMOs' won't work to provide information to these people. If we're going to have useful labels satisfactory to enable an informed choice, they will have to carry the relevant information.

Another complication with GM label wording

Proponents of mandatory labelling need to determine the most useful information to enable an 'informed choice'. Let's say a vegetable oil is 100% canola rapeseed oil, made from GM rapeseed. Vegetable food oils are composed of several different 'fatty acids'—stearic, palmitic, oleic, and linoleic acids are the most common. The label might say '100% rapeseed'. Instead, it could list the proportions of fatty acids in the standard rapeseed oil batch, or perhaps list the proportion in that particular batch of oil, or maybe list the actual proportions in that particular bottle. If the fatty acid composition is useful information for a label, why should it be limited to GM oil? It would seem only customers of GM products would benefit from the useful information. Why not make it mandatory for all vegetable oils, GM or otherwise?

What about processed foods with multiple ingredients?

That tin of baked beans with bacon in tomato sauce looks interesting. What label is applied to a product where several ingredients are potentially GM? The beans, the bacon, and the tomato are each of interest to at least some consumers. If we include the actual gene information for each ingredient on the label, there won't be much room left to indicate what's in the tin. Other than the 'novel' genes, of course. What do we do if the only 'novel' DNA in the GM beans comes from tomatoes and the only foreign DNA in the GM tomatoes is from beans? We're eating food from a tin where tomato genes and proteins are all mixed in with bean genes and proteins. The genes and proteins are hardly foreign or novel at this stage. If some of those genes got mixed together earlier in the process, does that exempt the product from labelling?

Labelling is not simply a matter of printing a stamp with 'contains GMOs' or 'contains no GMOs'. Greenpeace has kindly designed a GM logo they suggest be placed on all GM products. The logo itself is simple, easily identifiable, and seems innocuous enough, lacking any apparent visual emotional component. Unfortunately, despite Greenpeace's good intentions, the logistical problems and costs are not in making and affixing a label or logo to designate GM products. The greater problem and cost is associated with segregated production, harvest, transport, processing, transport to markets, storage, shelving, and advertising in the shops. Each of these steps requires an additional bureaucratic layer to verify and enforce regulations in addition to the duplication of resources all along the production stream.

Some people think we can do no wrong in having factual information provided on a label. However, it is possible to go overboard. According to the 27 March 1998 issue of *New Scientist*, a camera instruction booklet (Konica 110 Zoom) carries this safety warning: 'This product is intended for photography. Please do not use for any other purpose other than photography'. The mind fairly boggles at the possibilities. Why not include 'Not for internal use. Not to be taken orally' as some products now warn? Such statements on obvious products serve to stimulate the creative mind. What else would one use the product for? If not orally, how? Could an injured consumer sue for damages if the product was used aurally?

What else is in our foods but not on the label?

Even well-designed and informative labels on some products are incomplete. Bacteria live in milk and other foods. Milk is pasteurized to kill bacteria, but it doesn't get them all. Over time, the bacteria increase in number and cause the milk to sour. How can a label accurately reflect the bacterial population if it's constantly increasing?

Ageing affects chemical composition in fats and oils. Fungal infections affect fruit and vegetables. Bacteria affect eggs. Weather can have effects beyond age; freezing, for example, can cause chemical changes in foods. How can we label all these when the composition changes so much?

Furthermore, consider something as simple as wheat flour. You take a batch of wheat seeds and grind it up. Pure flour, right? But each batch of seed will have a different composition. Even excluding contaminants (with insects, fungi, and so on, accounting for a large proportion), different cultivars have different chemical compositions. After the farmer harvests the grain, the wheat seed is blended in the elevator with seeds from other farmers, other wheat varieties, and other contaminants. Then, the miller who makes the flour further blends it. Then it is blended again by the baker, adding in all sorts of things to make, for example, speciality breads. Then there are the ingredients no one adds intentionally, like the flour mites. How is it possible to keep track of all these blends? Or do we take a chemical composition after the final consumer product is made? But this only raises more questions. Do we analyse one batch? Or every batch? Who pays for all these additional analyses? The only question I can answer with any confidence is this last one.

Most foods will face this problem. As fats and oil age, they go rancid. This is a chemical reaction. New chemicals appear in the food that didn't necessarily appear on the label. If they did appear on the label, the amounts and proportions have changed. How do we regulate this changing composition on the label?

Fruits and vegetables age. As they ripen, then overripen, the chemical composition changes. New chemicals are produced, sometimes in substantial quantities. Remember the polygalacturonase enzyme in ripening tomatoes? (Chapter 2). Different batches of fruit, even from the local market, will carry different amounts of natural chemicals. One batch may have a tiny amount of some toxin from a minor fungal infection. Eggs might carry some *Salmonella* bacteria. There's no way to accurately tell 'how much', because it constantly changes. Are you sure you want to know these contaminants and compounds are in your foods? Edwina Currie tried to warn people about *Salmonella* in eggs but was told it only frightened people. What do we do? Proponents of blanket GM labelling assure us the public wants to know if there is one part per billion of rDNA in their foods. But apparently the public ought not to be told about bacteria in one out of 650 eggs.

If gene products are on the label, why aren't other things?

If a GM gene is present and reportable at, say 0.000 1%, then it is only sensible to account for all the other 99.999 9%. Even if the product is 99.5% pure (which, by the way, is very high), it means other things in there account for the remaining 0.499 99 %. This will include such yummies as arsenic, cyanide and a whole range of other 'natural' ingredients. Consider the L-tryptophan case from Showa Denko, described in Chapter 6. That product was 99.6% pure, according to the FDA analyses. The problem contaminants were present in fewer than 4 parts per thousand. The standard purity requirement for this product was 98.5%, meaning an approved batch could have 15 parts per thousand as contaminants.

In Chapter 5 we discussed ordinary contaminants in ordinary foods, such as flour and cereal grains. If there's such a strong demand to label GM foods, why isn't there any demand to label the far greater content of insects and rat shit in foods? Although the quantities are tiny, people still eat far more insect parts and faecal matter than rDNA or proteins from GMOs.

The 'may contain' trap

One alternative compromise is the 'may contain' wording. 'This product may contain GMOs (or nuts, etc.)' gets around the problems of uncertain identity and saves the various costs of continued monitoring from batch to batch. Unfortunately, it becomes meaningless and is potentially dangerous. My daughter has a nut allergy. At one time, there were no labels, so we avoided anything that looked as if it might contain nuts. Then labelling came along, and saved us a lot of anxiety about chocolate bars and other food items because they were labelled as having nuts—there was no question, those items were off the safe list for us. Other items were acceptable. This was useful labelling.

Then came 'may contain . . .' and we ended up worse off than before; products we earlier identified as being safe and nut free now said 'may contain nuts'. Better to be safe than sorry; they had to be struck off the safe list.

The reason for using this wording is obvious; by simply labelling everything as 'may contain' the producer claims no liability if someone sues them, and they don't have to perform any serious quality control as far as nuts are concerned (although many do). What it means to my daughter is that she now avoids many safe products she used to enjoy, even before any labels were used.

Other difficulties arise with the phrase 'may contain GMOs'. Consumers often interpret it as the company saying 'We don't know if there are any GMOs in this batch or not, and we can't be bothered finding out'. In reality, it usually means 'This batch of food is a blend from many sources, some of which use GMOs, and we have no way of knowing if a particular shipment includes product from a GM source or not.' Consumers see the companies as incompetent, uncaring, or uninterested, simply using the 'may contain' label for expediency. The food industry sees the impracticality of determining the source of every batch of every ingredient. Until there is sufficient consumer demand (i.e. willingness to pay) for segregated products (whether for nuts or GMOs), there will be no segregation.

Can we use negative labelling?

Another alternative to blanket GMO labelling is the 'negative label', in which a label guarantees the underlying product to be free of GM material. There is a legitimate place in the market for non-GM products to accommodate those consumers who wish to avoid GM for whatever reason. Unfortunately, advocates of negative labels (i.e. 'this product contains no GM ingredients') can't prove the assertion, because negatives can't be proved. In many jurisdictions, the onus is on the 'labeller' to prove the claim before the label is allowed. Even without the legal aspect, we need to recognize the difficulty in assigning such labels. Proponents of negative labelling need to address many of the same complications as for the 'positive' labels. How do we deal with vegetable oil, for example, containing no detectable DNA or protein, GM or otherwise? Can it be labelled 'contains no GM ingredients'? If so, what if it came from GM maize? Presumably, if the oil came from GM maize, then the product should not have a 'contains no GM ingredients' label, even if no GM ingredients are detectable. However, if you can't detect DNA or protein, how do you know for sure it came from GM material? Without a reliable means of detection, there's no legitimate means of enforcement. Dishonest processors will quickly debase the system by labelling 'contains no GM ingredients' on refined GM maize oil, knowing there's no way to detect the GM nature of the originating plants. Then they collect a premium for 'GM-free' oil.

In any case, occasional contamination will ensure no product can legitimately claim to be devoid of GM material. Perhaps we could devise a tolerance limit, say 2% or 5%, and have a label to the effect of 'contains minimal GM ingredients'. Or, better yet, 'organic'.

More impracticalities: where do we draw the line with labels?

In an Oxford University undergraduate biology experiment, students 'karyotype' themselves, using a simple and now obsolete method of looking at chromosomes from cheek cells swiped with a toothpick. As a lab demonstrator, my biggest concern was that someone would find a chromosomal aberration, but this was rare. Most people with gross chromosomal errors that might be detected in this lab exercise (e.g. Turner or Klinefelter syndromes) are already aware of it.

However, some other benign unusual features did turn up from time to time. I remember one student asked me to have a look down her microscope. I did, and then asked her 'Do you drink much coffee?' She went pale, and said, quietly, 'How do you know?' I pointed out her cheek epithelial cells, a large proportion of them binucleate. I explained that the caffeine in coffee (and other common drinks) can cause nuclei in cells to replicate, but the cell does not then divide to complete the mitotic process. A single cell ends up with two nuclei. It seems to be harmless. Nevertheless, it is a common genetic change induced by a very commonly consumed chemical.

People have a right to know this about caffeine, as well as about all the other quirks caused or exacerbated by the various things we consume. Does this mean we should now remove caffeine from the market? Or require labelling of all products with caffeine? It's worth a reminder that caffeine is a natural product, not synthesized by one of the big multinational companies in an effort to undermine the cells of an unsuspecting world.

Labelling of coffee presents many questions. How do we label coffee beans sold in bulk? Instant coffee powder? What about decaffeinated coffee—certainly not all of the caffeine has been removed. And what about the process used to remove the caffeine? Did they use that nasty mercury process, or the 'natural' process? While we're on the subject, isn't there caffeine in chocolate bars? Cola drinks? Even the ones labelled 'caffeine-free' probably have a little bit left behind. What about trade secrets? Coca-Cola doesn't tell us what's in their popular drink. How do we know they're not slipping something past us? Kentucky Fried Chicken is another example of a common food with unknown, undisclosed ingredients. Eleven different herbs and spices found in an ordinary kitchen—what does that mean? What else is in the chicken? What did the chicken eat? What else is in (or on) the herbs and spices?

Unfortunately, labelling is not the answer many people had hoped it would be. These complications are the tip of the iceberg. The move to use a label as a marketing tool or otherwise misleading marketing information is anathema to the whole concept of labelling.

Then there's the problem with bulk commodities such as maize, soya, or wheat. How do we label them? A processed food, such as a loaf of bread, has so many different ingredients it is impossible to provide a label documenting all of them. Most people are satisfied with the basics: wheat, yeast, water, etc. If we have to extend the label to define wheat cultivars, or yeast strains, why not also include source of the water? Every source of water will contain different amounts of minerals (such as arsenic) and other contaminants. How do we put that on the label?

Another problem is the differences in batches. Food producers often source different ingredients according to what's available at the least cost. Each batch of ingredient will have a slightly different chemical composition. The processor will ensure the final product is consistent in quality from batch to batch, but minor constituents and contaminants will vary and, for the most part, are immaterial to the overall taste and quality of the product.

What do we do about something as fresh and wholesome as local produce at the farmers' market? Do we just assume it's safe? How can we expect a local farmer to analyse and label these 'home-grown' products? Of course it is not feasible to conduct these analyses at the local level. Visual, olfactory, and tactile inspection is usually sufficient to tell if a plum from the local market is fresh and safe to consume. But plums and other market products can harbour massive amounts of fungal and bacterial, as well as non-biotic contaminants. They're still likely safe to eat, but shouldn't they still be labelled with the amounts of contaminants? Then there are the natural, non-contaminant ingredients in plums, the cyanogenic glycosides. I'm more concerned about them than a few fungi, bacteria, or pesticide residues.

If our motivation is to provide an informed choice to consumers, then it is logically consistent to require labels on these farmers' market products as well. If they are exempt because they are 'safe', then shouldn't other products determined to be 'safe', including GMOs, be exempt also?

'Best before . . .' when?

What about the 'best before' or 'use by' debate? The exact wording may differ slightly (I like 'enjoy before' and 'guaranteed fresh until 31 May' as if a built-in staleness switch is activated at midnight on that date). 'Best before' does not take into account the conditions of storage after purchase by the consumer. Some people like to keep certain products in the refrigerator, others will store the same product in a cupboard. Obviously the realistic 'best before' date will differ.

Personally, I prefer the custom practised in Yugoslavia when it was still a beautiful and peaceful country. The food producers there didn't use 'best before' or 'use by' on their perishable foods. They used a 'produced on' date. Consumers would quickly learn the realistic lifespan of the product under their own domestic usage and storage conditions. They would learn, for example, that the tofu processed in February would keep in their refrigerator without any appreciable loss in quality or taste until, say, next November. In contrast, if their personal preference was to store the tofu out on the counter, it would only last until sometime in September. Date of production is far superior to 'best before' information in such cases. Another advantage to the 'date of production' label, unlike the 'best before' label, is that it tells us how long the product has been sitting waiting for a purchaser.

The politically expedient compromise

The majority of GM products under development now will be labelled. Most will be labelled voluntarily by the company, because the product will carry some premium attribute for which the consumer is willing to pay extra. The consumer will actively seek out a GM reduced-calorie sugar product, so a conspicuous label will facilitate identification of the desired brand. The company will see it as in their own best interest to provide a prominent label. They will certainly charge a hefty and prominent premium. However, more mundane GM products will also be labelled.

I foresee a transition phase in which all GM products are labelled, in order to satisfy the 'public demand', until such time as the requirement is phased out as people become familiar with the safety of the GM products.

I'm not sure this is a good idea. It's like a patient going to the physician demanding a crutch in order to walk properly, although the physician knows the patient can walk perfectly well without a crutch. Too often the crutch is prescribed just to placate the patient. But is that the right course of action? Compliance may give the patient a sense of satisfaction in exercising control over the health care professional, a real sense of empowerment. But will compliance bring about a greater sense of dependence on the crutch, such that the patient truly can't walk without it? Would it not be preferable for the physician to convince the patient that they can walk without the crutch? Would the patient not be more empowered and more independent in such a case? Sometimes what we need and what we want are different. Is it the responsibility of the physician to pander to our wants, or is it to minister to our needs, even if we don't like what's being said? The latter, of course, necessitates a high degree of confidence and trust in our physician. Without it, little healing will occur, crutch or no crutch.

I do not think a blanket label on all GM products will serve a useful consumer purpose. My position is that it will wreak havoc with the label utility. However, it seems there is sufficient demand in Europe, particularly, that politicians will insist on such labels, to the detriment of their consumers. I see this as a short-term compromise required to allow GM commodities into the European marketplace. Soon enough, after consumers become familiar with the products and their relative safety, the mandatory GM labels will be seen for what they are—superfluous and deleterious to meaningful consumer information—and legislation will be modified along more sensible lines.

Apart from the consumer information issue, labelling has also been suggested as a way to track products in the market and domestically, in the event of a necessary recall due to some 'unexpected event or consequences' implicating the GM product. If epidemiologists find this attractive, would it not be sensible to label all products, GM and non-GM? Obviously, problems will continue to occur from time to time with various batches of food, but the introduction of GM products will not curtail such events in conventional foods. Perhaps a bar code on all food packages will extend the epidemiologists' database beyond GM foods to cover all potential food problems.

The small print

The common and most compelling argument in favour of indiscriminate GM labelling is that it enables an informed choice to consumers in the marketplace. We're seen how current labels can be misleading, misunderstood, ignored, or otherwise useless. Mandatory labelling of GM products will similarly not always enable 'informed choice' and may instead actually detract from an informed choice. I am fully in favour of informed choice by the consumer. But informed choice means full information and option for all consumers. Some consumers actively want the choice to be able to buy GM products. These people, 'early adopters' in sociological parlance, have rights also and should be just as important in our deliberations as those people who will choose against GM products. Consumers ought to have the right to an option to buy or not buy any particular approved GM product. Some 'consumer advocates' wish to restrict that option by banning GM products altogether, or by limiting the full information required to evaluate a product, to come to an 'informed' decision. To me, an informed decision is one taken by the consumer, not by me or some other 'consumer advocate' and imposed on consumers. A GM product lacking a label is less an assault on informed choice than is denial of consumer access to a product that has passed appropriate scientific review for health and environmental safety. Banning a product evaluated and judged safe by competent authorities denies informed choice to consumers.

Conclusion

In this chapter I have presented examples of situations to show that labelling is not always a simple exercise. These situations are all feasible and the complications have to be addressed now, before we ruin the advantages proper labelling provides to consumers. We need a strategy to enable labelling of products not currently available but coming though the development process, to be introduced to the market next month, next year, or in ten years. A scientifically sound labelling strategy will remain valid even if we can't today predict what those novelties might be in the future.

Future GM foods will not require statutory GM labels. Consumer-oriented 'value-added' GM products will shout from the shelves to attract your attention, so companies will ensure they're well marked, not only as GM but with the new attribute also. In the meantime, we do need mandatory labels on products, GM or otherwise, with a substantial change in nutritional composition. Low fat or low sodium is already well marked. But what about a food with increased fat or sodium? We need to know this information also, and it doesn't matter if the product was made from GM or conventional methods. We also need labels on products carrying new allergens, toxins, or other 'undesirable' compounds. However, we're not likely to see such products developed for commercialization anyway.

Product labelling is the single best achievement to emanate from the consumers' movement, in spite of the problems, some of which are outlined in this chapter. We ought to be working toward removing the ambiguous, misleading labels and instead expanding meaningful information. I'm cautious and suspicious of any activity further jeopardizing the usefulness of labels to consumers making informed purchasing decisions. Mandatory and blanket labelling of GM products debases labelling by contradicting the meaningful and informative benefits and simply contributes to the accelerating decline in label utility. We've seen how labels can be misleading, uninformative, or informative but useless. We've seen some of the practical problems in implementation and enforcement. We've seen that few people actually base their buying decisions on labels anyway, and how people least able to afford it, the poor, will pay the greatest price.

CHAPTER 13

'Waiter, can't I have a GM-free meal ?'

- Is it possible to avoid GM foods completely?
- Is organic production the alternative?
- If I want to avoid GM foods, what can I eat?
- Is there a better way to identify GM products?

Avoiding GM foods

In the stampede to avoid GM foods, the demand for organic and other 'guaranteed non-GM' foods has increased dramatically in recent years, and many institutions as well as individuals have taken the plunge. Schools and childcare centres are particularly prone to public pronouncements of rejecting any GM foodstuffs. In a remarkable example of modern leadership, the UK prime minister, Tony Blair, exhorts the nation to accept the benefits of GM foods, while refusing to deny reports that his wife has declared their own kitchen 'GM-free'. For some reason, other public institutions, such as prisons and psychiatric hospitals, have been slower to protect their charges from the perceived terrors of GM foods.

Australian childcare centres in Waverly, New South Wales made the local papers by declaring themselves GM-free. Food suppliers must guarantee their products contain no 'modified' ingredients. The mayor, Mr Paul Pearce, said 'Foods that can't be given that quality assurance will not be used'. Considering that no food can legitimately be given that guarantee, Mr Pearce neglected to indicate what the children would be fed as an alternative to food. Hundreds of food products in Australia contain ingredients derived from GM foods, and labelling is not required for derived ingredients. As we discussed in Chapter 12, labelling will not provide much assurance that a product does or does not contain GM ingredients. Negative labelling (i.e. 'this product contains no GM ingredients') is especially equivocal, as GMOs have been detected in a great many samples of supposedly 'GM-free' foodstuffs. How does it get there? Ordinary contamination for one, and uncertain test procedures for another. The basic technology used to detect GMOs is the polymerase chain reaction—PCR (discussed in Chapter 3), used to detect a particular DNA sequence. It is so sensitive it is able, in the right hands, to provide a DNA fingerprint from a crime suspect's single hair. PCR is so powerful it is often hard to master. Because it duplicates DNA sequences, even having the lab exposed to the DNA sequence for some unrelated purpose or for some other set of assays can be enough to contaminate and give false positive readings to other test samples.

In any case, guaranteeing that a particular foodstuff contains no GM ingredients requires the entire process to be managed, assessed, evaluated, segregated, and tested for no other purpose than to try to detect the appearance of GM contaminants. This might work fine when you provide a schoolchild with a fresh apple or carrot from the local organic market (which might hold its own peculiar risks), but what about other foods the children want and demand? One of the big food suppliers, Heinz, says some of their product lines contain 20 ingredients. However, although Heinz recognizes all of the ingredients have been assessed and evaluated as safe, they agreed to audit all their sources of ingredients in response to public queries. This is a typical company response. In order to maintain their good reputation as a high quality food producer and supplier, they will accede to public wishes and provide what is demanded. If the market demands GM-free processed foods, they are happy to fulfil that demand. As a company, they have no problem with using GM ingredients properly evaluated for health safety, but if there is a consumer demand for a GM-free line, they may see that as a market opportunity. Of course, the consumer will have to pay for the cost of such provision, plus a reasonable mark-up for profit. In the real world, 'consumer demand' equates with 'willingness to pay'. If consumers are not willing to pay extra for a product or service, it means there is no consumer demand. Producing, monitoring, and rejecting positive-testing batches of each of those potentially GM ingredients, and the cost of an entire new GM-free production facility, will incur substantial additional costs.

Why do we need a complete new production line? Cross-contamination. If you're going to offer a guarantee of GM-free, you have to eliminate sources of mixing with GM material. Any food processing line dealing with both GM and non-GM versions of the same product will experience cross-contamination. New production facilities will be built at considerable cost which will, of course, be passed on to consumers.

So why not require the new production line and facility to be dedicated to the GM version, with the additional costs accruing to the GMO consumers? Two reasons:

1   The demand for segregation emanates from the consumers of the non-GM versions. Those consumers content to consume the GM ingredients probably aren't concerned if some non-GM ingredient made its way into the GM version. It is the non-GMO consumers who are demanding a guarantee of segregation and non-contamination. They want the service, they pay the costs of providing that service.

2 The initial and capital costs accrue to the same company. The bottom line is
   that the company needs to recover the costs of the outlay. In practice, it is
   likely both GM and non-GM product lines will experience a cost increase, to
   share the load, as it were. In this scenario, the GMO consumers will actually
   be subsidizing the non-GM version, as it is unlikely the company will place the
   entire load on one version when they have two virtually identical product
   lines.

Until complete segregation or efficient labelling occurs and makes avoiding
GM products simple (I'm not holding my breath), some consumers seek a refuge
from GM products. What are the options? The most obvious one, organic production, warrants closer inspection.

The organic alternative

Many critics proclaim organic food production as the answer to the GM question. But is organic farming actually compatible with GM production, as
suggested by the USDA in their proposed US organic regulations? American
organic producers themselves do not think so. They responded by issuing the following statement:

The Organic Farmers Marketing Association (US) calls for a complete prohibition on the
use of Genetically Engineered ingredients, processing aids, enzymes, food additives and
derivatives from GE products in a certified organic handling operation (processing, pack-
aging or storing) of foods and fibers labelled and sold as 'organically produced'.

Now consider the their proposed definition of 'genetically engineered':

'Genetically Engineered' means made with techniques that alter the molecular or cell biology of an organism by means that are not possible under natural conditions of processes.
Genetic engineering includes recombinant DNA and RNA techniques, cell fusion, micro
and macro encapsulation, gene deletion and doubling, introducing a foreign gene, and
changing the positions of genes. It shall not include breeding, conjugation, fermentation,
hybridization, in-vitro fertilization and tissue culture.

This definition represents a common theme but is fundamentally flawed. The
first sentence of the definition prohibits '. . . techniques that alter the molecular
or cell biology of an organism by means that are not possible under natural conditions of processes.' I'm sure the drafters of this definition meant to include
many or all current GMOs, but almost all of them are possible (albeit unlikely)
under natural processes. The subsequent two sentences are largely self-contradictory. It prohibits 'introducing a foreign gene' yet allows 'conjugation' and
'breeding', which by their nature introduce foreign genes. Life is a continuum,
not a series of discrete boxes. Saying an organism has never carried a particular
inserted gene implies the recipient species is a discrete box, bearing no genetic
relationship (except, perhaps a common language) with the donor organism.

This is an example of the type of human arrogance many environmentalists rightfully charge against scientists. A species designation is indeed a human applied concept. In nature, all species are closely aligned—remember, humans share thousands of genes with a nematode worm. Also, many genes have a common ancestor. It is likely that the recipient organism already has a similar gene, or one that is native, but has been inactivated over the course of evolutionary divergence. The concept of speciation is a human-designed one, not a natural one. The US Organic Farmers Marketing Association, and many others, are trying to fit 'genetic engineering' into a human-designed pigeonhole. Nature doesn't always recognize or comply with our human desire to categorize and segregate everything and happily ignores our arrogant ignorance.

Organic production does provide an alternative to GM, so organic producers ought to be fully supportive of GM technology. The presence of GM foods will ensure a slice of the market (those consumers wishing to avoid GM) for organic producers. Eliminate GM and a substantial organic market share dissipates with it.

Is organic food safer?

Surely, supporting organically produced and other health foods can save us? There is indeed a place in the market for organic products, with or without GM. Organic produce may carry fewer pesticide residues than conventionally grown produce. But is that all you're concerned about? What about other things— insects, manure, fungal spores, and toxins are all common contaminants of foods. Are these unpleasant things present in greater or lesser amounts in organic products than conventional or GM?

According to Dennis Avery of the Hudson Institute the highly respected US Centers for Disease Control in Atlanta noted 2471 cases, including 250 deaths, of infection by the unpleasant *E. coli* strain O157:H7 in 1996 alone. These bacteria live in manure. Manure is used as a fertilizer in organic farming systems. Organic foods were implicated in about a third of the confirmed O157:H7 cases despite the fact that organic food constitutes only about 1% of food consumed in the US. According to the FDA, organically produced foods suffer higher rates of biological contamination, including tuberculosis bacteria and aflatoxin-producing fungi.

Add to this the previously mentioned *Salmonella,* along with *Listeria, Campylobacter,* and *Clostridium,* the agent that brings us botulism. All of these naturally occurring, non-GM organisms are part and parcel of our foods—especially organically produced foods, where their control is limited.

Unfortunately, completely clean uncontaminated food is not an option, it's simply not on the table. I know I prefer to consume the small quantities of regulated and approved pesticides in conventional foods than unknown quantities of 'natural' toxins, manure, bacteria, fungi, and whatever else. Many people enthusiastically support organic production, and I support their right to choose.

But the choice ought to be an informed one. The fact is that organic foods carry more 'organic' contaminants than conventional or GM foods. Although the extent of the risk is under considerable debate, the evidence implicating organic products as potential health hazards is compelling and warrants, at least, rigorous further scrutiny.

Organic products can also carry undesirable amounts of non-contaminants, such as excessive fat, sugar, or sodium. The British Heart Foundation warns against organic foods and other diet fads, arguing instead people ought to become more aware of their entire food intake, not just one component. According to the Foundation, some organic foods are actually dangerous.

Is organic production sustainable?

Organic production is supposed to represent a return to simple, sustainable agrarian production practices. No nasty chemicals contaminating our land, animals or crops. Just good, wholesome food they way we had in the 'good old days'. It is sold as being environmentally, economically, and agronomically sustainable. Sounds idyllic, but how realistic are these claims?

Does organic production really contribute to environmental sustainability, or is it depleting nutrient reserves from the soil? Is it capable of economic sustainability, where the farmer makes a reasonable financial reward independent of government assistance? Will it be able to provide enough food to meet the demand of a burgeoning world population, estimated to increase 20% over the next twenty years in the face of rapidly diminishing farmland?

We won't know about environmental sustainability of organic production until the long-term studies are complete. We won't know about economic sustainability of organic produce until consumer demand proves a willingness to pay the additional costs associated with organic production. There's no question, however; organic systems simply do not provide the same volume of food as conventional farming systems. There is considerable debate over the sense, let alone the sustainability, of producing less food for an increasing population, but that is not an issue for discussion here. There are, however, questions about organic production systems. Advocates for the organic movement like to give the impression that organic food is produced without synthetic or artificial pesticides. Natural alternatives to the nasty synthetic chemicals have to be carefully developed and utilized. B.t. toxin, a 'natural' insecticide, is often used by organic producers as an alternative to the 'unnatural' chemical insecticides. But this is the same B.t. used in insect resistant GM maize, soya, cotton, and other plants. It's the same product whether applied on the plants by an organic farmer or produced inside the plants by the B.t. gene.

Organic farmers in Canada recently held a conference and detailed the maturing of the industry. Organic production was inhibited for some time because of various insect and weed control problems, along with the immature infrastructure. However, these enterprising farmers have since established a sustainable organic farming system. They had organic seeds and crops, organic weed control, organic pest control, and a segregated marketing and distribution network in place. They had overcome all the obstacles to environmental and agricultural sustainability. All they needed now to achieve successful economic sustainability, they claimed, was generous government subsidies.

Some organic production systems are still lacking. Many organic producers see the organic movement as a market opportunity and have moved into organic production to serve a market niche as well as, they hope, contribute to a more environmentally sustainable practice. I fully support this group and wish them well, knowing they have an uphill battle. Honey is an example of a difficult organic product. Honeybees have to forage among flowers growing near the hives. They can't read the signs telling them that some plants might be GM. Honeybees also become infected with nasty parasites such as varroa mite. Unlike Asian bees, European honeybees—the mainstay of hives in North America as well as Europe—have little natural resistance to the pests. Varroa mite infestations can kill the bee unless treated, and the only effective treatment is a non-organic chemical. Although there is promising research into organic alternatives for varroa mite control, at present an organic honey producer must choose between treating the bees with a chemical or watching the bees, along with the business, slow to a crawl. Either way, production of organic honey drops with the bees.

One complaint from organic producers is that GMOs might contaminate their crops. An organic producer of oilseed rape in the UK claimed his crop was contaminated by pollen from nearby GM rape (I'm willing to wager it was less than the allowable tolerance for organic production, in which case the crop technically wasn't contaminated at all). Having pollen from a GM crop certainly would seem to jeopardize the 'organic' standard, as GM seems anathema to organic production. GM seems to exemplify everything the organic movement opposes: big multinational domination, intensive agricultural practices, pesticides, and chemical overutilization. However, the end-product, the oil that finds its way into the grocery shelves, is remarkably similar whether its production has been GM or organic. In both cases, the composition of the product can be clean, nutritious, and free of pesticides.

If organic produce is to be rejected because it has been contaminated with GM pollen, can an organic crop also rejected for having been contaminated with conventional, pesticide-treated pollen? If organic producers can sue GMO growers for contamination, can GMO growers sue organic producers for similar contamination? Pollen does tend to flow both ways. And at least some consumers might wish to avoid the biological contaminants of organic produce.

As we've seen earlier, oilseed rape pollen can travel considerable distances. Professional farmers—seed growers—use an isolation distance of 400 metres between oilseed rape fields to minimize (not eliminate!) cross-pollination. The isolation distance varies widely depending on the species (even within oilseed rape there are different species to take into account), wind, insect populations in a given season and region, wind, weather, and so on. Some crop species, including soya bean and linseed, have virtually no outcrossing.

Spot checks show the majority of organic produce is contaminated—sometimes with GMOs, but more frequently with other contaminants, such as pesticide residues. The tolerance for contaminants in organic production is typically about 5%, or one out of twenty. In theory, that means an organic farmer with twenty fields can spray one of them to obtain a clean but certified organic crop. Fortunately, no organic farmer admits to this activity.

We need to put the issues into perspective, to relate GM with alternatives, both conventional and organic. We accept a general contaminant tolerance in organic production of 5%. Is there a difference if a shipment is 95% organically certified wheat and 5% conventional wheat? What if it's 95% organic and 5% GM wheat? What if the shipment is 95% conventional and 5% GM wheat?

Long-term effects of consuming 'organic' produce

One major current concern over GMOs is the 'long-term effects'. On the surface, it seems like a legitimate concern. We want to know what might happen in the 'long term' if we approve GMOs. But it loses clarity when we delve deeper.

'Long term'—does it apply to product or process? Health or environment? Both? We need to remember we aren't working in a vacuum, all is relative. If it is fair to ask this question of GMOs, it is equally fair to ask the same question of organic products and even many common foods. Potato, maize, squash, and other New World crops are relatively recent additions to the European human diet. What is the long-term effect of eating organic food? We can't be sure of the long-term effects of consuming organic produce; it hasn't been around long enough in its current form. Historically, people who consumed foods grown by what we now call 'organic methods' had substantially shorter lifespans. We know this because people living in the days when organic production was the only method had a short lifespan. In contrast, people who consume GM foods have no such shortened lifespan. Is there a connection between organic food consumption and shorter life? We don't know for sure. Just because there's a statistical association or correlation doesn't mean there's a causal connection.

Similarly, what is the long-term effect of growing organic crops on our land? Is it really as sustainable as proponents would have us believe? Some experts say organic production extracts more nutrients from the soil than are being replenished. We won't know for sure until the long-term studies are complete. Using that same rationale, some organic supporters call for a moratorium on GM production until long-term studies are complete. Using the same argument to support two opposing conclusions doesn't seem logically sound. Why not expand GM production and curtail organic production until the long-term studies are complete?

From my perspective, both GM and organic production have been around long enough to conclude there is no inherent danger in either one, but specific products of either may be hazardous. Neither is immune to lapses in food safety;

no system is. So far, GM has been more fortunate, in that no one has been harmed from eating GM foods, whereas organic production has harmed innocent victims—at least 250 deaths in one incident alone, as noted above. We seem to have a choice. Conventional foods have more pesticide residue contamination; organic foods have more biological contamination. Choose your poison.

Before we abandon the GM ship, let's make sure we're not jumping on to a less seaworthy craft. I support the orderly and properly regulated development of both GM and organic systems. Both have positive attributes, both have dangers to overcome. Neither is the single answer to world hunger or malnutrition, but both can play a role.

Health foods and speciality items

What is the cost of a 'health food'? Take, for example, linseed, which is growing in popularity as a healthy additive to multigrain breads and other baked goods.

The main product of linseed, flaxseed oil, is touted as having various medicinal properties (for which there is, by the way, some legitimate scientific evidence). A recent sale at my local 'health and nutrition centre' offered 90 capsules of 1 gram each for just under $9, or about 10 cents per gram of oil ($100 per kilo).

The farmgate value of flaxseed varies considerably from year to year, but typically a farmer is paid about $9 per 25 kilogram bushel of flaxseed (about 36 cents per kilogram). The oil is only about 45% of the seed weight, so the farmer is paid $9 for

$$25 \text{ kilograms} \times 0.45 = 11.25 \text{ kilograms}$$

of flaxseed oil. The farmer gets about 80 cents for delivering enough flaxseed to make a kilogram of oil, which costs $100 per kilogram in the shop.

Extracting the oil from the seed and putting the oil into capsules also has a cost, as does distribution and marketing. But the difference between what the farmer gets paid and what you pay is phenomenal. Consumers pay far too much for these products. Someone is making a fortune from you, and it isn't the farmer.

In Australia, I could buy a small bottle of linseed oil to coat my cricket bat (another potentially hazardous item carrying no warning label!), containing about 100 grams, for $7.95. Obviously, this works out to $79.50 per kilogram (although perhaps I could negotiate a better unit price if I were to ask for a full kilogram). An art supply shop sells linseed oil for blending pigments at a similar price. Where does this money go? Australia is self-sufficient in linseed oil, so they didn't have to import it. The farmer gets a share of the proceeds, about $9 per bushel of linseed (highly variable, depending on the market) from which approximately 11.25 kilograms of linseed oil is extracted. Linseed oil is squeezed out of the seeds and cleaned, bottled, labelled, and distributed; it's one of the most simply and inexpensively processed farm commodities.

Doing the calculations, about 8 cents out of the $7.95 goes to the farmer, who produced 100% of the product labelled '100% linseed oil'. Of course, the processor, bottler, marketer, distributor, wholesaler, and retailer all deserve a share, as they're all involved in providing you the consumer with the final retail product. But 8 cents is just 1% of the retail price.

In England, I found a health food shop in Oxford selling linseed at £1 for 500 grams, or £2 per kilogram. Much better value for money, but there's no processing involved as there is to obtain the oil—this is the same seed as harvested by the farmer, with perhaps some cleaning to rid some of the larger pieces of dirt and rat shit. And it's still over ten times what the farmer gets paid for providing it.

I buy linseed oil or flaxseed oil a kilogram at a time, not for $100 from my health food store, and not for $79.50 a kilogram from my sporting goods shop or art supply shop, but from my hardware store for $5 per kilogram. The farmer still gets 80 cents for the kilogram, but at least this is now a healthy 16% of the retail cost of the product, and my saving up to $95 on the purchase enhances my own financial health. I could consume the oil to remain healthy, or coat the oil on my cricket bat for it to remain healthy, but in fact I use the oil primarily to seal my driveway. The ancients were right. It is truly a 'most useful' product.

Herbal remedies and foods, natural foods

Herbal remedies are popular among people dissatisfied with the medical establishment, because either the conventional therapy isn't working to their satisfaction, or else they don't like the industrialization of health care. Supporters of herbal and 'alternative' treatments are lobbying to have easier access to the products, because current regulations are so restrictive. The Canadian government is under pressure to establish a new agency to regulate herbal and homeopathic products. The agency would require manufacturers to show the product is 'safe', but wouldn't have to show the products necessarily work. A committee of the health department says 'traditional usage' should be sufficient to permit over-the-counter marketing of such products as St John's wort as a cure for depression. However, St John's wort has not been shown to be effective as an antidepressant in the type of scientific tests required of new pharmaceutical products. Meanwhile, scientists in the USA have found evidence that St John's wort causes infertility and mutations in sperm. Apparently this side effect was not noted in 'traditional usage'.

Clever marketers in Australia are selling a herbal cigarette to schoolchildren as an alternative to marijuana. It contains neither tobacco nor marijuana, so is essentially unregulated. The distributors can't keep up with demand from teenagers wanting the claimed and advertised 'real buzz' and feelings of relaxation in a legal smoke. And, since it's 'herbal', it must be healthy, right?

Does it strike you odd that the same groups that decry and demand more stringent regulation of GM products are often the same ones who decry and demand less regulation of 'natural foods' and 'herbal remedies'? Surely, if there were a health and safety concern, the source of the problem, whether GM or 'natural' shouldn't matter, it should be investigated and regulated.

Yet, because of intense lobbying from some of these groups, in 1994, the USA passed a law stating the FDA must prove a health food unsafe before it can be taken off the shelves. Since that time, the US dietary supplement market has recorded a large increase in the number of product introductions. These products are advertised to prevent cancer, slow ageing, and improve memory. Although many of the supplements are legitimate and beneficial, others are suspect and lack scientific data to support the claims of the manufacturers. Many consumers shell out large sums of money in the mistaken belief that 'If it weren't true, they wouldn't be allowed to make the claims'. The USA is not the only jurisdiction where citizens labour under such naive delusions. Many countries have a large industry in 'health products' with misleading health claims in advertisements. Why are these allowed?

According to the Associated Press, the US Food and Drug Administration has recorded over 2500 reports of adverse side effects and 79 deaths associated with dietary supplements since the passage of the 1994 legislation. The industry in the US has started to take some measures to compile a listing of potentially dangerous supplements, and may even suggest wording for warning labels, but it is unlikely they will say 'This product is a placebo. It has no documented beneficial effect, but may be as hazardous to your health as it certainly is to your financial well-being'.

Some activist groups, operating on the pretext of providing a public service by warning of the dangers of GM, often cite (incorrectly, as we've seen in Chapter 6) the deaths of 37 people in the Showa Denko L-tryptophan dietary supplement contamination case. I have not been able to find any of these groups warning us of the other dietary supplements responsible for 79 deaths. If they are sincerely concerned over public health issues, why have they not used their considerable media machinery to warn us of these other potentially lethal dietary supplements claiming more than double the number of lives in the Showa Denko L-tryptophan tragedy?

I want to avoid GM foods. What do I eat?

If, having read this far, you still want to avoid GM foods, OK. Here's the plan. First, you have to accept that no system can guarantee 100% efficiency at avoiding GM material. Even those items marked 'organic' or 'contains no GMOs' are suspect, as we've seen. Aim instead to minimize your GMO intake. And you still need to identify the rationale for your concern. Are all GM-derived products to be eschewed, including meat from animals fed on GM grain? Or do you wish to forego only specific GM products, such as GM fresh fruit? If the latter, your wish is relatively easy to fulfil. If the former, more difficult but still feasible.

Let's take the most extreme case and assume you want to avoid GM material as much as humanly possible. Emigrate to a desert island and take up residence in a remote mountain tree. Failing that (or in addition), familiarize yourself with approved GM products and avoid them. Each country maintains a public database listing of approved GMOs. Regularly consult the listing for your area (see the website addresses in Chapter 16). Use the GM labels as a guide. UK sources have compulsory labels, while the US and Canada ones are largely voluntary. But remember, labels can be misleading and misinformative, whether they claim the product contains or does not contain GM ingredients.

Organic products are less likely to carry GM components than conventionally produced foods. Individual food items are less likely to be GM. Keep a listing of approved GM foods to avoid any whole or fresh fruits and vegetables you might encounter. The only fresh food item approved for sale in the UK is the Flavr-Savr™ tomato. This tomato went defunct several years ago, so if you see any in a high street shop, it will provide an indisputable testament to the veracity of the claim of prolonged shelf life. In the US and Canada, fresh GM fruits and vegetables may include tomatoes, potatoes, squash, radish, and Hawaiian papayas. These, fortunately, are among the GM products where labelling will be most efficient—or least inefficient.

Meat is almost certainly GM-free, unless you're concerned about what the animals were fed, in which case you're about to become a vegan.

Processed foods, especially those with multiple ingredients, are more likely to contain ingredients derived from soya or maize, both of which are suspect, especially if they come from the US or Canada. These are not always evident, hiding in products as diverse as bread and margarine.

Refined products, such as vegetable oil, may not be a concern as they have, at most, only trace amounts of DNA or protein, even if they do come from GM plants. If trace amounts are a concern, avoid soya bean, rapeseed/canola, maize/corn, or vegetable oil blends, usually labelled (unhelpfully) simply as 'vegetable oil'. Go instead for pure olive, safflower, or sunflower oil—none of these plants is GM yet. For the same reason, refined sugar is GM-free, as it lacks DNA and protein, but if it is a concern, buy cane sugar, not the beet version.

Highly refined products, such as lecithin from GM soya, are identical to ordinary non-GM versions. Such products cannot be independently detected as GM, as they have no GM DNA, protein, or other GM characteristics. Before you decide to avoid these 'derived from' products, check the range of items you'll be scratching from your list. Soya products are especially pervasive, just take a look at an industry site, for example, Central Soya. You might decide such products are acceptable after all.

Hard cheese, unless the label specifically states it is made without GM components, was almost certainly made with enzymes from GMOs. Bread may lack soya and maize derivatives, but remains a GM possibility, as the UK has approved a GM yeast. However, the company has voluntarily kept the product off the market, fearing a consumer backlash rejecting the bread and depressing sales. Brewer's yeast has also been modified, but not on the market in the UK for similar reasons. The brewers didn't even ask for approval, presumably fearing the same consumer reprisals as for GM bread.

In general, avoid convenience foods, snack foods, and highly processed foods. Eat more fresh fruit and vegetables; they're usually not GM unless labelled and most of us don't eat enough of them anyway. Dump the tofu and anything else made with soya, including those awful veggie burgers. (I'd recommend this even if they weren't GM.)

Moving to other GM products, if not quite foodstuffs, we have ascorbic acid (vitamin C). If you supplement your diet with vitamin C or multivitamins containing vitamin C, you'll have to stop as most now comes from GM sources. Eat a fresh orange instead. They're still not GM but most people overdo vitamin C anyway.

Since we're considering the extreme case of wanting to avoid any GM components, you'll also have to give up insulin if you're diabetic. And dornase alfa (Pulmozyme) if you have cystic fibrosis, factor VIII if you're haemophiliac, and other treatments if you have certain forms of lymphoma or breast cancer, as all these medicines are products of GMOs. And as more and more medical treatments incorporate GMOs, it will be increasingly hard to avoid them. The best answer is to stay healthy.

Finally, as we now have GM versions of natural fibre crops like cotton and flax, don't eat your shirt.

You're probably saying to yourself 'This all seems pretty silly. Isn't there an easier way?' Yes, there is. We could scrap the knee-jerk GM labelling laws and demand a mechanism by which each consumer can identify exactly which products fit specified criteria. If it's to avoid all GM products, fine, we can provide a comprehensive list. If it's to avoid only Monsanto products, GM or not, we can do that, too. Some consumers might not object to GM, but wish to avoid products of mutation breeding. We can accommodate those consumers as well. What is this mechanism?

An alternative to indiscriminate GM labels

Instead of trying to figure out how to put meaningful labels on products, we can satisfy part of the demand for knowledge of not only contents but also process by establishing a public database for all products and all processes. It could record all of the contents, in percentage form, with a measure of variation from batch to batch. It could record the method of production, regardless of the method, so people could chose to select or avoid a particular method. Consumers who don't like GM products or production will be able to eschew them. Consumers who don't like mutation breeding will be able to avoid those products. Want to boycott Monsanto? Easy. The database could be published and maintained on the Internet and made available to everyone through public libraries. Unfortunately, the product database is imperfect. It would not capture the generic blends of unknown sources, or products that vary widely from batch to batch. It would also not capture 'secret ingredients' like Coca-Cola or Kentucky Fried Chicken recipes. In these respects it is not inferior to the indiscriminate GM label programme. Most of us will be satisfied knowing that, if it's on the market, it's probably safe. Just as we are now.

Information on specific GMOs is widely available already. In the European Union, massive dossiers detailing the intimate secrets of every GMO are available in a public database. The US and Canada also document their GM products. At present, the technical information is available to the public, but is scattered and not always (in fact, not usually) in an easily readable or understandable format. The public databases are typically not set up to easily compare one GM product with another. By combining the detailed information on all products in one user-friendly database, and including similar information on all food products, regardless of method of development, we can all decide for ourselves which products we wish to purchase or avoid. We would be able to make direct comparisons for all manner of information, from caloric content and nutritional composition to method of development and source company. As a consumer, this is the information I would like in order to make meaningful comparisons.

'Consumers have a right to make an informed choice!' is almost a worldwide chorus 'So we demand mandatory GM product labels' as if labelling is the only route to informed choice. It is not. Meaningful and practicable informed choice is possible through a common and comprehensive database of all commercial foodstuffs. Indiscriminate GM product labels fail to meet the goal of the informed choice. Indeed, they will debase that noble objective. However, a standardized public database for all commercial food products will meet the demand. Let's press for one!

CHAPTER 14

'The chef does not share his recipes': intellectual property and GM technology

- What's all the fuss over 'intellectual property'?
- Classical plant breeders never had legal protection, did they?
- Just what is a patent, anyway?
- Is it true that farmers can't grow their own seeds any more?

Historically, consumers have not been too interested in patents, copyrights, trademarks, and other means of intellectual property protection. When we buy a product, royalty, or licence, fees are built into the cost—they're invisible to us, so we don't even notice them, although we are probably vaguely aware they exist, and that companies place great emphasis on patents and such. Then the news of Terminator provided a wake-up call. Now, it appears, the companies will be able to force farmers, particularly those in the poorer developing countries who are least able to afford it, to buy patented seed year after year. According the rumour, even traditional varieties grown for generations could be subject to patent and private sector monopoly, and recent legal contracts like Monsanto's technology use agreement (TUA) would reduce farmers to being like indentured employees, unable to own even the seed they sow.

Intellectual property protection of food crop varieties ranks among the most contentious and misunderstood issues associated with biotechnology. Traditionally, plant breeders had no intellectual property rights whatever. Their new crops were freely available and germplasm—seed—was freely given to others, even to competing breeders. Plant breeders' rights (PBR) is a relatively recent innovation to recognize and protect the legitimate skills of plant breeding, but is quite limited in scope and not well understood, even by many plant breeders. Life-form patenting, especially, is fraught with misunderstanding to a degree seen only by GM technology in general. Finally, a seed contract limiting a farmer's traditional rights is an alien concept but fast becoming reality down on the farm. In this chapter we try to clarify some often befuddling issues of intellectual property as they relate to living things.

Plant breeders' rights (PBR)

Until recently, plant breeders enjoyed protection of their registered varieties only according to international convention based on the Union for Protection of New Varieties (UPOV). UPOV was initiated in Europe in 1961 and has since spread around the world. Many countries enacted legislation to deal with **plant breeder's rights** (PBR). Even those countries without statutory rights or who are not official signatories to the convention adhere, by and large, to the provisions of UPOV because they are refreshingly sensible and benefit everyone in the long run.

According to the principles of UPOV (specific details vary according to jurisdiction), a new plant variety can be protected from blatant genetic piracy. If the new variety (as registered in the local jurisdiction) meets the requirements of being distinct, uniform, and genetically stable (DUS) (see Chapter 4), it can qualify for international protection. An unscrupulous seed dealer cannot then buy a bag of your new variety, take it across a border and re-register it under their chosen name for commercial release in the new country. At least, they can't do it legally, although it does occur from time to time.

UPOV includes a **farmer's exemption**, meaning that farmers can keep a portion of seed grown in one season to provide seed for a subsequent season. Whether or not they can do other things with that seed, for instance sell it to a neighbour, depends on the jurisdiction. There is also a **research exemption**, meaning that *bona fide* researchers can acquire samples of seed for research purposes, and breeders can use the seed as a parent in a breeding programme. Conceivably, they can't simply pretend to breed with it, for example by selecting a minor trait and re-releasing the selection as a new variety. This has not been a problem in practice, not because breeders are inherently honest but because by the time the spurious 'new' variety has gone through the motions—it still takes several years—the parent variety is likely obsolete or at least near the end of its commercial life. It's just as easy to legitimately use the initial variety as a parent and develop a truly improved variety.

Plant breeders hold to a traditional creed. Historically, breeders enjoyed easy access to each other's varieties and germplasm to use as parents. By the time of variety release, the breeder already has several years' head start with a potential successor variety, as he or she will have been using the breeding line all along. A good breeder can, in this respect, keep at least one step ahead of the competitors and so has little concern for the legitimate use of a variety by a competitor. Also, the competitor is often breeding varieties for a different geographical location, a different market, so the relationship between breeders is often more collaborative than competitive, especially when they share germplasm back and forth. The culture and spirit of plant breeding has traditionally been one of cooperation and collaboration wherever possible. This, unfortunately, is changing rapidly with the advent of more powerful (read: more lucrative) means of intellectual or genetic property protection. To most breeders, this means patents.

Patents

The USA has a couple of 'junior' plant patent statutes, the Plant Variety Protection Act, to cover seed-reproduced varieties, and the Plant Patent Act (PPA), which covers vegetatively propagated varieties, those propagated by cuttings or runners or whatnot. Although they provided certain rights to breeders, they were not 'true' patents, hence the term 'junior'. No jurisdiction allowed ordinary utility patents (the implied 'senior' patent) for living organisms. Then, in 1980, two worlds collided—the patent world and the world of biology. Ananda Chakrabarty developed a strain of GM bacteria designed to digest crude oil; the intention was to use the bacteria to help contain and degrade oil spills. The US patent office initially refused to grant the patent, because living organisms, even microbes, were 'not patentable subject matter'. The appeals made their way up the line, until, in a landmark decision, the US Supreme Court decided in the Chakrabarty case that the US Patent Act did indeed allow utility patents on his bacteria. Living organisms can be patented inventions as long as they were truly new (i.e. not existing in nature), useful (interpreted broadly), and a product of intellectual ingenuity (i.e. not obvious). In this case, the GM bacteria 'invention' fit the criteria—it did not previously exist in nature, it was useful, and it was not an obvious step. The US patent office began to recognize bacteria and other microbes as suitable patent matter, but not higher organisms such as plants or animals. The scope expanded in 1984 when Ken Hibberd and his coworkers from Minnesota were refused a patent for a line of maize. Hibberd appealed, and, in a stinging rebuke for the commissioner of patents, his application was allowed, as were other patent applications covering higher plants held in abeyance, including one of mine.

Because of the Hibberd case, scientists may seek US patent protection for higher plants, animals, cell lines, genes, and, in fact, 'Anything under the Sun', so long as it meets the other requirements for utility patent protection. Other countries also expanded their utility patent coverage, allowing, in some cases and jurisdictions (including most of Europe), patents on higher organisms.

Here's where the misunderstandings come in. The requirements for obtaining a patent generally (i.e. not limited to the USA, but in patent offices in many countries) include the following.

- **Novelty.** The invention cannot have been already in existence. This is a requirement everywhere, and a major unnecessary cause for concern. Some people think the big companies will be able to go into a developing country, steal the local plants, and patent them, thus depriving local farmers from growing the crops they've traditionally grown. Such a scary scenario simply cannot happen under patent law. It might occur under some other draconian regime, but not under patent law. Furthermore, an issued patent is disallowed if the invention was later shown to be already in existence anywhere in the world, not just in the country where patent protection was being sought. The novelty requirement is fairly easy to satisfy. Inventors usually know if their invention is already out there somewhere.

- **Utility.** The invention must be useful in some respect, and it doesn't have to be an important respect. Most inventions can be useful as a doorstop, if nothing else, and can be described as such. Utility is usually the easiest of the criteria to satisfy. An inventor who cannot think of any possible use for the new invention is unlikely to invest the funds to pursue patent protection. Why bother?
- **Inventiveness.** The invention must have been non-obvious to one 'skilled in the art'. This is usually the hardest criterion to satisfy, as many truly inventive items are obvious in the retrospective vision of a patent examiner. Once you have the invention in your hand, it might be apparent how to generate it. The applicant has to convince the patent examiner that the invention involved an unusual procedure or an ingenious logical connection no one had made before, and that it would not be obvious to another person with similar expertise.

An additional, technical requirement is that the invention has to be described in adequate detail to allow another person of ordinary skill to reproduce the same result. This requisite is part of the deal. Patents are rewards from the state for sharing a new invention with the public, so the disclosure must allow others access to the invention.

An issued patent protects an invention for up to twenty years from the initial filing date. It gives the patent holder the right to exclude others from making use of the invention for that period. To correct another odd but popular misconception, a patent does not automatically give the right to use the invention to the patent holder. This may seem contradictory—what's the point of a patent if you can't use it yourself? What this means is that you can't use your own invention if it necessarily infringes another patent. If your invention builds on another patent, you have to ensure you have the right, through a licence or other permission from the patent holder, to use the underlying patent in the exercise of your own. Most patents nowadays build on the intellectual property of others. One of my recent patents is like this. It describes how to use the particle gun to make transgenic linseed plants. But I cannot practice my invention in the USA without a licence from DuPont, who own the patent on the particle gun machine. By the same token, DuPont cannot use their machine to make transgenic linseed plants without a licence from me (or rather, from the University of Saskatchewan). I'm sure we'll be able to work something out.

Usually, such cross-licensing is common but unseen by consumers. When you buy a new mobile phone, computer, or almost any consumer item, a portion of your cost goes to royalty payments to dozens or perhaps hundreds of different patent holders. Having patents on new foods and food processes is traditional. We pay royalties whenever we buy a new foodstuff or new method to prepare or package an old foodstuff.

Another misconception concerns jurisdictional authority. A US patent is in force only in the USA. Likewise, a patent issued in Australia has no force in the USA, Europe, or anywhere except Australia. An inventor who wants wide-ranging protection must file in each jurisdiction. Some countries do not allow patents on living organisms. Canada does not allow patents on higher life forms, but does allow microbial strains. In 1983, Pioneer Hi-Bred tried to patent a soya bean variety, produced using conventional breeding methods, in Canada, but the patent examiner tossed it out as 'unpatentable subject matter'. Pioneer asked the Patent Appeal Board to re-evaluate the application. They did, and they also tossed it out, an action also supported by the Commissioner of Patents. Undeterred, Pioneer took the legal route, presenting their case to the Federal Court of Appeals. The appellate court also decided Pioneer's arguments didn't amount to a hill of beans and tossed them out. Persistent if nothing else, Pioneer took the final step, appealing to the Supreme Court, who also tossed them out.

Patents vs. UPOV

How do patents for plant varieties compare with the rights under UPOV?

UPOV is limited to plant varieties. Utility patents cover an invention, whether a plant variety, a mousetrap, a method for baking bread, or an improved version of a previously patented method for baking bread.

Rights under UPOV require the new variety to be DUS. Patents must be adequately described as well as meeting the other statutory requirements outlined above. Since plant varieties cannot be verbally described the way a sewing machine can, this requirement for description can be met, at least partially, by a deposition of a seed sample of the invention or variety in a seed bank or other depository where the public, including your competitors, can access it. They may not be allowed to commercialize the invention without your consent during the lifetime of the patent, but they are allowed to use it for research purposes.

Under UPOV, farmers have an exemption allowing them to replant saved seed year after year. There is no such exemption under a utility patent.

Breeders are allowed to use varieties protected under UPOV provisions in breeding and research programmes. Researchers are allowed to use patented inventions for research purposes, but cannot commercialize the results of the research programme without a licence as long as the patent is in force. This is an important distinction.

One other little-known distinction: you cannot obtain UPOV protection for a plant 'discovered' in a field. It has to be a product of intentional breeding. You may be able to patent a new improved plant discovered in a cultivated field, as long as the other requirements are met.

Breeders in the USA have the option of protecting their varieties under any and all of their procedures, providing they can satisfy the specific requirements of each. Breeders in Europe, by contrast, must choose one method of protection. They cannot obtain both patent and UPOV protection on a plant variety as American breeders may. The European breeders get around this by applying for UPOV protection on the variety and for a patent on a germplasm, describing the invention not as a variety but as the underlying variety breeding line carrying novel traits. Splitting hairs, perhaps, but protection of germplasm is more powerful as many crop varieties could be generated using the same parental germplasm. They can then preclude others from using the germplasm, but spin out any number of new varieties using their patented germplasm as a parent. They then seek UPOV protection on each new variety.

The utility of utility patents

Patents are not designed to limit availability of new and useful inventions. On the contrary—they are a reward for public disclosure of a new invention. Without patent protection, a company will have no incentive to conduct the research needed to develop an inventive idea. Why would you spend the money and time to do so when, without protection, a competitor simply takes your invention, reverse engineers it, and sells it in competition with your own? The competitor can sell it at less cost, because they don't have to recover any of the development costs. So, faced with this likelihood, the company with the great idea simply shelves it. The work doesn't get done. The invention never makes it to the marketplace, and we consumers don't get the opportunity even to consider buying the product. Without patent protection, we are denied access to potentially useful products and intellectual advances.

A valuable idea or invention need not be protected by a patent. An alternative to a patent is a trade secret. Some companies don't like patents because they expire in twenty years. So instead of disclosing and obtaining a twenty-year monopoly reward, they keep the invention a secret and maintain a monopoly indefinitely. Recipes for Coca-Cola and Kentucky Fried Chicken are examples. It seems to have worked for them, as they've been in business far longer than twenty years. However, trade secrets offer no protection if the secret becomes public knowledge. If I acquired the secret recipe to Cola or KFC, I could open a competing brand offering a virtually identical product at lower cost and seriously cut into their business, and it would all be quite legal.

Trade secrets might work for speciality products like Cola or KFC, but don't offer much protection for self-replicating inventions like plant varieties. A competitor could legally buy one bag of seed and start an identical crop variety, offered at lower cost. Is this fair?

Confusion reigns

There are a multitude of misconceptions and misunderstandings concerning intellectual property protection. They arise because of different statutes in different countries, differing intellectual property case law, and evolving regulations. With the world becoming a smaller market, there is considerable effort to harmonize international trade. Even the US patent office, after the World Trade Organization's (WTO) 1994 General Agreement on Tariffs and Trade (GATT) agreed to alter several provisions of its patent law to fall in line with most of the rest of the world. The WTO is also behind the agreement on Trade-Related Aspects of Intellectual Property Rights (TRIPS), which requires member countries to establish a legal mechanism to protect plant varieties and animal breeds, via patents or other means. Yet another international negotiating group, the Convention on Biological Diversity (CBD), has as one of its objectives to distribute and share the benefits of the exploitation of biological diversity, especially germplasm. The discussions of this group collapsed in Cartagena, Colombia in 1999, partly because they couldn't agree to define starch or oil as a living modified organism (LMO) as some delegates were demanding. They finally concluded a deal in Montreal, but the implementation will take years. The Food and Agriculture Organization of the United Nations is also in the fray representing their version of 'farmer's rights'. With all these acronyms, it's no wonder we're all confused.

Technology use agreements

After the patent on glyphosate expired, Monsanto faced the predicament of capturing value, or 'Return on investment' from GM Roundup™-Ready crop varieties. Turning to contract law, Monsanto came up with the controversial **technology use agreement** (TUA). This is a contract specifying that farmers do not own the seed, they just grow it under contract and have to deliver all the grain in accordance with Monsanto's wishes. A farmer cannot keep any seed to re-plant next season, and cannot sell any to neighbours. Monsanto is allowed to come and inspect subsequent crops to ensure the farmer isn't growing any illicit Monsanto seed.

The TUA removes management capacity from the farmers, turning them into Monsanto contract workers. Some farmers have no problem with this: they read the contract and agree to its provisions, abide by them, and are happy making the increased money. Others are unwilling to cede their freedom and either buy seed (GM or non-GM) elsewhere or continue to grow their own saved seed. Some farmers want the Monsanto seed but don't like the TUA, so ignore the contractual provisions they don't like. Farmers enjoy making their own management decisions, even the wrong ones. Agricultural education programmes try to teach farmers the value of using certified seed each year. Fresh, clean seed is preferable to 'saved seed' for a number of reasons, the chief one being that it increases a farmer's net income. Many farmers haven't figured that out yet, and continue to grow 'saved' seed year after year. That's their choice and privilege; if they want to limit their income by growing saved seed, there's no law against it.

Monsanto already has several farmers in court over violations of their TUA. Suing farmers is not a good way to ingratiate yourself into an agricultural market or community. Most farmers are individuals and as such take things like lawsuits personally. Monsanto, on the other hand, is a multinational corporation. To big companies, lawsuits are often simply a way to come to closure on a dispute with another party. Monsanto and DuPont are constantly in Court against each other. Sometimes the big companies work on a project together, and sometimes, like any relationship, a collaboration falls apart. After some attempt to negotiate a settlement, the lawyers for each side say, 'We can't agree on a resolution, and we can't spend much more time on it. Let's litigate, let the courts decide for us so we can bring this issue to closure and then we can both go back to work on other things'.

Monsanto is an agricultural chemical company and, until recently, most of its customers were other companies in the chemical business. It didn't have too many direct dealings with individuals. The litigation route seemed to work fine in a dispute with another company; there is little personal animosity, and it is seen as an expedient route to closure. Litigating against an individual, however, is always a personal attack. And Monsanto against any individual farmer can only be seen as a David and Goliath altercation.

Not all farmer-oriented intellectual property contracts will be as restrictive or their enforcement as draconian as the Monsanto version, but we can expect to see more of them attached to seed. Along with global warming, the agricultural community will have to deal with yet another change in their environment, this one legal.

Legal disclaimer

The GM debate sometimes encounters issues relating to intellectual property. The recent developments in intellectual property law around the world were not created by, nor do they exclusively relate to, GMOs or GM technology. This chapter provides some background information to help in evaluating the intellectual property issues and components arising from time to time in the international GM debate. The information provided here is not intended to be comprehensive, nor is it a legal document. Readers interested in specific aspects of intellectual property law are directed to proper legal counsel in the appropriate jurisdiction.

CHAPTER 15

Just desserts

- Where is the public GM debate going?
- Will GM provide any real benefits to consumers?
- What's happening to our food?
- What's happening to our environment?
- What can I do to protect myself, my family,
  and my environment from these new technologies and products?

Where are we going?

Is the public debate over GMOs simply another battle between luddites and techno-rats? A hundred years ago our society argued about the safety of artificial ice, and whether ice from a mechanical freezer was as safe as ice harvested from frozen lakes or rivers. Some argued the synthetic ice was unnatural and so could not possibly be as 'safe' as lake ice. The technocrats of the day argued the artificial ice was chemically identical and performed various tests to show it was indeed as safe as natural ice. Now, with the benefit of time and experience, we know the 'artificial ice' is not only as safe as natural ice, but actually safer, as it lacks the contaminants, natural as well as artificial, found in the rivers and lakes. But relative safety was not the reason artificial ice gained market acceptance and we happily consume artificial ice today. Are we, a century later, replaying the same argument over GMOs?

We can expect continuing problems as long as fears and politics instead of science drive regulation of GMOs. Certainly a better-informed public debate will contribute to less political expediency and more sensible, true science-based regulation to address the real risks and hazards associated with GMOs. Can we learn nothing from history? The extensive and costly regulations quickly implemented in the UK in the aftermath of the *Salmonella* scare of the late 1980s had almost no effect on the incidence of *Salmonella* a decade later. To quell public fears, MAFF subsequently assured us its bureaucrats and their regulations had BSE well under control. Subsequent events proved they didn't. Hasty and spurious regulations made by politicians and bureaucrats simply to appease public concern may meet short-term political objectives but don't necessarily address the real scientific issues. Consumers end up paying the price, literally and figuratively.

As we've seen, there are real reasons to be concerned with GM as well as conventional foods. There are health reasons: a highly allergenic Brazil nut protein in a grain legume was a pea-brained idea to begin with. Potatoes modified to produce additional known toxins might never have been intended for public consumption, but they were real enough to scare people.

There are also legitimate environmental reasons for concern. An aggressive plant like rapeseed carrying stress resistance genes perhaps ought not be released into the delicately balanced ecosystem and intense agricultural environment of the UK. But what does it matter if the product was developed using GM or conventional methods? The potential adverse effect on the environment is the same in both cases. Why do we continue to target the *process* when the risk is associated with the *product*?

Bird populations, particularly in the UK, are diminishing and have been since long before GM crops came along. The decline is caused not by GM technology but by intensification of agriculture, especially prevalent in Europe. We don't know for sure if the GM crops will exacerbate the problem or alleviate it. We might direct GM cropping to reduce pressure on birds and other wildlife. Without proper management, the indiscriminate or improperly regulated release of GM crops in the UK will contribute to a continued intensification of agriculture, the true culprit of reduced biodiversity.

There are other reasons to object to GMOs. If, after reading this or other sources you find you cannot accept GMOs, then I don't think you should be forced to accept them. Alternatives already exist, even without going organic, and market demand will provide more. While I respect and support your right to avoid GM food, I don't think you should expect other people to conform to your view. You have the right to choose for yourself. Other people have the same right to choose for themselves.

Some people object to GMOs because multinational corporations dominate the technology, and they don't like multinational corporations. This view is entirely legal and legitimate. If you are in this camp, don't buy GMOs, or anything else, from multinational companies. But don't forget, not all GMOs come from multinational companies. Will you also reject the GMOs from the public sector and small companies? And the multinationals make far more consumer products than GMOs. Do you support the big multinationals by buying cars, clothing, or kitchen utensils? Support the companies and institutions you like, whether big multinational, small local, or public institutions. Consumers already patronize their favourite manufacturers. It's not unusual to encounter a person who says, 'I don't like company X, so I don't buy any of its products'. The reason for the dislike is often unstated but ordinarily based on an unpleasant past experience with the company or their product. Similarly, perhaps it's not as common but it's still not unheard of for someone to say 'I buy all my Y products from company Z. I can trust them to give good quality for a fair price'. Consumers in each camp are making

individual purchasing decisions on the basis of personal preference, often enough
based on misunderstanding but legal and common nevertheless.

Some people reject GMOs because the products represent the arrogance of
mere mortals who think they as humans can improve on nature (or God's plan,
if you prefer). I chuckle to myself whenever I review a research plan intended to
improve on nature. We humans might know far more about nature than we did
just a few years ago, but we've just scratched the surface of all there is to know, or
even of what we need to know to deign to set out to improve her. How, then, can
I be party to this genetic manipulation business without being seen as hypocritical myself? The starting assumption is incorrect. Genetic modification is not
intended to improve on nature. It is intended to help produce more food per unit
of area, or of energy input, than is currently the case. I work to develop GMOs
not to improve on nature, but to augment nature to be able to sustain our
increasing human population.

Nature has no plan for agricultural systems based on high chemical inputs and
low biodiversity. Nature has no place for massive administrative bureaucracies
and immense financial subsidies. The current intensive agricultural industry is a
human creation. English Nature, an environmental watchdog, is concerned that
biotechnology will contribute to the intensification of agriculture. They are concerned, for example, that herbicide-resistant GM crops will be too effective,
eradicating all manner of plants, including those serving as food and habitat to
wildlife. I share this concern. But there are mechanisms to deal with it. One, mentioned earlier, enables farmers to benefit from the enhanced productivity of GM
crops by taking a portion of farmland out of production, allowing it to return to
a semi-wild state, similar to the 'set-aside' programmes. Under this scenario, the
farmer benefits from increased production on fewer acres, biodiversity benefits
from having more park and reserve land, and consumers benefit both from having less expensive, cleaner food and from the satisfaction of knowing there's
more wildlife in the rural settings.

English Nature and I diverge when they, along with various other groups,
argue GM crops will increase chemical usage. Yes, some GM crops are designed
to have certain chemicals applied, but those certain chemicals do not add to but
replace other, often older and nastier chemicals. Other GM crops are designed to
decrease chemical usage. The GM *B.t.* crops, for example, enable farmers to
reduce the amount of insecticide needed and currently applied to conventional
crops. We won't have to wait long to see which view is correct. Data from early
USDA studies show a reduction in overall chemical usage with GM crops. In
seven of twelve regions surveyed, the use of pesticides was significantly lower, the
other five were unchanged. In no case was there in increase in pesticide usage.
Will English Nature change its mind and support GM crops if the early reports
are verified? Time will tell.

English Nature and others are wrong if they think banning GM crops will eliminate or even substantially reduce the chemicalization and industrialization of
agriculture. These phenomena were well entrenched long before GM technology

came along, and society is unlikely to support a massive swing to organic production, vegetarianism, subsistence farming, and higher food prices concomitant with a return to 'traditional' agrarian practices. But must we choose between two extremes? Surely there is a sensible middle ground, where we identify and restrict the nastiest chemicals, minimize other chemicals, and employ approved crops and sustainable agronomic practices.

If left to nature, the human population would not have been able to reach its current figure of six billion. Without the dramatic increases in food production over the last generation, largely dependent upon chemical inputs (in the era ironically named the Green Revolution), we would face food shortages far more extensive and devastating than we already do. Scientists love to argue and debate the natural sustainable human population level, but are generally agreed it is far less than the current figure. It may be true that world food distribution, not production, is the true cause of malnutrition and famine. Food redistribution requires a long-term political solution. While we wait, people starve. GM technology is a tool we can use immediately to help feed people.

I disagree with GM proponents pushing the 'feed the world' argument. I do not see GM technology, or any single technology, eradicating hunger and malnutrition. But producing substantially more food, and more nutritious food, is a powerful weapon to help in the fight. Even the Nuffield Council says it would be unethical *not* to use GM.

What will happen in the short term?

The battle to ban GM technology worldwide is essentially over. Thousands of GMOs have been created in hundreds of labs around the world. Several GMOs are in international commercial production, growing on vast acreage and already present in a wide range of foodstuffs. Some GMOs are microbial, providing pharmaceuticals such as human insulin, or food ingredients, including enzymes used in cheese manufacturing. Others are whole or processed foods like GM tomatoes or soya products, respectively. Even predominantly industrial commodities such as cotton and linseed are available in GM varieties. GM technology is already entrenched in the world market and claiming a larger share every year. Expecting a ban on GM technology at this stage is unrealistic.

With GM technology entrenched and the first GMOs already in the international market, our only feasible influence is on future products. For this we need to know what's coming next.

Technology and GM products

The first wave of GM foods was dominated by major crop species expressing novel pesticide resistance. They involved genes for simple traits relatively easy to isolate and modify at a molecular or biochemical level. Also, and equally conspicuously, the genes were controlled by private companies.

Second generation GMOs, those with more complex attributes and more attractive to consumers, are being developed. They include quality enhancement and speciality products. Crop varieties with value-added attributes will make a huge difference to our global economy within a few years. Countries will become less dependent on imports of many commodities as local species are modified to produce commodities currently imported. Cocoa butter, for example, is used widely in the manufacture of various foods and cosmetics. Canada cannot grow cocoa trees (no matter how many Arctic flounder genes might be inserted), so all of the demand for this common ingredient has to be satisfied by imports. However, Canadian farmers grow linseed very successfully. Linseed varieties capable of producing not linseed oil but a cocoa butter-like oil will become available, permitting a domestic supply. Each country will support similar developments in other crop species better suited to a local agricultural environment.

Other 'value added' traits include plants modified to produce high value chemicals, such as pharmaceuticals or expensive industrial chemicals. Scientists are also developing crops with better nutritional composition, either by enhancing the nutrient or reducing anti-nutritional components:

- more nutritious rice
- potatoes that absorb less oil in frying
- sugar beets with modified, lower-calorie sugars
- oilseed crops, such as canola and soya, with reduced saturates, providing 'healthier' oil.

Almost all food products will have improved storage quality and longer shelf lives.

Apart from foods, we can expect improvements in other consumer products:

- cotton and flax with better fibre characteristics
- improved ingredients for cosmetics and personal hygiene products
- flowers with a much greater range of colours and longer 'vase life'.

There are several reasons for the shift into these second generation traits:

- Our technology has advanced to the point where we can deal with more complex genetic traits. The first wave GM products were necessarily restricted to simple, single gene traits, such as pesticide resistance. Technological advances will continue, enabling access to composite, multigene traits.
- The early and enabling GM technology was developed largely in public sector labs, but private industry was driving commercialization of GMOs. Monsanto had a financial incentive to generate Roundup-Ready™ crops, for example, as AgrEvo had in developing Liberty™-link crops. As the largest pesticide companies now have GMOs resistant to their respective products on the market, they

need to find new products. These companies have active research programmes developing more 'value-added' second and third generation GM products.

- The high cost of regulatory compliance for GM crops relative to conventional products drives the developers to value-added GM products. Traditional breeders have long given us various herbicide-resistant crops. Triazine-tolerant canola resulted from a natural mutation and is considered 'conventional'. It is probably as safe as GM canola, but doesn't trigger the additional regulatory scrutiny of a GMO. The cost of regulatory scrutiny to place a mutation-bred variety on the international market is about the same as any other conventional crop variety. The cost of putting a transgenic crop on the market is much higher than for a conventional variety with a similar attribute. Because of the high costs of regulatory compliance for a GM compared with a conventional cultivar, transgenic technology is simply not cost effective for products that could be generated conventionally. However, there is much less discrepancy between the regulatory burden on a GM-generated pharmaceutical vs. an equivalent conventional pharmaceutical.

- The cost of regulatory compliance is often reduced with a GM value-added trait as opposed to a GM commodity crop. There is less environmental concern where the GMO will not be cultivated or released into the environment. For very high value commodities, such as a particular novel pharmaceutical, GMOs contained in sealed labs or glasshouses may satisfy the entire world demand. Without the need for environmental release, the regulatory compliance of environmental issues becomes easier and less expensive.

- Security of intellectual property is simpler because high value speciality products are generated in much smaller quantities than high volume bulk commodities. Most plants, GM or otherwise, are self-reproducing. An unscrupulous competitor could buy one bag of seed and acquire the proprietary technology indefinitely (even if illegally). To guard against such theft, high value commodities may be delivered, in the seed, in a vertically integrated, 'closed-loop' system. That is, the company maintains all the germplasm and product in-house. Such systems are much easier to monitor for illicit activity, because the seed and the product need never leave the company's control or even their physical possession. High value commodities produced on a smaller scale are also easier to trace.

- Newer GM products will attract consumer demand. At present, the end-product customer has little interest in whether a crop is resistant to insects, as long as the food product presented for retail purchase is (or, rather, appears to be) insect-free. There is no 'pull' or demand from the consumer to acquire these pesticide-resistant new crops. Instead, first generation GMO commodities were 'pushed' onto the market by the developers who have the inventory and need to sell it. This will change considerably when a GM product carries an attribute the final consumer wants, either directly (e.g. an enhanced quality product) or indirectly (e.g. lower price, based on increased production efficiencies).

- Consumer concern lessens as the technology is more removed from the product. There is little public concern over the insulin produced by genetically engineered bacteria because we consumers have no idea how pharmaceuticals are produced anyway; we are removed from the process. On the other hand, we are close to foods, especially whole food items. We know what a tomato is, how it grows and how it should taste, so we are more suspicious when a 'new' tomato appears in the market. Value-added products are typically extracted from the actual transgenic organism that produced them. The consumer might inject the product of GM technology into their bodies, but they don't have to touch the actual GM organism. This distance reduces consumer concern and thereby lowers socio-political regulatory anxiety.
- Higher value products will generate a greater return on investment for companies. The cost of inserting a gene into an organism is about the same regardless of what attribute the gene confers. Bulk commodities (such as grains and oilseeds) are low in value, bought and sold by the tonne. A speciality chemical is high in value and may be priced, in some cases, by the milligram. As the technology and cost of developing each is similar, why expend resources to develop a lower value commodity when a high value product could be generated instead? So, given the return on investment, it makes sense to devote research and development resources in higher value products.
- Finally, and in general, as the GM products become more commonplace, we consumers become more familiar with GMOs and concentrate on real, as opposed to imagined or hypothetical, risks to environment or health. This increased comfort will reduce the overall anxiety to society and allow more sensible and focused public debate leading ultimately to more appropriate regulation of all products, GM as well as conventional.

The marketplace

My crystal ball doesn't give me such a clear view of the marketplace at it does of technical developments, largely because of the vagaries of the market. However, the general impression is that there will be several stages of market evolution over the next few years. I see as a first step some supermarkets providing tomatoes in three separate bins, largely in response to public concern over GMOs. One bin will be labelled 'GM tomatoes', a second bin 'conventional tomatoes', and the third 'organic tomatoes'. This will be repeated for many or most products on the shelves, at substantial cost to the supermarket which, of course, passes those costs on to consumers.

Although the cost of regulatory compliance will be highest for the GMO, the product price will have to be competitive with conventional products. One reason the Flavr-Savr™ failed was that it was too expensive and didn't offer a premium in taste, quality, or freshness to warrant consumers spending the extra money. To be successful, the costs of GM products have to remain competitive with the 'substantially equivalent' conventional product. A small segment of consumers is known as 'early adopters'—these are people who are excited by new technology and willing to pay a premium just to be among the first. They are the ones who buy state-of-the-art computers every six months, or high-end stereo equipment before it's even available from regular retailers. However, their numbers are probably too small to sustain substantially higher prices, especially when the GM product is essentially identical to the conventional product.

Continuing my prediction, there will be a consolidation within a few years. The GM bin and the conventional bin will coalesce, as people come to accept GM technology and products as 'substantially equivalent' to their conventional counterparts. The organic bin will still be there, but now battling for its survival against the now considerably lower priced competitor. Eventually, we'll see a return to the old-fashioned single 'tomatoes' bin. The organic bin will be eliminated, the others replaced by a 'sustainable' bin, containing produce developed and grown using sustainable methods. 'Sustainable' will be a hybrid between what is now organic and what are now the intensive agricultural practices of European Union farmers. It will entail reduced but not eliminated pesticide use. The pesticides will be less harmful than those currently employed, developed with greater regard for environment and safety of non-target species. The product will be more nutritious, containing fewer anti-nutritional components and fewer contaminants. GM will cease to be an issue of intense public debate. And, yes, the big companies will still make most of the money.

Are you concerned about fish genes in tomatoes?

Trying to make sense of molecular genetic technology can be bewildering and frustrating. No wonder. We start with a highly specialized technical foundation of uncertain stability, then try to build on it a structure using the only available materials—misinformation, misunderstanding, and mistakes, all the while wrapped in that vaguely disconcerting feeling we're doing something unethical. I'd be surprised if you're *not* anxious. If you need any validation, it is this: you can't be expected to make rational sense of an irrational situation. The GM situation as described in the public forum is largely irrational.

This book gives you the tools to delve behind the façade and build your own foundation, find the real substances, ignore the false, and construct your own edifice.

And so we return to our starting point. We've exploded the scary myths of fish genes in tomatoes, Brazil nuts genes in beans, and rapeseed plants becoming superweeds immune to all herbicides. At the same time, we appreciate that fish genes could, technically, be inserted into tomatoes, or that legumes could be genetically modified with Brazil nut genes. We know rapeseed plants with a novel herbicide resistance are in commercial production, and we've seen they are still under control by any of various other herbicides. We're concerned that GM potatoes might be toxic to Scottish rats, yet American humans have been eating GM potatoes for years will no apparent ill effect.

How do we as consumers apply the knowledge gained?

Identify your concern

Try to determine if your concern is process- or product-based. If you are worried about process, consider what other molecular genetic technologies are suspect. Are pharmaceuticals produced from GM acceptable? Is using PCR to detect GMOs in shipments acceptable? If they are, identify the crucial differences between using GM technology to make food and using it to make medicine. I can't think of any scientifically sound rationale to distinguish them.

Identify and ignore the spurious scare stories and instead concentrate on the real hazards. The phantom Brazil nut gene in soya bean didn't cause any harm because it did not exist; no legume carrying a Brazil nut gene was ever released. It might have been, if common sense and proper scientific scrutiny had not identified the risk at an early stage.

If your concern is with a product, not the technology or process for making the product, ask how the product is hazardous. Concentrate on the hazardous product, not the method of delivery.

Keep the issues in perspective

Be sure of the product you're concerned about. Is it the whole food, complete with intact genes, or a processed product, with denatured or destroyed genes, or is it a derived product, such as oil or starch, devoid of genes altogether? Are all soya bean products hazardous, or just GM ones? Consider the differences between a whole soya bean, soya bean paste, and soya oil.

Compare GM products with conventional technology and products. Antibiotic resistance genes in GMOs jeopardize therapeutic agents less than patients 'forgetting' to take their full course of antibiotics. Conventional or organic foodstuffs are not always safer, nor do they carry fewer contaminants than GM foods.

When considering a new GM product, learn how it differs from the parent and from the current alternative. Consider GM *B.t.* maize. We need to compare the GM maize with the parent variety of corn and we need to compare the current form of insect protection used on the farm. *B.t.* toxin, whether sprinkled on crops by organic farmers or inserted directly into the plant using GM, is toxic to insects, both pest and non-pest insects. If we want to protect insects from *B.t.* poisoning, we need to ban *B.t.* in all its forms, including the 'organic' version.

Identify the real risks associated with GMOs

Some potential GM products are both hazardous and unnecessary. Genes for allergens (e.g. Brazil nut storage protein) ought not to be, and probably won't be, introduced into common foods. If they are, they will be tightly regulated and comprehensively labelled.

Some GM products might be environmentally benign in some regions, hazardous in others. Cultivation of GM herbicide-tolerant rapeseed might be acceptable in parts of Australia or the Americas but perhaps not in parts of Europe.

Other GMOs might be acceptable, but with stringent management, such as the use of insect-resistant *B.t.* crops, where management is required to minimize damage to non-pest insects or evolution of resistant insect pests.

Question regulatory processes.

If a GM canola is intended for cultivation in the UK, a full environmental assessment might be appropriate. Oil from the same crop, but grown elsewhere and shipped in, doesn't need the same degree of assessment, as oil does not pose the same potential hazards. GM cotton is unlikely to pose any environmental risk to the UK, as it cannot grow there no matter how many foreign genes are inserted.

New technology

Critics say this technology is 'new' and untested over the long term. GM technology is not all that new. Consider other recent technical developments: mobile phones, personal computers, even the Teletubbies. Genetic engineering has been around about as long as microwave ovens, longer than these other modern developments. GM risk assessments since the early 1970s gives a better indication of hazards than many other technologies. There have been no environmental disasters or health issues attributable to GM or GMOs, despite their being grown on millions of acres and consumed by millions of humans over several years. If we demand a moratorium on GM (until we can determine the 'long-term' risks), we must also demand a moratorium on these other technologies. Certainly, there are identifiable problems in all of them. We didn't expect mobile phones to increase traffic accidents, we didn't expect home computers to create 'Internet widows'. And we didn't expect children's TV programmes to promote controversial 'alternative lifestyles'.

A GM plant starts with about 25 thousand genes, all found in nature and all commonly eaten. To that base we add one or two other genes, also found in nature and commonly eaten. The difference is we now have them in the same organism, where before they were in different ones. Some opponents like to claim that we've never seen this combination of genes before, and the combination might be harmful. Traditional plant breeders constantly generate new combinations of genes, too, but instead of adding one or two to the mix, they add another 25 thousand. Nature is also constantly generating new combinations of genes. Few are ever harmful.

This does not mean all GMOs are completely safe. All new products, including GMOs, must be evaluated for risk, and any identified risks assessed.

Food safety

Of course we are concerned with food and feed safety of GMOs. But when we scrutinize products for safety, why do we exempt non-GM products? We've seen some examples of problems caused by some 'health' foods, organic foods, and natural remedies. Yet none of these potentially hazardous products receive anything like the regulatory scrutiny of GMOs. Why not? We assume 'natural' products are safe. As we've seen, the assumption is, unfortunately, wrong. All products, GM and otherwise, ought to be reasonably scrutinized for food and feed safety. Do we really want to jump out of the GM frying pan until we know the heat of the fire below?

If we eliminate GM foods because of potential hazards, we must also eliminate conventional foods presenting the same hazards. Many common foods carry anti-nutritional factors. Potatoes, legumes, fruits are a great source of a range of naturally occurring toxins, from lectins to cyanide. Let's ban them these foods outright. So what if millions of people then suffer increased hunger? At least we reduce the risk of their suffering from the toxins. But, of course, humans already know how to deal with naturally occurring toxins, most commonly by cooking or simply avoiding the parts carrying the toxins. By the same method, toxins in GM foods, whether introduced or natural, might also be detoxified by cooking or avoidance.

The environment

We're worried about the environment. Of course we need to scrutinize GMOs for any adverse environmental impact. But why only GMOs? Conventional products introduced into new environments have caused problems. Why are they now either exempt, or receive a small fraction of the regulatory attention of GMOs? Surely, if something is potentially hazardous, regardless of its provenance, it should be carefully scrutinized prior to release. At the same time, we need not overregulate. We can save taxpayers money and time, once sufficient and appropriate data are collected, by making a decision.

Bureaucracy

Paying for a bureaucracy to scrutinize well beyond the point needed to come to a reasonable determination is like paying a large additional premium to insure your house well beyond its value when the insurance only provides replacement costs. The wasted additional resources might have gone instead to something more useful. More importantly, it gives us a false sense of security.

A speaker at a recent meeting said the only way to restore public trust in the British bureaucracy (especially MAFF) is to have more regulations. No! Credibility and trust are earned only through *appropriate* regulation and transparent application. More is not always better; surely quality is preferable to quantity.

Satiated at last

So we come full circle. Were you concerned about fish genes in tomatoes? Of course you were. Your concern led you to read this book. Your concern might also have been influenced by uncertainty, even ignorance, of the risks. For many consumers, the first real awareness of GM was a direct encounter with a GM product in the market. No wonder we often feel this technology was imposed on us quickly and covertly, as a *fait accompli*, without an adequate opportunity to debate the matters beforehand. Perhaps we feel impotent to stop it. This combination of concern, ignorance, and powerlessness leads inexorably to fear. We fear the unknown hazards we cannot control. Fear, in turn, grips our attention, disabling our usual capacity to solve problems efficiently and effectively. At the extremes, we are unable to move, paralysed with fear.

Having read this book, let's revisit the initial questions. Are you still concerned? We've exploded some myths, we've exposed some real hazards. You now have the tools, the technical knowledge, to fight the fears.

Use the tools to recognize, and disregard, the constant attempts from every quarter to manipulate your thinking. The media attract you with either sensational headlines—they sell better than a well-documented analysis—or superficial snippets, which are, like sugar, tasty little morsels but neither nutritious nor sustainable. We're left unsated, hungry for more. The companies reach out with their advertising, puff pieces designed by expensive agencies and the marketing department. Sometimes I look at the ads and wonder if there is any communication between the product development team and the advertising office. Activists use whatever means necessary to grab your attention, from scaremongering to stunts. However, all of these sources do convey useful information. You just have to use your tools and dig for it. Then combine this with information from more credible and reliable sources.

With a supply of factual information from varied sources, you can properly evaluate your position. Devoid of fear and thinking clearly, identify the source of concern and evaluate rational tenability. Compare a questionable technology (GM) with current or acceptable technologies to identify any fundamental differences. Compare a questionable GM product with a comparable but conventional version, again seeking any fundamental differences. If you find substantial differences, compare the risks. Is a GM herbicide-resistant rapeseed variety really more hazardous than a mutant herbicide-resistant rapeseed variety? Does the degraded DNA in a GM tomato paste pose a risk of escape to devastate the environment any more than that of ordinary tomato paste? Is oil from a GM maize more toxic than normal maize oil, when both have identical chemical composition and both lack DNA and protein? If you remain opposed to GM as a technology, you should now know why and be able to defend your position, if only to yourself. At the same time and on the same grounds, you might need to re-evaluate your current acceptance of some essentially similar technologies. If you decide to accept a GMO, you do so aware of any associated risks and how to manage them. Use of *B.t.* to control insect pests requires management. But this is true whether the *B.t.* is in a GM plant or sprayed by an organic farmer.

Whether we support or oppose them, GMOs are already with us and will only increase in both number and impact. Our best course of action is to learn the facts behind GM technology and each GM product, as well as their conventional alternatives. Then we can ignore both the scaremongers and the soothsayers, and consider the risks and benefits of genetic technology from different perspectives and in proper context. The only way to keep from being overwhelmed is by using your tools to learn the facts and decide for yourself.

You may well still be concerned about GMOs. But your concern now, as opposed to earlier, is based on a solid understanding and assessment of the real risks of GMOs and their current alternatives. Thus enlightened and armed, you can now feel confident in your position to accept or reject any product, whether conventional or GM.

Last but not least—the tip!

Whenever possible, I try to avoid providing direct advice, preferring instead to let people decide for themselves (my occasional aspersions on the insipidity of tofu are based not on health concerns but are rather an appeal to apply common sense and good taste). However, I leave you with the following explicit advice. Constant media coverage of food scares notwithstanding, six billion people eat something every day without undue harm to themselves or the environment. The tragic incidents of harm from food are extremely rare. This doesn't mean we should ignore legitimate food safety concerns, but rather that we should place them in proper perspective.

What is the single greatest food-related threat to your health? Is it GMOs? Synthetic pesticides? Natural toxins? Food poisoning through human negligence? Contaminants in organic food? *Salmonella* or other nasty bacteria? Allergens? None comes close. The greatest real damage is chronic anxiety over diet.

Instead of worrying—almost always needlessly—over whether or not your food supply is safe, or if you're eating too much pesticide, or not getting enough fibre, or too much cholesterol, or to little polyunsaturated fat, simplify your life and diet. Eat balanced and varied meals. Stop worrying so much about your food; it's almost certainly healthier than you are. If, on the advice of your physician, you need to monitor intake of sodium, saturated fats, tofu, or whatever, then do so. Otherwise, forget the food fads, fearmongering, and fabricated fashion model fantasy ideal. They lead you to obsession and overwrought concern. If you don't look like a model today, you're unlikely to achieve that unrealistic goal by next year. Save your money and grief. If you need to lose weight, consult your physician, not the 'miracle diets'. Don't anguish with guilt over the occasional fatty, salty, or sugary snack. Moderation and variety are the key. Not only will you relish a diverse selection of tasty nutritious foods, but the occasional anti-nutritional components, whether natural or synthetic, will be diluted and compensated by the volume and balance provided by everything else. Enjoy your meals. *Bon appétit.*

CHAPTER 16

Post-prandial delights: some resources

Tangible

Bill Bryson, *Notes from a big country. Doubleday.* New York, 1998.
Matt Ridley, *Genome,* an 'autobiography' of a species in 23 chapters. Fourth Estate, London, 1999.
James Walsh, *True odds: how risk affects your everyday life.* Santa Monica, CA, Merritt, 1996.

Virtual

A selection of some interesting websites (note that the content or even the existence of websites can change without notice).

Government: GMO regulatory sites

UK

DETR (Department of the Environment, Transport and the Regions) homepage *http://www.detr.gov.uk/*
DETR: ACRE (Advisory Committee on Releases to the Environment) homepage (carries GMO public register list for UK releases) *http://www.environment.detr.gov.uk/acre/index.htm*
DoH (Department of Health) report on health implications of GM foods *http://www.doh.gov.uk/gmfood.htm*
House of Commons Select Committee on Science and Technology *http://www.parliament.the-stationery-office.co.uk/pa/cm199899/cmselect/ cmsctech /286/28602.htm*
House of Lords Select Committee report *http://www.parliament.the-stationery-office.co.uk/pa/ld199899/ldselect/ldeucom/11/8121501.htm*
MAFF (Ministry of Agriculture, Fisheries and Food) novel foods *http://www.maff.gov.uk/food/foodnov.htm*

MAFF: ACNFP (Advisory Committee on Novel Foods and Processes)
(Regulation 258/97)   *http://www.maff.gov.uk/food/novel/nfrregn.htm*

USA

EPA (Environmental Protection Agency) (microbials)
   http://www.epa.gov/opptintr/ biotech/
FDA (Food and Drug Administration) (biotechnology information)
   http://vm.cfsan.fda.gov/ ~lrd/biotechm.html
FDA (biotech final consultations)   *http://vm.cfsan.fda.gov/ ~lrd/biocon.html*
USDA (US Federal Department of Agriculture) (biotechnology information)
   http://www.aphis.usda.gov/bbep/bp/
USDA (status of petitions)   *http://www.aphis.usda.gov/biotech/petday.html*
USDA: APHIS (Animal and Plant Health Inspection Service) (regulates the
   introduction and cultivation of GM plant material)

Canada

Canada agriculture and environment approvals for plants with novel traits
   (GMOs)   *http://www.cfia-acia.agr.ca/english/plant/pbo/okays.html*
CFIA (Canadian Food Inspection Agency) (Agriculture)
   http://www.cfia-acia.agr.ca/english/plant/pbo/ dir9501e.html#A8
Health Canada (novel foods approvals)   *http://www.hc-sc.gc.ca/english/
   food.htm#novel*

Biotechnology industry sites

AgrEvo   *http://www.aventis.com/*
AgWest Biotech (Canada)   *http://www.agwest.sk.ca*
Biotechnology Industry Organization (USA)   *http://www.bio.org/*
DuPont   *http://www.dupont.com/index.html*
EuropaBio (EU)   *http://www.europa-bio.be/*
Genentech   *http://www.genentech.com/Company/timeline.html*
Monsanto (USA)   *http://www.monsanto.com*
Novartis   *http://www.seeds.novartis.com/*
The BioIndustry Association (UK)   *http://www.bioindustry.org/*
Zeneca   *http://www.zenecaag.com/*

Biosafety and biotechnology information sites

American Council on Science and Health   *http://www.acsh.org/*
Belgian Biosafety Server   *http://biosafety.ihe.be/*

CAB International   *http://agbio.technet.com*
CBD (Convention on Biological Diversity)   *http://www.biodiv.org/biosafe/*
InfoBiotec Canada   *http://www.cisti.nrc.ca/ibc/home.html*
Information Systems for Biotechnology (USA)   *http://www.nbiap.vt.edu/*
Institute for Crop and Food Research (NZ)   *http://www.crop.cri.nz/*
International Center for Genetic Engineering and Biotechnology
   http://www.icgeb.trieste.it/biosafety/
John Innes Institute (UK)   *http://www.gmissues.org/*
National Agricultural Biotechnology Council (USA)
   http://www.cals.cornell.edu/extension/nabc/
National Agricultural Library (USA)   *http://www.nal.usda.gov/bic/*
Nuffield Council on Bioethics (UK)   *http://www.nuffield.org/bioethics/publica-tion/pub0010805.html*
OECD Biotechnology database   *http://www.oecd.org/ehs/service.htm*
Rowett Institute (UK)   *http://www.rri.sari.ac.uk/press/*
Royal Society (UK)   *http://www.royalsoc.ac.uk/*
United Nations Environment Programme International Register on Biosafety
   (Switzerland)   *http://irptc.unep.ch/biodiv/*

Medical research search information

NCBI Genbank and other databases (DNA and protein sequence searching)
   http://www.ncbi.nlm.nih.gov/entrez/query.fcgi
Swiss Institute of Bioinformatics   *http://www.expasy.ch/*
US National Library of Medicine   *http://www.nlm.nih.gov/*

Patent search

Canada patent search   *http://Patents1.ic.gc.ca/intro-e.html*
International World Intellectual Property Organization(WIPO)
   http://pctgazette.wipo.int/
US, Europe, and Japan patent search   *http://patent.womplex.ibm.com/*

Contents of tobacco smoke

Government of British Columbia and Canadian Council for Tobacco Control
   http://www.cctc.ca/bcreports/

Soya products

Central Soya   *http://www.centralsoya.com/*

Articles on another controversial food technology— irradiation

Pennsylvania State University *E. coli* Reference Center
http://www.ecoli.cas.psu.edu/ecoli/index.htm

News and press releases relating to GM food and GMOs

The Millennium Environment Debate   *http://www.millennium-debate.org/gmfood.htm*
Die Zeitung (Germany)   *http://www.netlink.de/gen/Zeitung/1999/home.html*

Mainstream news servers with search feature

ABC (USA)   *http://search.abcnews.go.com/index.html*
BBC (UK)   *http://www.bbc.co.uk/search/*
CNN (USA)   *http://www.cnn.com/INDEX/services.html*

Various views of other organizations

Biodemocracy and the Organic Consumers Association
   http://www.purefood.org/
Church of England   *http://www.cofe.epinet.co.uk/view/index.html*
English Nature   *http://www.english-nature.org.uk/start.htm*
Friends of the Earth   *http://www.foe.co.uk/camps/foodbio/*
Greenpeace (international)   *http://www.greenpeace.org/~geneng/*
Institute of Food Science and Technology (UK)   *http://www.ifst.org/*
Natural Law Party (Canada site)   *http://www.natural-law.ca/genetic/geindex.html*
Natural Law Party (USA site)   *http://www.safe-food.org*
Natural Resources Defense Council   *http://www.nrdc.org/nrdc/*
Soil Association   *http://www.soilassociation.org/*
Union of Concerned Scientists   *http://www.ucsusa.org/agriculture/*

Glossary and abbreviations

Agrobacterium tumefaciens   A soil-borne bacterium with the unique natural ability to transfer DNA into organisms of another biological kingdom to transform them genetically.

Bacillus thuringiensis (B.t.)   A bacterium with the natural ability to produce a crystal protein toxic to certain insects, mainly Lepidoptera (caterpillars, butterflies) insects. Available since the 1950s. Farmers use the *B.t.* toxin to control insect pests in crops. Crops transformed with the relevant gene from the *B.t.* bacterium produce the same toxin.

Clone   An identical copy (noun); to make identical copies (verb), usually of a gene, another piece of DNA or an organism.

Cultivar   Contraction of 'cultivated variety'; often used interchangeably with variety.

DNA   Deoxyribonucleic acid, the physical molecule consisting of long sequences of the bases A, T, C, and G, the arrangement of which determines the genetic characteristics of the organism or cell containing it. All organisms other than viruses use DNA as the carrier of genetic information.

Enzyme   A protein with a specific duty; usually facilitates chemical reactions.

Eukaryote   All higher organisms, including plants and animals; they share similar genetic organization.

Gametes   The 'sex'cells, sperm or egg; each cell has one set of chromosomes. They combine to make an embryo with two sets of chromosomes, one from each parent.

Gene A unit of biological information, carried on a sequence of DNA. A recipe for a particular protein.

Genetic engineering   Inserting genes from one source into another using molecular techniques.

Genetic modification (GM)   No accepted technical or political definition, but widely used to denote the insertion of DNA from one organism to another, usually by molecular technologies.

Genetically modified organism (GMO)   The plant, animal, or microbe resulting from a genetic modification.

Genetic pollution   A phrase fabricated to elicit a negative emotional response, yet lacking a scientific heritage or definition.

Homologue/homology   If the DNA base sequence of two pieces of DNA are similar, they are said to be homologous. Many genes are homologous across many species.

Intron   A stretch of DNA inside a gene recipe, but not actually contributing to the final protein product. Found only in eukaryotic genes.

Landrace   A primitive and ancient plant variety.

Lecithin   A common food additive derived from soya bean, but present in many organisms, including animals.

Lectin   A class of chemicals with pesticidal properties, produced by many types of plant species.

Living modified organism (LMO)   Any product of GM, resulting in plant, animal, microbe, or derived materials, such as starch, oil or fibre.

Locus   The position in the genome. Analogous to a specific page in a recipe book.

Meiosis   The process of genome halving, followed by cell division, so daughter cells get one copy of each chromosome, making gametes.

Mitosis   The process of genome doubling followed by cell division, so each daughter cell gets two sets of chromosomes.

Mutation   A change in the DNA, regardless of cause.

Pathogen   A disease-causing agent, often a bacterium like *Salmonella*.

Protein   The product of a gene recipe. Usually an enzyme, but also can provide structure.

Prokaryote   Simple single-celled organisms, such as bacteria.

Recombinant DNA (rDNA)   Artificially splicing pieces of DNA together, usually using specialized enzymes. Synonymous with genetic engineering.

Restriction endonuclease, restriction enzyme   Any of an entire group of highly specialized enzymes capable of cutting DNA or RNA at particular base sequences.

RNA   Ribonucleic acid, chemical and biological relative to DNA, serving several other purposes but carrier of genetic material in only a few simple species, all viruses.

Transformation, genetic transformation   The act of inserting genetic material into a cell or organism.

Transgenic   Adjective for an organism carrying foreign or artificially inserted genetic material. Also **transformed.**

Variety   Genetically distinct, uniform, and stable crop strain. See Cultivar.

Index